VACCINATION

and

NATUROPATHIC MEDICINE

VACCINATION
and

NATUROPATHIC MEDICINE

in their own words

Edited by Sussanna Czeranko, ND, BBE
Foreword by Jim Sensenig, ND
Epilogue by Jared Zeff, ND
Afterword by Alex Vasquez, DC, ND, DO, FACN

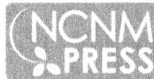

NCNM PRESS

Portland, Oregon

© 2015 by NCNM Press
Managing Editor: Sandra Snyder, PhD

Cover photograph: Henry Lindlahr, M.D., taken from *Nature Cure Magazine*,
which he began publishing in November, 1907.

Published by NCNM Press
National College of Natural Medicine
49 SW Porter Street
Portland, Oregon 97201, USA
www.ncnm.edu

NCNM Press gratefully acknowledges the generous and prescient financial
support of HEVERT USA which has made possible the creation and
distribution of the *In Their Own Words* historical series.
The HEVERT COLLECTION comprises twelve historical compilations which
preserve for the healing professions significant and representational works
from contributors to the historical Benedict Lust journals.

Production: Fourth Lloyd Productions, LLC.
Design: Richard Stodart

Printed in the United States of America

ISBN: 978-0-9969863-0-4
Library of Congress Control Number: 2015959806

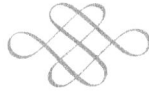

It often happens that the universal belief of one age—a belief from which no one was, nor without an extraordinary effort of genius and courage could, at that time, be free—becomes to a subsequent age so palpable an absurdity that the only difficulty then is to imagine how such a thing can ever have appeared credible.

—John Stuart Mill

It takes courage, vision, conviction and purpose to challenge the status quo. This book is dedicated to all those who took up the challenge of questioning vaccination.

TABLE OF CONTENTS

The objections to vaccination after its introduction into western medicine, and as it is still practiced in conventional medicine, are straightforward. It is potentially harmful and often not effective. Those doctors and practitioners who advocate the treatment and prevention of disease through the maintenance and restoration of health have always found the techniques of vaccination to be objectionable. Experience in the naturopathic approach to medicine teaches that the best way to prevent disease, including infectious disease, is to maintain robust good health in so far as possible and when needed to use treatments that pose no harm. These must be the goals of any rational medical system. It may be difficult for the modern reader to understand how good health and increased resistance to disease can protect one from *germs* since we have been told for over a hundred and fifty years to fear these invisible microbes as the cause of our ills. The naturopathic understanding of the cause of disease calls into question the validity of the *germ theory of disease*, a key departure point for the naturopathic professional from the conventional belief that we are at the mercy of microbes. This is not merely an academic question; rather, it forms the basis for the very argument in support of vaccination and for the fear-based beliefs in recommending them, and even for mandating them.

As you read through these pages, it will become clear that many doctors within the dominant school of medicine contended that vaccination can be harmful. Many of our own forebears present cases which document such harm and support this concern. The text of these articles documents how doctors of this earlier time clearly saw vaccination as a deliberate *poisoning of the blood* and questioned how it was possible that injecting potential toxins into the body could improve a patient's health. They and many others, including the anti-vaccination societies and the general public, not only challenged the rationale of such techniques, but also railed against their compulsory use.

Recurring arguments in this persisting conversation and debate are that such objections to vaccination belong in the past and that medicine has advanced since then, not only in terms of vaccine production and distribution, but also in terms of the validity of the science substantiating its use. However, these are dubious assertions. There is little doubt that medical technology has advanced and with it increasingly sophisticated ways to measure, analyze and intervene in one's body, but still the therapeutic rationale of treating symptoms with suppressive therapies in conventional medicine has not changed. In addition, the principles that govern health as documented eloquently in this volume remain as valid as ever. Thus, the concept of optimal health as the best treatment and prevention is at odds with the idea of injecting foreign substances into someone to ward off disease.

As well, and echoed eloquently in these pages by the early naturopathic physicians and those allied with their philosophy and practice, is the persisting concern about the potentially harmful effects of vaccination. In our own era these concerns are at an all-time high as the public continues to question the assertions of the dominant school of medicine and its powerful ally—the pharmaceutical industry. The belief that vaccinations are safe and effective obtains only if one takes the public health view that the collateral damage for the technique is acceptable in light of its perceived benefit. Just as the early naturopathic doctors cautioned, one need only read the package insert for most vaccinations to see that they are *not* always safe or effective. As reported in these pages, and consistent with today's research, many who are vaccinated are not protected; vaccinations do not always confer immunity (nor long lasting immunity for that matter), and those who are vaccinated may actually be carriers of the microbe spreading disease by infecting others (here invoking the conventional model of infectious disease).

The writers presented in this volume were quite prescient. They were concerned as much about the potential damage of vaccinations as they were about the adverse impacts and unpredictability of the microbial material itself. In recent years in this regard, significant research has shown that some microbes can evolve to evade the vaccination and there is evidence that the microbes from the vaccine may indeed colonize the patient. In fact, the stakes for vaccine damage are so high that it eventually became extremely difficult in the United States to sue a medical practitioner or a vaccine manufacturer for damages sustained from a vaccine. Under the 1986 *National Childhood Vaccine Injury Act*, Congress granted immunity to these groups because of the rising number of lawsuits alleging vaccine damage and the concomitant fear of vaccine manufacturers not providing vaccines. Instead of filing a medical injury lawsuit, an individual's sole remedy for vaccine damage is through the "vaccine court" or the United States Court of Federal Claims. Vaccine court is an administrative proceeding overseen by the United States Department of Health and Human Services. In spite of the assertion that vaccines are safe, the vaccine court has awarded since its inception more than $3.2 billion in damages to Americans for certain childhood vaccines. In my own practice of nearly forty years, I have seen dozens of children who were "normal", healthy children, meeting all of their developmental milestones, with no health problems until immediately after a vaccination. The changes in their behavior ranged from mild to severe neurological impairment, including diagnoses (made by conventional physicians) from attention deficient disorder to autism.

The doctors in these pages also point out that, despite the argument that vaccination was believed to greatly reduce or eradicate certain infectious diseases, much has been documented from their era to the present that suggests or proves otherwise. These undeniable outcomes are more likely due to better sanitation, hygiene, clean water supplies, and other public health measures, and not to the vaccinations themselves. Naturopathic doctors also recognize that one must go beyond the external environment and address the internal environment as well.

In recent years, reminiscent of the assertions of these early physicians, multitudes of studies have shown, for example, that various essential nutrients including Vitamins A, C, D and E, as well as zinc and selenium, each individually and in combination is effective in reducing the incidence of influenza and other so-called infectious diseases. As I write these words there is news in the press of studies showing that one who gets more than six hours of sleep at night has half the risk of "catching" the common cold as someone who gets less than six hours of sleep. Here again this simple way of intervening to prevent and cure illness, by sustaining good health and optimal function, is both explicit and implicit throughout these pages, in the very words of our naturopathic elders from the era of Benedict Lust, Henry Lindlahr and others whom you will meet here.

The early naturopathic doctors appear to have had no quarrel with the concept of active immunity. However, naturopathic and homeopathic physicians as well as indigenous healers have long known that there are methods which confer such immunity without any risk whatsoever. The naturopathic school of medicine argues that resistance to illness is conferred by good health. It is a matter of historical record that with every *infectious* disease and every epidemic there are those who are exposed to the "germ" with few or no consequences and those who succumb to the *disease* manifesting in serious symptoms or even death. Whether it's the bubonic plague of the fourteenth century, small pox of Shakespearian England, the 1918 global *flu* epidemic, or the Ebola scare in North Africa in the early twenty first century, there were many thousands or millions of deaths, but there are also those thousands or millions who survived. The difference is obviously in the individual and in our understanding of susceptibility and resistance. Simply stated, all living organisms, flowers, horses, children and, yes, *germs*, require the proper milieu or medium for their growth. Without an environment to support microbial growth, there can be no *infection*. Further, doctors of rational medicine have successfully treated many diseases now thought of as being caused by bacteria or viruses before microbes had been identified. This raises the obvious question discussed by critical thinkers since the discovery of microbes: *Does the microbe cause the tissue changes we call disease, or do the dis-*

ease conditions provide the proper environment for the proliferation of the microbe?

Also referenced in these pages are the practices and fundamentals of the homeopathic school of medicine from which our predecessors understood that immunity could be developed through the use of medicines which mimic the disease symptoms or through the use of microbes administered orally in infinitesimal doses. These procedures are similar to vaccination, and are equally, if not more, effective and without any harm at all.

The naturopathic pioneers cited in these pages were very familiar with the arguments for and against vaccination as it is performed in conventional medicine today. Despite the oppressive measures taken in those early days to establish vaccination with impunity in the community, the doctors cited in these articles did not hesitate to raise questions about its safety and its effectiveness, and further to challenge it as a mandatory medical procedure administered without consent. Theirs was a logical response given the knowledge that there are other safer, more effective, and less costly ways to enhance immunity than vaccination. Their bewilderment about why this was not common knowledge and why this was not known to the dominant medical community even to this day is a question, they insisted, of economics and politics, not of science and medicine.

Jim Sensenig, ND

Preface

Vaccination And Naturopathic Medicine is one of the twelve books that comprise The Hevert Collection. Each title consists of articles selected from the Lust journals from 1900-1923 (and occasionally when English articles are available, from 1899). The Rare Book Room at National College of Natural Medicine is the home of these unique, precious original papers. Published by Naturopathy's founder, Benedict Lust, across fifty years [1896-1945], the Lust journals coalesce the concerns, ambitions and vision of the emerging, young naturopathic profession. In the early days, *The Naturopath and Herald of Health* offered a voice to many NDs, MDs, DCs, DOs, and over thirty different groups who aligned themselves with the Naturopaths. The Hevert Collection is a celebration of our naturopathic history and makes available in the words of our naturopathic pioneers, their voices on what was important in Naturopathy in the early 20th century.

Fifty years of publishing is indeed a long time; it's a lifetime of dedication, editing and writing. Benedict devoted his life to Naturopathy and left behind a rich tapestry of literature that we can benefit from. Benedict did not do anything in small measure. He embraced journalism with ferocity and astute observation. He founded three principle journals and two of these underwent numerous name changes. *Amerikanischen Kneipp-Blätter* [1896-1899] an adaptation of a German publication was his first foray into publishing and was later renamed *The Kneipp Water Cure Monthly* [1900-1901]. As his horizons expanded from Father Sebastian Kneipp's water therapies, Benedict incorporated Adolf Just and Louis Kuhne and others into the new naturopathic healing paradigm and the next journal reflected those new interests.

The Naturopath and Herald of Health [1902-1915] became the first naturopathic journal ever to be published and it too soon underwent a name change to *Herald of Health and Naturopath* [1916-1922] in 1916. Then in 1923 this same journal became simply, *Naturopath* [1923-1945] retaining this name even after Benedict's death in 1945 and afterwards when his nephew, John Lust, assumed responsibility for the Lust publications. The third journal, *Nature's Path* [1925-1960's] preserved its original name throughout its entire lifespan. After Benedict's death, the journals also retained his photo and recognized him as the founder of the journals and of Naturopathy. Benedict's publishing career has made it possible to produce these twelve volumes for the Hevert Collection.

In 2010, before the Hevert Collection, a preliminary version of the current Vaccination book in a spiral bound format was published, *In Their Words: Vaccinations, a Naturopathic Historical Perspective*. It contained

44 articles. The book in this improvised form used original documents from the Lust journals and it soon became apparent that it needed to be revised. Inclusion and exclusion of articles were often dependent upon being able to legibly duplicate the original, and not always on the merit of their content. In this new collection, there are fifty-eight robust articles selected from 1900 to 1923, highlighting the animated conversations amongst the early doctors who had strong opinions about the political and social implications of compulsory vaccinations. In *Vaccinations and Naturopathic Medicine* there is a wide range of voices challenging vaccinations. The line up of articles reflects not only the accumulating objection by medical professionals, but also the broad range of those across the spectrum of the medical professions and civil society who were concerned and determined to speak up. There are 29 by M.D.s, 20 by Naturopaths, 3 by politicians and /or lawyers; 2 by scientists, and 4 by Anti-vaccination organizations who were invariably founded and led by Medical Doctors.

Since the introduction of vaccination by Jenner in 1796, the outpouring of dissent built and persisted across more than two centuries. Many doctors raised their voices in protest against vaccination, reasoning that vaccinations needlessly maimed and killed innocent people. The same doctors demonstrated the importance of sanitation in disease control and provided credible examples that the low incidence of smallpox hinged not on compulsory vaccination programs, but rather on sanitation and hygiene. The argument that vaccinations saved lives was and remains unresolved. Many of the medical doctors from the regular school attested and witnessed first-hand that people did indeed die from the smallpox vaccine. We may be inclined to conclude that the doctors a century ago were simply over reacting and alarmist in their opposition; however, the statistics speak volumes that their concerns were well founded. In their own words, many of the doctors in this volume were more afraid of vaccination than of the actual diseases for which the vaccines were developed. This same literature points out that treating diseases such as smallpox was entirely possible using natural treatment guidelines. You will also find in these pages protocols that were used successfully for whooping cough, diphtheria, smallpox, scarlet fever, infantile cholera and the dreaded measles.

Further, a careful read of the work of our pioneering forebears will demonstrate that we haven't evolved within the last two hundred years in regards to the germ theory and vaccination. Indeed, a number of the examples and specific cases cited in these articles may well remind us of a recent event in the USA. The American Center for Disease Control [CDC] asserted that low vaccination rates were responsible for a measles outbreak in Disneyland, California [December 2014–February 2015]. The 159 measles cases linked to the Disneyland episode resulted in no deaths; yet during the past ten years [2004–2014] there have been 108 documented deaths in children receiving the measles vaccine, juxtaposed in the same period with there having been zero deaths from contracting measles. What the early Naturopaths knew was that it was far easier to treat smallpox and the other infectious diseases if one followed the laws of Nature. Natural treatment that included dietetics, water therapies, sanitation and hygiene supported the body to eliminate the conditions of disease and restore health.

Although articles appear each year from 1900 to 1923, the majority of the vaccination pieces were published between 1909 and 1913. In 1913, one sees a shift in the dialogue from vaccinations to medical freedom contextualized within the naturopathic community. August A. Erz, for example, published a book, *Medical Laws vs Rights and Constitution* in 1913, which Benedict Lust re-published in his journal allotting many successive pages in each issue. It was with great regret that I could not include whole articles from Erz because of their 20 to 30 page lengths.

Vaccination has occupied a continually shifting historical position; sometimes it has the golden seal of approval and then in a blink, it is condemned as dangerous, only to revert back to good and the cycle persists. We are currently seeing the biomedical community embrace vaccinations as its sanctified miracle against the germs which surround us. At the same time, we are recognizing the importance of the human microbiome and the invaluable contribution micro-organisms have in human health. Some theories persist, such as Koch's Germ Theory. Another example is the work of Metchnikoff and Béchamp whose countering theories of germs recognized their essential role in human life. These debates have persisted for centuries and will likely generate literature for centuries more.

In this book, you will discover the history of vaccination from the perspective of the early pioneers. You will read statistics. You will learn about the Anti-Vaccination League of America and its struggles and victories. Pay close attention, as well, to Henry Lindlahr's account of vaccination and see if it still fits for you in the 21st century. Discover champions and doctors who worked selflessly to educate their patients to choose health. Of the hundreds of vaccination articles found in the Lust journals, there was not one that presented a neutral opinion. All of the articles were polarized against vaccinations and in particular, compulsory vaccination of children.

You will find in *Vaccination And Naturopathic Medicine* examples of patient care and the protocols used to treat infectious diseases. Contemporary reliance upon antibiotics is reaching a plateau, and perhaps even an end point, or at least a place in medicine when we cannot place our entire trust in a drug that sometimes backfires. You will discover treatments that are simple and surprising. These protocols may seem unfathomable and perhaps even impossible for treating disease. Let me tell you a secret which was known all over the early naturopathic neighborhood. The early Naturopaths did not have much in the way of gadgets, nutraceuticals were non-existent, and antibiotics weren't invented yet (had they been, they would have been completely out of the question). They used water and knew how to manipulate water to achieve the healing reaction desired. They endorsed fresh air, sunshine, dietary measures, exercise and hygiene. With their understanding of Nature, they were able to treat diseases quite successfully that Allopaths attributed to germs.

I want to thank everyone who has breathed life into *Vaccination And Naturopathic Medicine*. Behind the glossy book cover are hundreds of typed pages which were patiently transcribed by many magnificent students at NCNM. In fact, there are over 1000 articles typed from the Benedict Lust journals in preparation for the books in this collection. I want to acknowledge every NCNM student who typed or proof-read articles while navigating his or her intense course loads and juggling personal lives. I bow with gratitude to **Adam Dombrowski, Alla Nicolulis, Anemone Fresh, Delia Sewell, Jenny Curto, Karis Tressel, Katelyn Mudry, Kirsten Carle, Lauren Geyman, Marie Benkley, Meagan Hammel, Meagan Watts, Olif Wojciechowski, Rebecca Jennings, Tristian Rowe,** and all those whom I am inadvertently missing here.

And, as this book project continues, my appreciation for the invaluable organizational help that I had received from **Dr. Karis Tressel** at the commencement is a daily reminder that book making is an undertaking of an entire community. I am deeply grateful for her profound love of the traditions and history of Naturopathy and her loving tenacity with this project.

I so much enjoyed working with each and every student who sacrificed scarce, precious study and leisure time for the hard work of meticulous research and transcription. As you launch yourselves into the Naturopathic profession, never forget how special and important your work has been. You have chosen a path of sacred work. You will be loved and cherished by your patients because you listen and truly care. Remember to trust Nature's power of healing, the *Vis medicatrix naturae*! Pay careful attention to your patients and they will feel enlivened and grateful to have found their way to you.

I am grateful for my colleagues who have added their voices to *Vaccination and Naturopathic Medicine*, especially doctors Jim Sensenig, ND, Jared Zeff, N.D., and Alex Vasquez, DC, ND, DO, FACN. Jim Sensenig, from Connecticut, is a modern day elder of the profession whose foreword graces this book. He has sustained for forty years the same kind of remarkable commitment as students and graduates at the beginning of their careers. He has been full throttle at building the Naturopathic profession all these years. Instrumental in every corner of professional formation (to name a few: key architect of the AANP, the CNME, the eventual AANMC; key negotiator in the early licensing efforts across the United States; former Dean at NCNM; lecturer at Southwest College of Naturopathic Medicine; award winner from NCNM, CCNM); in family practice for over three decades), his work embodies the very essence of Naturopathic principles and philosophy.

Jared Zeff, ND is a champion in the Naturopathic profession, providing leadership and stewardship of our precious naturopathic principles and values. It is one thing to read and talk about the wonders of Naturopathy and another to put into practice our philosophical values with each and every patient. To embody the essence of Naturopathy means to fearlessly use water as a medicine; it means confidently using food, herbs, sunshine, and fresh air as medicine. We have in Jared a Naturopathic Physician who doesn't mince words when he says that vaccination causes harm, a conviction he holds based on his decades of clinical experience with his patients. Thank you, Jared, for your courageous voice.

Dr. Alex Vasquez assimilates and shares his tireless, formidable academic medicine inquiry and scholarship with fellow health professionals, spanning a vast literature of diverse and relevant medical subjects. He too is fearless about standing behind his beliefs and his work. Earlier this year when I was working on *Vaccinations and Naturopathic Medicine*, news of legislation which proposed to impose compulsory vaccination in Oregon alarmed many physicians in our state. We were disturbed that our otherwise progressive state would contemplate such a draconian initiative. I contacted colleagues with my concerns and with lightning speed Alex responded, providing an abundance of research and documents regarding vaccination and its effects. The ensuing collaboration of medical and naturopathic doctors yielded a wealth of information for doctors and their patients regarding vaccination. Being part of Alex' network of like-minded, esteemed colleagues is a personal and professional privilege.

His position on the vaccination issue quickly puts us in mind of the work of our naturopathic elders a century ago. Their concerns also arose from clinical experiences of the dangers of vaccination. Today, a growing scientific literature clearly and unquestionably corroborates the perils of vaccination. I am deeply grateful that Dr. Vasquez shares clinical data and astute, broad knowledge from which he accesses the facts of the matter and then shares those findings so generously, coherently and systematically. Alex, never stop doing what you do.

Dr Alex Vasquez holds three clinical doctorates: DC, ND. and DO. He has authored many definitive textbooks such as *Integrative Orthope-*

dics (2012), *Integrative Rheumatology* (2014), and *Musculoskeletal Pain: Expanded Clinical Strategies* (Institute for Functional Medicine, 2008), among many others, and is a frequent contributor to professional magazines and medical journals such as *British Medical Journal* (BMJ), *The Lancet, Annals of Pharmacotherapy,* and many more. He is the Chief Editor of *International Journal of Human Nutrition and Functional Medicine* (Int J Hum Nutr Funct Med.ORG).

I am very thankful for the unrelenting support of the Hevert Corporation here in America and in Germany. Thank you and my most gracious accolades to Americana and Wolf Aulenbacher and the Hevert family in Germany for believing in the impossible. Yes, we can create 12 books that are an exquisite testimony to the power of Naturopathy. Much gratitude, as well, to the unwavering, behind-the-scenes support of the Board of NCNM, Dr. Sandra Snyder, Susan Hunter, and Jerry Bores who understood from the beginning the importance of this project.

The precision and beauty that Fourth Lloyd Productions, Nancy and Richard Stodart, my designers, bring to this book are wonderful. We're now at book six and we have travelled through many conversations and details to bring this book to life. Thank you both for the exquisite care that you took with every minute detail!

The best of all, I want to thank, heart to heart, my patient and beloved husband, David Schleich, who inspires me in this journey of revitilizing the past. David becomes my tangible connection to the 21st century when I become lost in the previous one. I could not do what I do without you.

Lastly, I am so indebted to the men and women of the profession who lived a hundred years ago and have left behind a trail of wisdom and passion that fills me with confidence and gratitude for their contributions to a literature that I can read when I want. You may find that some of the sentences can be a mile long or embellished with words no longer in our current vocabulary, but this is on purpose. These articles have been carefully transcribed and edited to ensure that you are taken back into time. So, settle back in a comfortable chair and enjoy these articles chosen from the past and from our elders in their own words.

Blessings,
Sussanna Czeranko, ND, BBE
Portland, Oregon, December, 2015

On my arrival the appearance of the little patient gave me the impression that my help had come too late. The body was a mere frame-work of bones covered with loose skin; the face was wrinkled and old-looking, the eyes dull and lusterless, half obscured. The whole body was cold to the touch, particularly the hands and feet; the pulse thin and thread-like, often scarcely perceptible; in short, the whole appearance was the reverse of reassuring.

—Otto Wagner, 1900, 45

We condemn a system which makes medical heterdoxy a social crime; we condemn a system which is the principal hindrance to the development of the noblest most humane, most useful of all arts.

—J. T. Robinson, 1909, 117

Naturopathy claims that germs of themselves alone cannot create disease—if they could, humanity would soon be extinct. Disease germs are present everywhere, on the food we eat, and the water we drink, and air and dust we breathe, and on the money we handle. Can you imagine anything fouler and more thoroughly saturated with disease germs and bacteria than our beloved money?

—Henry Lindlahr, 1910, 130

The system of compulsory vaccination is founded upon a hypothesis too preposterous for a moment's serious argument. It arose from the curious dogma that a healthy person is a focus of disease; and that not having been diseased (i. e., vaccinated) he would be the propagator of disease (small-pox) to those who had been diseased (vaccinated) and thus "protected." If vaccination protected the vaccinated, they would have no occasion to fear infection.

—John W. Hodge, 1910, 467

The scab from a running sore is scraped away and the pus or running matter is collected and this is what vaccine virus is that is put into your healthy bodies. This is a direct violation of the principle of asepsis in surgery, which is advocated by scientific medicine and which stands for this: that no foreign organisms shall be permitted to go into any cut part on the human body, and aseptic medicines are used in all operations to prevent what is done in vaccination.

—Joseph P. Rinn, 1911, 207-208

A barrel of ignited turpentine could not have flared up with more startling effect than did the epidemic of smallpox in the face of the vicious vaccination crusade.

—John W. Hodge, 1912, 224

Vaccination represents an honest effort on the part of the medical profession to find a preventive for a simple, yet loathsome disease. This effort, however, like many others of its kind, has not only failed to meet the expectation of its discoverer, but has left in its wake, a blighting curse which it will require many generations to remove. Were it not for the fact that vaccination has been enforced by legislation, we would not now be discussing it except as an antiquated medical experiment akin to leeches and blood-letting.

—Charles W. Littlefield, 1912, 12

In his classical work on "History of Epidemics in Britain", Dr. Creighton tells us that in all the great epidemics of smallpox, which have scourged civilized nations since the adoption and establishment of vaccination, it has been the vaccinated, not the unvaccinated, who were first seized by smallpox, which disease subsequently spread from them, as foci of infection, to the unvaccinated.

—John W. Hodge, 1912, 225

Real immunity is overlooked and lost sight of in the mad chase after imaginary ones, such as serums, antitoxins, and vaccines. The use of these measures to cure or prevent disease diverts attention from genuine immunity, from the means that ought to be employed to secure such immunity.

—Helen Sayr Gray, 1912, 383

If the prevention theory were true, then no person could possibly ever have smallpox in any form after vaccination.

—August Andrew Erz, 1913, 835

Someday our wise and learned will realize that there is a heap of difference between preventing disease and preventing or suppressing reactions.

—William Freeman Havard, 1918, 867

Germs are scavengers. Their duty is to break down substances in the body that need to be removed. So long as we live according to the laws of Nature, no germ will or can injure us.

—Per Nelson, 1920, 136

No man can violate this unfailing and unalterable law of Nature, which is older than the race itself, and expect to escape suffering the penalty by simply swallowing some poison drug. If we could do that, then the law of God would be completely subservient to the caprice of the will of man, and the price of drugs would soar so high that only the rich could afford to buy them.

—Benedict Lust, 1923, 580

INTRODUCTION

The vaccination debate is widespread today, and has a galvanizing effect in our era not unlike on the early Naturopaths entering the new twentieth century. Concerns about the very theory of vaccination, and also about safety and efficacy helped rally the profession to recognize and proclaim the importance of following Nature's laws, about medical freedom and about choice in health care a hundred and ten years back. Their collective, cumulative voice was not unlike what we experience in contemporary North America in the middle of the second decade of another new century. For a long time now the idea and practice of vaccination conjure up strong opinions among health care providers, both pro and con. Politicians what the early Naturopaths called "the laity" weighed in quickly and often. Just as back in the day of Lindlahr and Lust, surrounding issues about health choice accent the worry about safety and effectiveness.

The early Naturopaths fought bitterly against compulsory vaccination when this public health net cascaded out of the nineteenth century right into communities all over North America in the early twentieth. This collection of articles, by no means an exhaustive compilation, but rather a modest, representative selection of articles found in Lust's journals, voices such concerns of our forebears, raising alarm bells then which reverberate to the modern era in the media and the medical literature. Whereas the concern about vaccination brought together Naturopaths and many more Allopaths than one might expect from our perspective in this century, a century ago, today, the issue of vaccination has been dividing and fracturing the naturopathic profession. Some align with vaccination and others choose to oppose its use. Similar fault lines are also seen in the allopathic communities.

As you read through these articles, you may well experience as I did the moral conviction and deep commitment to the laws of Nature our elders exhibit. As you reflect further upon the writings of these pioneers, you will soon discern their astute reflection on this complex topic, and the brilliance and courage of their response to elements of the autocratic imposition of vaccination. In some ways, this book distills out for us the essence of Naturopathy, manifesting all of its strength as a natural therapeutic model. Disease, and especially infectious disease, was not avoided, feared or considered hopeless by the early Naturopaths; rather, they saw such presentations as an opportunity to practice medicine using the gifts of Nature to help heal patients. And heal they did.

The first two articles get right to the point and strike home with their clear message. Naturopaths did *not* blink when faced with dreaded and feared childhood diseases which claimed so many in 19th and early 20th centuries, such as measles, scarlet fever, diphtheria and infantile cholera. Always, they turned to natural methods of helping the body to overcome disease and malady. The early Naturopaths who confronted these diseases in their patients did so with confidence and with their splendid tools, such as the simple protocols used by Father Kneipp. The hay-flower shirt and the salt-shirt invented by Kneipp offered relief for children suffering from measles, and other childhood diseases. (Lust, 1900, 28; Kneipp, 1903, 237) In this regard, Benedict Lust counsels his colleagues, "One does not need to feel frightened on account of [the rash accompanying diphtheria], for the rash is a natural consequence of the process of healing." (Lust, 1900, 28)

Otto Wagner in his short article outlines a case of infantile cholera which can only fill us with awe. Having no antibiotics, no heroic medicine, nor an urgent intervention in a hospital emergency room, Wagner used simple baths, enemas and diet to cure a six month old infant of cholera within a matter of days. His first impression of this tiny patient was that the infant was a "framework of bones covered with loose skin; the face was wrinkled and old looking, the eyes dull and lusterless. ... The whole body was cold to the touch, ... the whole appearance was the reverse of reassuring ." (Wagner, 1900, 45) By his third visit to the bedside of this very young patient, Wagner states, "The child could be regarded as saved. There was no more vomiting, stools took place 3 or 4 times a day ... sleep and appetite were good, appearance fresher." (Wagner, 1900, 46) This prognosis comes 4 days after the initial consultation. Very spectacular considering that infantile cholera was essentially a death sentence for infants. This documented account is not unusual in the literature, and even more significant given the profile of the doctor, whose reliable accounts of such cases had wide circulation and profound credibility in this era. Otto Wagner held the Director position at the famed palatial sanitarium that Friedrich Eduard Bilz established in Radebeul - Dresden, Germany.

Bilz, for his part, was a devout follower of Father Sebastian Kneipp. He had written a two volume encyclopedia numbering over 2,000 pages and built one of the most successful sanitariums in 19th century Europe. It was in this context that another Naturopath, Wagner, documents the revival of a dying child, restored back to health with cold water compresses, baths, enemas and a simple diet. Kneipp and such followers were famous for such miraculous cures and today Wöerishofen stands prominently, testament to the wisdom of Kneipp more than a century after his death.

The medical feats established by Kneipp and his followers spread to all continents. Infectious diseases could indeed be treated and cured with confidence and success, just as Kneipp demonstrated, by using ingenious, intuitive variations of Nature's elements of water, sunshine, fresh air and a healthy diet. In his article, "Children's Diseases", for example, Sebastian Kneipp describes the use of the salt shirt treatment and fenugreek tea for scarlatina and measles. Kneipp viewed childhood diseases as a detoxifying process and health promoting. He states, "It is a well-known fact that children who have recovered from either of these two diseases [scarlatina, measles], are much healthier and feel much better than those who have not had them." (Kneipp, 1903, 237)

Thus it was that the introduction of vaccination as the singularly reliable method of preventing infectious diseases was not unchallenged. In fact, Edward Jenner's solution to disease was met with mounting opposition, including the creation of Anti-Vaccination organizations. One of the first such organizations in the U.S. was the Anti-Vaccination Society of America. We discover in the April 1901 issue of *The Kneipp Water Cure Monthly,* a notice appearing with its written constitution. Its primary purpose was to educate the public about vaccination with provocative descriptors warning that vaccination was "a disease and death-producing agency". (Blue, 1901, 116) Each month a publication was distributed to its membership. In 1910, a second group called the Anti-Vaccination League of America began to publish its meetings and events in the *Naturopath*. This group had as its objective "to secure the abolition of all oppressive medical laws, and ... to give aid and assistance to societies or individuals engaged in the movement for freedom from compulsory vaccination." (Anti-Vaccination League, 1910, 549)

One of the members of the Anti-Vaccination Society and second Vice-President, Dr. A. J. Clausen, MD, delivered a speech to its St. Paul, Minnesota members. As a medical doctor, he was appalled that compulsory vaccination could even exist under the American constitution. He argued, "If there is anything a man owns, it is his own blood and just as a man has the unquestioned right to choose his political party, religion, physician, and to say whether or not a surgical operation shall be performed on his body, just so he has the right to reject vaccination." (Clausen, 1901, 158)

From its inception the naturopathic profession collaborated with the Anti-Vaccinationists many of whose members were from the medical (or allopathic) profession. Illustrative of this shared position, Lust documents the outcome of a meeting of the Naturopathic Society of America at which E. B. Foote, MD (the Treasurer of the Anti-Vaccination Society of America) reported victory on the Stewart Bill, Number 235 in the New York Assembly, a legislative initiative about compulsory vaccination. One of the Society's members was able to retract a few lines to prevent these mandatory vaccinations. Lust comments, "At least we may congratulate ourselves that the vigilance of a few has protected the many from a very imminent danger of the worst sort of compulsory vaccination law." (Lust, 1903, 127)

Prevention was recognized early by the nature doctors to be instrumental in curbing the incidence of contagion and diseases. Dr. A. L. Wood, MD's article in *The Naturopath and Herald of Health* recounts the dysentery epidemics in the Lake Champlain district as a result of impure water supplies along with a similar crisis in Brooklyn, New York. He extolls the virtues of distilled water and compares it to "Nature's distilled water in the form of rain". (Wood, 1902, 131) Filtered and distilled water were both advocated by the Naturopaths to prevent infections. Impure water containing bacteria was remedied with the use of a water distiller and there were many advertisements of various distillers in *The Naturopath and Herald of Health*. The notion of prevention, then as now, was grounded in access to healthy water in this case, along with the Naturopath's advocacy for clean air, good food and hygienic living space.

The Naturopaths did not deny that bacteria introduced into the body caused illness; however, they recognized that when the human body succumbed to an overload of micro-organisms, it was their view that perhaps the problem was not the bacteria, but the underlying conditions that bacteria favoured. They contended that acute symptoms arising from the presence of bacteria in a body were the body's attempt to restore health. In this regard, Dr. Carl Strueh, MD cites examples of mechanisms of the body protecting itself and maintaining homeostasis. He reminds readers, "Bacilli by themselves are never the cause of illness; they are everywhere in Nature; they are always swarming about us, but they never settle in our organism and multiply if there be nothing to do for them, i.e., if they do not find dead material on which they can subsist." (Strueh, 1904, 82) Strueh viewed vaccination as an interference with such natural protective mechanisms of the body. He states, "So-called preventive vaccination (immunization) [enables] the disease, i.e., the predisposition, or the morbid material in our system [to be] preserved." (Strueh, 1904, 82)

Morbid matter, in fact, lies at the center of the naturopathic etiological paradigm. Naturopathic doctors have long anchored their approach in life style counseling to help patients navigate the dangerous terrain of fast food, GMO foods, stress, late nights, sedentary life habits and many related behaviours which accumulate unrelentingly into chronicity, morbidity and mortality. In the early literature morbid matter referred to "indigestible food and faulty diet ... unhealthy, damp, dark dwelling places, often dirty, and never aired, ... too little exercise." (Lust, 1905, 13) Morbid matter and poor life style choices were faulted as the cause of diseases, for example diphtheria. Benedict Lust cites morbid matter as a major cause and provides a detailed account of patient management. The therapies used by Sebastian Kneipp and Louis Kuhne are prominent in his protocol.

In a following article, "Diphtheria and Antitoxine", Dr. Schulze brings to our attention the fervent efforts by the Allopaths to discover a solution or *antitoxine* for diphtheria. Proponents of the antitoxine claimed it to be only effective in the early stages of the disease which confounded men such as Schulze who points out the unpredictable and precipitous onset of diphtheria. He states, "No other disease approaches so treacherously and breaks out so suddenly in its fully characteristic developed form, before the least suspicion has been entertained of the presence of the danger." (Schulze, 1905, 17) Schulze's paper presents questions and leaves a message of caution. He recounts details of a newspaper story of a medical doctor's use of the antitoxine on his own son. Upon receiving the injection, "in an instant the boy was a corpse". (Schulze, 1905, 17-18) The inclusion of this article in Benedict Lust's journal was crystal clear. Lust, having seen personally the success of naturopathic modalities for the treatment of diphtheria, must have cringed witnessing the allopathic pursuit of dangerous vaccines. He wanted his membership to be forewarned and aware of the adverse possibilities that vaccines entailed.

Another medical doctor brings her voice to the vaccination discussion. Dr. Ellen Goodell Smith, M.D., bursts the bubble of misconception that vegetarians are safe from contracting smallpox. As a vegetarian, she recounts her brush with the illness and briefly describes her treatments. Her attending physician remarks, "Your baths, packs and fasting could not have been improved and you do not need a drop of my medicine." (Goodell Smith, 1906, 159) The water cure applications used by Dr. Goodell Smith demonstrate that it is possible to cure smallpox without resorting to vaccination. Her case demonstrates that smallpox, treated using Nature's methods, was not synonymous with death.

Yet many died from smallpox and more often than not under the care of allopathic methods. Vaccination for the prevention of smallpox seemed reasonable in such a cascading scenario. Yet, questions regarding its use appear and re-appear in *The Naturopath*. One medical doctor opposed to compulsory vaccination had formulated a logical argument that continues to be heard even to our present day. Dr. Leverson, M.D. states, "If [vaccination] really does protect from smallpox, then those who are vaccinated are protected and can incur no danger from the unvaccinated." (Leverson, 1906, 260) From this perspective, compulsory vaccination of those who objected was unequivocally wrong.

Another objecting medical doctor, C. S. Carr, M.D., questions the dishonest tactics used by the Public Health Boards in establishing statistics in favour of vaccination and to cover up its failures. Carr exposed the practice by the Public Health Boards in their statistical findings by pointing out that their methodology included vaccinated people who contract smallpox in the group of un-vaccinated. The discrepancy had huge implications for the illusionary success of vaccination preventing smallpox.

Carr reveals, "It was frankly stated by the health officer to charge that if these people had been *'successfully vaccinated'* they would not have had smallpox. Therefore, he felt entirely justified in classifying them as *'never vaccinated'*." (Carr, 1907, 222)

Smallpox was a much feared disease and so too was pertussis (whooping cough), a highly contagious, respiratory tract infection caused by a bacterium (Bordetella pertussis). The treatment of whooping cough by Allopaths and by Naturopaths differed both in application and outcomes. Benedict Lust remarks upon the allopathic failure to treat whooping cough: "The treatment of this sickness by the Allopaths, as they themselves will frankly admit, is in no way satisfactory. Their only remedies are the following ones: belladonna, hydrocyanic acid, inhalations of the nitrate of silver and bromide of potash, infections of morphia and so forth." (Lust, 1907, 355)   Lust concludes his article with Kneipp's water applications and directions on the treatment of whooping cough that used water therapies as well as herbal remedies. It is easy to understand that some of the Allopaths chose to cling tightly to vaccination as a means to contain infectious diseases.

In the early 20th century compulsory vaccination was limited to smallpox. Those parents who had children vaccinated had more to fear than one vaccination shot. Vaccinated children who did not manifest signs and symptoms as a result of their vaccination were subjected to more vaccination injections until the vaccine 'took'. Proof of a vaccination that *took* was visible at the injection site. Dr. Walter Elfrink, Secretary of the Anti-Vaccination Society of America explains, "The Health Department refuses to accept the certificates of physicians in good standing, and insists that every pupil must exhibit a typical scar not smaller than a ten-cent piece before he can be admitted to the schools." (Elfrink, 1908, 95) The public outrage against compulsory vaccination in such a political climate was supported by doctors from both the naturopathic and allopathic trenches.

Compulsory vaccination enforced by the American Medical Association was seen by Dr. Robinson, M.D. as "the greatest evil that confronts the American people today [and] is [an] evil monopoly". (Robinson, 1909, 116) The monopoly Robinson references was that the A.M.A. exerted in its enforcement of vaccination against the will of the people, thus attracting many foes and protestors. It did not take long for people to speak their minds and to rally and expose the tyranny of the Allopaths who had chosen political means to power. Called many names and branded as diabolical and villainous, the A.M.A. did not win the support of the people and sometimes of their very own members. Robinson adds emphatically, "These medical trust pirates pretend that their object is to protect the people against the imposition of quacks and impostors, judging from the size of the medical fees and the wholesale butcheries in our hospitals infirmaries, the people will not appreciate such protection." (Robinson, 1909, 116)   A significant proportion of voices that we witness in *The Naturopath* actually come from Allopathic medical doctors who determined compulsory vaccination to be nefarious and inexpiable. For medical doctors opposed to vaccination, *The Naturopath* was a vehicle to make their views known. These medical doctors exhibited a social conscience that motivated them to speak out and help inform the public.

More views of the dangers of vaccination were presented in a paper by another M.D., William D. Gentry. Determined to influence the Committee on Education of the House of Representatives of the Illinois Legislature, he spoke on the subject of compulsory "vaccination and revaccination of all inhabitants of towns or cities, the vaccination of inmates of almshouses, reform and industrial schools, hospitals, prisons, jails or any institution which is supported or aided by the State." (Gentry, 1909, 633)

Gentry's purpose was to educate the members of the House of Representatives about the dangers of vaccines and to reassure these politicians that more efficient and preventive approaches against smallpox than vaccination. His address to his members of State may have fallen on deaf ears, though. After all, he was also alerting this group of politicians of the misdeeds of some of its supporters. "A great amount of money is being made by men and women in the business of producing virus of various degrees of effectiveness in producing disease, and in vaccinating, whose business and income will be greatly increased by having this Bill become a law. These are the individuals who are using every influence in their power to persuade you to approve and recommend this Bill for passage." (Gentry, 1909, 634) Today, Big Pharma has the attention of the government and continues to reap the financial benefits of compulsory vaccination in America.

Related to this burgeoning debate about compulsory vaccination was the dialogue about germ theory. Hereward Carrington, writing on the subject of fasting and diet, revisited the theories of the plague that decimated the world in the Middle Ages. Indeed, throughout the Lust journals, naturopathic contributors were compelled to make the distinction from the germ theory and what they considered to be the real cause of disease. Carrington states, "Orthodox medical science contends that the germs cause the disease; many nature-curists contend, equally firmly, that the foul conditions of the disease rendered possible the presence of the germ. Doubtless there is much truth in both of these views." (Carrington, 1909, 356)   Carrington reminds us that perhaps one important fact is omitted when viewing the plague and germs and that is the person's individual health. He continues, "There can be no doubt ... that this question of the state of the individual's health is relegated to a very unimportant and subsidiary position, when it should hold a very important, if not preeminent one." (Carrington, 1909, 356)   Carrington contended that hygiene and diet need to be considered in treatment plans for patients.

Long before the Ivan Illich published *Medical Nemesis: Limits to Medicine (1974)* [London: Calder & Boyars, 1974], in which he warned that the medicalizing of the human life continuum had converted millions into lifelong patients and in which he postulated the notion of "iatrogenic disease" (side effects, complications arising from treatments or procedures, medical errors, unnecessary treatment for profit), doctors practicing medicine throughout the 19th and 20th centuries have observed an unexplained surge of new disease presentations as a result of vaccinations.

Another medical doctor who rose to the forefront of those opposing the enforcement of vaccination was Dr. John W. Hodge, M.D., who had a practice in Lockport, New York. Hodge wrote often in *The Naturopath* and his articles touched upon every imaginable aspect of the intrusive nature of vaccination. Over time, vaccinations were implicated with diseases such as cancer, syphilis, tuberculosis and others. The complicity of tuberculosis and smallpox vaccinations arose, for example, with the practice of using cows infected with tuberculosis to propagate smallpox vaccines. Cows and calves were the primary source for the smallpox vaccine. Hodge explains, "These inoculation experiments prove conclusively that tuberculosis is communicable through vaccination; and as cows are peculiarly subject to tuberculosis, both in its latent and active forms, we can never be certain that the so-called "calf-lymph used by vaccinators is free from the subtle and insidious foe: tuberculosis." (Hodge, 1910, 76) Hodge noted that the causal relation between smallpox vaccination and the incidence of tuberculosis was most marked in countries with high vaccination use.

Another who was a leading voice about the danger of vaccination was Henry Lindlahr, M.D. Lindlahr wrote numerous articles on vaccination, four of which are included here, in a series called "The Anti-Vaccination Crusade". Reading these four articles, a student and practitioner of Naturopathy can arrive at a comprehensive understanding of the essence and roots of naturopathic practice. Lindlahr encapsulates the philosophical differences which set Naturopathy apart from and renders it superior to its detractors, and he does so without apology. He speaks with conviction and tutors us in the laws of Nature.

In the first of his series, he challenges Dr. Koch (the originator of the Germ Theory) and his failed Tuberculin serum. He enlightens and entertains:

Naturopathy claims that germs of themselves alone cannot create disease—if they could, humanity would soon be extinct. Disease germs are present everywhere, on the food we eat, and the water we drink, and air and dust we breathe, and on the money we handle. Can you imagine anything fouler and more thoroughly saturated with disease germs and bacteria than our beloved money? (Lindlahr, 1910, 130)

To understand the difference between Naturopathy and Allopathy, one must first understand the differences between acute and chronic disease. Lindlahr makes these distinctions crystal clear for us.

If Henry Lindlahr were given the choice, he would choose to have smallpox in the form of the disease rather than to be subjected to a smallpox vaccination. In the following article, he explains why. He illustrates with the example of his son who had contracted smallpox and describes in great detail his protocol. This is where his teaching shines and illuminates, generating one of those precious *"Ah ha"* moments in naturopathic medicine. Lindlahr declares,

All acute diseases are natural processes—as we express it—the result of Nature's healing, cleansing efforts, which run a certain well-defined, orderly and natural course. There is a stage of incipiency followed by stages of intense acute activity during which Nature endeavors to burn up, tear down and eliminate by means of fever heat, sores, catarrhal discharges, etc., the morbid matter and poisons from the system. (Lindlahr, 1910, 258)

Why is the disease preferred? His edifying answer comes next: "If during any one of these stages Nature's orderly processes is hindered, interrupted or suppressed by ice bags, poisonous drugs, antitoxin, serums, surgical operations, or mental effort, the disease condition is arrested and made a permanent one." (Lindlahr, 1910, 258) By creating a chronic smallpox in the body with vaccination, one is predisposed "to the development of all kinds of chronic diseases". (Lindlahr, 1910, 387) Lindlahr reiterated the concerns of his colleagues of new chronic diseases manifesting after vaccination: "Undoubtedly this systematic and almost universal contamination and degeneration of vital fluids and tissues accounts in a large measure for the steady increase of tuberculosis, cancer, syphilis, insanity and for a multitude of other chronic destructive diseases unknown among primitive peoples, free from the blessings of syphilization, mercurialization and vaccination." (Lindlahr, 1910, 387)

In this regard, Lindlahr was horrified, for example, with the repetitive vaccinations children received if the vaccinations did not "take". He recounts a news story in the Chicago papers, "The case of a girl who had been vaccinated ten times without *results* and then admission to the public schools was refused to the child because she was *not properly vac-*

cinated." (Lindlahr, 1910, 491)   When vaccinations did *take,* Lindlahr considered that these children were the lucky ones because they were able to expel the vaccine more successfully.

John Hodge was one of the most outspoken on compulsory vaccination and especially in children. His views of the doctors who politicized their position to gain entry into schools and to profit from vaccination were searing and exposing. Hodge elucidates, "In commenting on this wholesale execution of healthy children by doctors who intentionally propagate a filth-disease (cowpox) under the pretense of sanitation, I pointed out the fact that vaccination with the medical faculty is a matter of business, and not one of philanthropy." (Hodge, 1910, 465)   The injection of pathological and purulent matter into healthy humans lacked ethical integrity on the part of the politicians and doctors bent on enforcing vaccination at all costs. Hodge continues, "The introduction of the product's diseased animal tissues—miscalled *calf lymph*—into the circulation of healthy human body is contrary to the teachings of modern surgery and sanitary science, and has no justification in either science or common sense." (Hodge, 1910, 466)   Not only can we find appalling the ethical conflict which the monetary gain accruing to medical doctors promoting wholesale vaccination, but also shocking were the ensuing chronic diseases (associated with vaccination) that Lindlahr references.

Related association of cancer with vaccination prevalence was also viewed with suspicion. Theories and papers were written to find the links. F. M. Padelford, for example, writes, "While there may not be any direct relationship between vaccination and cancer, yet the practice of inoculating generation after generation with the complex product known as vaccine lymph may ultimately so modify the metabolic processes that cancer is likely to develop." (Padelford, 1910, 660)   The discovery of "a resemblance between the inclusions found in cancer and those observed in smallpox and vaccinia were the first to call attention to the analogy between the two processes". (Padelford, 1910, 659)   As scientist exploring the connection between chronic diseases such as cancer, it is not hard to see why he and many others including Naturopaths questioned the safety of vaccination.

In his 1910 article, "Public Health Tracts" Benedict Lust illustrates the gulf between the medical intentions of vaccination and the experience of the people receiving those injections. Lust says, "The doctors discovered that vaccination, with four good marks, prevented smallpox for life—*The people find that it does not."* (Lust, 1910, 661) Lust continues citing the most probable cause of the decline in smallpox, "*The people are discovering that defective drainage, overcrowding, badly constructed dwellings, ill-ventilation, un-wholesome food and deficient water supply are the exciting causes of smallpox epidemics.*—The doctors must be compelled to make the same discovery."* (Lust, 1910, 662)

Improved sanitation, a cornerstone of preventative medicine for the early Naturopaths was their trumpet cry around the question of compulsory vaccination. They did not submit to the notion that vaccination was responsible for the elimination of smallpox epidemics. Their proof came from the municipalities that did something about epidemics using the wisdom of Nature: clean water, clean air and healthy food and homes. In this connection, the Naturopaths pulled a rabbit out of the debate hat with the example of Leicester, an industrial town in England, with a population of 250,000. John Hodge showed with statistics gathered by Dr. Millard, the medical officer of health in Leicester, how vaccination had a devastating effect on this town and verified that smallpox could be eradicated if a focus on public sanitation was practiced. Hodge states clearly,

> Surely the experience of unvaccinated Leicester has clearly demonstrated that vaccination, if it does anything at all, increases liability to smallpox, and renders it more fatal, and that the only effective plan by which to abolish the 'dread disease' (smallpox) from a municipality is to do as Leicester did. This is: abandon vaccination and devote attention and energy to sanitation and to the isolation of such few cases of smallpox as are wont to occur in the absence of 'preventative' vaccination. (Hodge, 1911, 27)

Leicester established proof that with widespread sanitary measures, mortality from smallpox could be reduced drastically. Another caveat with Leicester was that the danger of contracting smallpox in vaccinated people was fraught with morbidity and mortality. The prevalence of facial pock marks was rare in those not vaccinated, unlike the disfigurements found in the vaccinated. Hodge wrote about Leicester and its success in employing sanitation to counter the smallpox epidemic. He applauds the triumphs of hygiene:

> Leicester stands out conspicuously at the present day, a shining example to the whole world of the fact that prophylaxis against smallpox is to be realized through the attainment of health by means of personal hygiene, isolation and municipal sanitation and not by the inoculation of diseased products of man and beast into the healthy human body. (Hodge, 1911, 32)

Hodge boldly extols the heroic efforts of Leicester. Here was a substantial English city whose experience demonstrated clearly that smallpox could be controlled with simple hygiene. Despite the well-publicized outcomes in Leicester, though, the Boards of Health in America continued to enforce and advocate vaccination as the preferable prevention. The literature documents that in communities with lax laws people would eschew vaccination. The reaction from the medical community was to continue reassuring the public that vaccination did not pose any danger. In this regard, Samuel Saloman cites William Osler's position on sanitation versus vaccination in this debate. Osler claims, "Sanitation cannot account for the diminution in smallpox and for the low rate of mortality." (Saloman, 1911, 171) As well, Saloman addresses the related concern that other diseases could be transmitted through vaccination and the new terminology to diffuse and confuse the public. He writes, "Olser denies that syphilis and tuberculosis may be invaccinated; he concedes though that tetanus may be and undoubtedly is introduced into the system with the vaccine." (Saloman, 1911, 172-173) Osler continues, "If a vaccinated person is brought in contact with smallpox and escapes infection, set his escape down to successful vaccination; if he takes the disease, put it down either to unsuccessful vaccination or to *spurious vaccination*." (Saloman, 1911, 171) So went the ping pong rally of the different sides of the vaccination camps, each side proffering evidence to disprove the other.

Another investigator looking for answers was Joseph Rinn. He cites examples of how vaccination failed in protecting against smallpox even though medicine insisted on its infallibility. Rinn states,

> Dr. Adolf Vogt, professor of hygiene and sanitary statistics at the University of Berne, one of the greatest statisticians on medical science in Europe, proved in arguments presented to the Royal Commission of Great Britain in its investigation of vaccination resulting in the abolition there of compulsory vaccination, that a previous attack of smallpox and vaccination that took made a person more susceptible to another attack than if they had never had smallpox or been vaccinated. (Rinn, 1911, 207)

Using statistics and medical records, Rinn discloses the vaccination failures with data from three countries: Great Britain, United States and Japan. The mortality rates in each of these countries did little to promote the vaccinationists cause.

Meanwhile, in the United States men and women recognized that the political forces behind compulsory vaccination laws needed to be opposed. Compulsory vaccination attracted many, and from all sectors of society. Major Thomas Bourden of Connecticut, for example, wrote an open letter to the Governor and members of the Legislature of the State "to fairly weigh the evidence which will be presented". (Bourden, 1911, 304) In his letter, Bourden used numbers to strengthen his case. He alleged, "Nearly 100 deaths from vaccination have been reported in the press of the country during the past year, and most of them from lockjaw; yet, there is no doubt that the half has not been told." (Bourden, 1911, 304)

In *The Naturopath* news items appeared regularly, tabulating the number of deaths occurring due to vaccinations. The account of one such death stole the hearts of Americans. It was the story of a "sweet little girl ... Lucille Sturdevant [who] died 13 days after being vaccinated". (Lust, 1911, 312) The story of this child's death was heartbreaking. An only child, when Lucille died both of her parents was utterly destroyed with their grief. Lust relays the story and her fate:

> On May 15, 1902, she was in school 35, Buffalo, N.Y., and two public vaccinators, accompanied by two policemen, visited the school to engraft cow virus into the children at $1 a head. Though Lucille was only six years old she objected, saying she had been vaccinated and that she would go home, but would be vaccinated if she must. In spite of this, the officers threatened and forcibly vaccinated her. (Lust, 1911, 312)

She died of blood poisoning 13 days later.

Sad stories such as Lucille Sturdevant's sent alarms and parents rose up with more conviction to defeat compulsory vaccination bills within their State. In Berkeley, California, a group of parents removed their children from the public school and "an anti-vaccination school was opened on August 7, 1905, for all the children whose parents were opposed to vaccination". (Antonius, 1911, 429) These parents belonged to the California Anti-Compulsory Vaccination League and together they were able to change the laws so that "children need not be vaccinated, provided the parents sign a certificate that they are opposed to the practice of vaccination, and that it is the duty of the school board to furnish every parent with one of these blanks [exemption forms]." (Antonius, 1911, 429) The struggle to win their State Legislature was no easy task. California's Governor, Dr. G. C. Pardee had the power to veto efforts to modify compulsory vaccination laws, which he did in fact do.

Just as people were divided on the merits of vaccination so were medical doctors. Another doctor, one who did not leave behind a name, published his reasons for opposing vaccination. This unknown author recounts what he considered to be the vulgarity "of purposely infecting the body of a healthy person in this era of sanitary science with the poison from a diseased beast, under the senseless pretext of protecting the victim of the engrafted disease from the contagion of another disease!" (Unknown author, 1911, 449-450) He explained that a widely available medical lexicon provided its readers with information to discern and determine the knowledge base, use and context of terminology. In this regard, the anonymous writer exposes the medical doctors' use of the word, "calf lymph", in the context of vaccine to mean a natural body fluid, when in fact "the so-called *pure calf lymph* used by vaccinators is a pathological product, derived from a lesion on a diseased calf." (Unknown author, 1911, 450) There are many students of the contemporary orthodox medical profession in our current day who would contend that allopathic medicine still sanitizes its medical jargon to deceive the patient.

In allopathic medicine, a readily documentable pattern to dilute particular medical terminology in an effort to convey harmlessness and safety is common, and even rampant. Words with original derogatory or worrying connotations are constructed, altered or tweaked to become words that are neutral and sanitized, as our anonymous writer from over a century ago contended. Let us consider several examples from the literature. Vaccination, as a word is still in parlance, has been largely replaced in medical messaging and media with the word 'immunization' in an effort to distance medicine from the not forgotten shadows of vaccination. The word, 'immunization' connotes a natural body function and by using 'immunization' instead of 'vaccination', the medical establishment handily guides the public to think of their body's natural immune system. The word 'vaccine' itself is another example of morphing one medical term into another medical term with a completely different meaning. Vaccine is understood to be an injectable drug for preventing infectious diseases. Originally, however, so-called vaccine (actually an adjective meaning "pertaining to cows, or from cows") was an injectable fluid derived from the festering pustules of intentionally diseased animals and used to provide protection from smallpox. A quick review of the etymology, then, of the term, would cloud for the lay person the word 'vaccine' with a patina of alarm, and even repulsion.

Just recently, I was attending a naturopathic conference on cancer and listened to a Naturopath refer to a new cancer vaccine, as if vaccine equated to a desirable remedy for cancer. When did cancer become an infectious disease? We know that the causes of cancer have been variously documented as deriving from genetic factors, environmental toxins, life habits, and drugs themselves, including vaccination related etiologies. The early Naturopaths knew early that chronic diseases were generally not a result of acute infectious diseases. Every time we use the word 'immunization' or 'cancer vaccine', we are defaulting to this recurrent pattern of a type of medical-speak, and more often than not endorsing the strategy established by the Allopaths to minimize concern and opposition with terminology which rhetoricians would label euphemistic, accomplishing neatly an avoidance of harsh or unpleasant connotations.

Another medical doctor concerned about vaccination, Dr. Charles Littlefield, was the chair of the Washington State Branch of the National League for Medical Freedom. We find in *The Naturopath* a record of a debate he participated in with Dr. F. S. Bournes, former Health Officer of Seattle, Washington. He begins,

> Vaccination represents an honest effort on the part of the medical profession to find a preventive for a simple, yet loathsome disease. This effort, however, like many others of its kind, has not only failed to meet the expectation of its discoverer, but has left in its wake a blighting curse which it will require many generations to remove. Were it not for the fact that vaccination has

been enforced by legislation, we would not now be discussing it, except as an antiquated medical experiment akin to leeches and blood-letting. (Littlefield, 1912, 12)

Littlefield was keen to shed light on vaccination by reviewing historical events and by analyzing Dr. Jenner's work and claims. Littlefield notes, "Jenner began by claiming that vaccination made a person immune for life, but the facts of observation soon resulted in the term of immunity being shortened to fourteen years; then it was made seven, then two, and in the Spanish-American War, six weeks was the limit of immunity." (Littlefield 1912, 14)

Dr. Charles Creighton was another medical professional who spoke out against vaccination. He had been an eminent pathologist who had pro-vaccination views. When asked to write an article on vaccination for the *Encyclopedia Britannica*, he conducted "a most exhaustive study of the subject, and it was not long before the conviction forced itself upon him that vaccination was not only useless in preventing smallpox, but dangerous in practice". (Littlefield, 1912, 14)

Another prominent statesman, Alfred Russel Wallace, Britain's celebrated explorer and naturalist, also voiced his opinions on the vaccination question. Wallace is particularly known as having formulated independently, and prior to Darwin's publication of *On the Origins of Species*, his own theories of natural selection. He travelled extensively during his career and vaccinations were not foreign to him. Wallace recounts:

I was vaccinated in infancy, and before going to the Amazon I was persuaded to be vaccinated again. My children were duly vaccinated, and I never had the slightest doubt of the value of the operation—taking everything on trust without any inquiry whatever—till about 1875-80, when I first heard that there are anti-vaccinators, and read some articles on the subject. (Wallace, 1912, 41)

After a chance meeting, Wallace began investigating vaccination and made a complete 180 degree turn after his findings. He recounted his experiences as a member of the Royal Commission on Vaccination in England and disclosed his worry about the futility of raising awareness among officials responsible for the laws regarding vaccination. Compiling a comprehensive pamphlet of relevant statistical arguments made specifically for the House of Commons, he was disappointed that "not one of the six hundred and seventy members gave even that amount of their time to obtain information on a subject involving the health, life, and personal freedom of their constituents." (Wallace, 1912, 42) Wallace's dismay resulted in the completion of yet another publication. He states, "I *know* that in no work I have written have I presented so clear and so conclusive a demonstration of the fallacy of a popular belief as is given in this work, which was entitled *Vaccination a Delusion: Its Penal enforcement a Crime, proved by the Official Evidence in the Reports of the Royal Commission.*" (Wallace, 1912, 42)

Wallace was not alone in his distress about the political process. The Honorable Charles Miller, member of the Iowa State Legislature, wrote in 1912 an article for *The Naturopath* in which he raised the alarm about medical inspections in public schools, then pervasive in many States. On first glance, providing medical checkups of school children appears to be philanthropy at work; yet Miller questions the motives of exposing defenseless school children to unsolicited medical interventions at the expense of unwilling parents and children. Miller cites an example of 60,000 school children in Chicago being examined by doctors belonging to the American Medical Association. Miller discloses:

> When we consider that the sixty thousand children were the grist of the first inspection, and that it was followed by other grists at monthly intervals, and consider it in the light of the figures in a doctor's trust fee bill, no wild flight of the imagination is necessary to transport us quickly from the realm of noble philanthropy where the "political-doctors" would have us dwell as we contemplate their undertakings, into a realm of high finance where sordidness seems all the meaner for the cloak of benevolence with which it garbs itself. (Miller, 1912, 85-86)

The A.M.A. advocate doctors were quick to position themselves in public schools, positioning their work with vaccination as being for the public good, vaccination used as a preventative to germs. That this very widespread activity was demonstrably profitable for the doctors engaged in the welfare of school children is a matter of record, and not of speculation. The media helped enormously fan the flames of fear for germs. John Hodge explains,

> So much has been written in the sensational press about disease germs and the efforts of health departments to protect the dear people against the assaults of these microscopic enemies, which official doctors tell us swarm in the air we breathe, in the water we drink and in the food we eat, lurk on the lips of lovers of millions, billions, trillions, quadrillions, quintillions, sextillions, and so on ad infinitum, that one is led to inquire where will this craze about germs end? (Hodge, 1912, 173)

Hodge does not deny in his writing the existence of germs and their pathogenic potential. Rather, he raises awareness in an effort to counter the tactics of fear mongering. Continuing, he writes, "The superstitious fear engendered by bacteriologists, aided by shallow and sensational newspaper writers is developing into an instrument of power and possible oppression which health boards, being political bodies, know but too well how to manipulate to their own advantage." (Hodge, 1912, 173) Hodge had not always been of this opinion. The germ theory that Robert Koch hatched was completely acceptable by Hodge when he first became a doctor. In his own words,

> I was confidently assured by my parents and teachers that everybody who had been once vaccinated was thereby rendered forever afterward proof against smallpox infection. From my earliest recollection I had confided in the Jennerian rite more implicitly than in my clerical tenet or religious creed. I never entertained the slightest doubt as to the alleged value of the vaccine operations, taking everything on trust without any inquiry whatever. (Hodge, 1912, 223)

Then, by his own account, he graduated and became a doctor, only to witness the tactics and political maneuverings of Health Boards in their campaign to wholesale vaccination programs to entire populations without hesitation.

The record shows, in this regard, that when vaccination was administered to whole cities and enclaves, the unexpected occurred; namely more smallpox outbreaks, such as in western New York State as a case in point. Hodge writes, "Following the wake of the public vaccinators in that vigorously conducted vaccination crusade, smallpox of a severe type spread throughout the city of Lockport like wild fire on a prairie until the city was in the throes of a raging epidemic of the *dread disease*, while it lasted for many months, cost the city thousands of dollars and left a number of deaths to its record." Hodge observed an increase in smallpox outbreaks after vaccinations were conducted. He continues his narrative,

> The Lockport experience was an eye-opener to me. From that time on I studied the subject of vaccination as I should have studied it before and as every physician should study it, with a mind open to conviction; and I became actually appalled on discovering how fearfully and how wonderfully I had been deceived and how grossly I had deluded my trustful clients by inflicting this ruinous rite upon them. (Hodge, 1912, 225)

This eastern U.S. doctor also wrote prolifically on the subjects of vaccination and the vivisection practices. His western U.S. colleague, Helen Sayr Gray, ND, weighed into this disclosure with considerable wit and passion. Helen Gray, practicing in Portland, Oregon did not leave behind any published books and only a few precious articles that reveal her witty sense of perception. Like Hodge, Gray was aggrieved by the practices of medical doctors. She describes the confusion in vaccination hype,

> Doctors, like various other people, are very proficient in appropriating credit and transferring blame. When death or impaired

health results from vaccination, its advocates have a number of scapegoats that they put the blame on. When a vaccinated person contracts smallpox, the doctors say that he was not vaccinated successfully or not recently enough or not prior to exposure, or they reassure and console him by telling him that he would have had a severer or perhaps a fatal case, if he had not been vaccinated. (Gray, 1912, 382)

For Helen Sayr Gray, "Health is the only immunity against disease." (Gray, 1912, 383) For others, the prevention of disease balanced on the needle point of vaccination and was heralded as a triumph of medical science. The magic potion used in vaccination had more to cover up than make public in Dr. Gray's opinion. What was the composition of the much acclaimed and virtuous vaccine, she wanted to know? Transparency in the vaccination industry, as the documented history of this dimension of medicine reveals, has not ever been a strong trait. Just as contemporary populations are often oblivious to the adjuvants added to the current vaccine concoction, the lexicon used by the early vaccinationists disguised the overall composition of the vaccine. The Anti-Vaccination League of America did not shy from revealing how vaccines were made nor from demystifying the term, "pure calf lymph". The procedure that calves were subjected to is nothing short of criminal.

The calf is tied down to an operating table, the stomach is shaved for twelve to fifteen inches square, and about one hundred incisions are made. Into these incisions, one drop of glycerinated lymph ... is allowed to drop and is thoroughly rubbed in. Fever sets in, and the animal becomes exceedingly sick. In a few days the vesicles appear, the scabs form. (Anti-Vaccination League of America, 1912, 614)

Naturopaths of this era knew about these violent and septic conditions, and considered that a vivid imagination and exceptional tolerance were essential in order to believe that vaccines could belong to modern medicine. In fact, many health care professionals from the naturopathic and the allopathic communities considered vaccination to be a process characterized by ignorance and superstition. (Zurmuhlen, 1912, 725) Charles Zurmuhlen, MD asks, "The whole immoral serum traffic can be summoned up in one sentence: do we improve the healthy human blood by injecting the serum from the blood of half rotten animals into it? Only fools and Allopaths believe that we do!" (Zurmuhlen, 1912, 726)

Each new disease presentation fanned the vaccination debate flames. August Andrew Erz, an Osteopath well known to the Naturopathic community at the time, presented many arguments against vaccination. He attributes adverse effects and new diseases to vaccines. Erz states,

'Varioloid' is a term invented by the profession to conceal the failures of vaccination, and means *smallpox-like.* According to the vaccination law no person can rightly have smallpox after vaccination, because vaccination prevents smallpox; but he may have, by kind permission of the profession, varioloid—which is in plain language, smallpox that occurs after vaccination. (Erz, 1913, 835)

Erz does not mince words, "The mitigation theory is but another sub-terfuge, and actually implies another confession that vaccination does not protect. If the prevention theory were true, then no person could possibly ever have smallpox in any form after vaccination." (Erz, 1913, 835)

August Andrew Erz' 1914 book, *The Medical Question, The Truth About Official Medicine and Why We Must Have Medical Freedom* ignit-ed even more broadly the ruckus about medical freedom. Others added their voices including politicians and lawyers who collectively informed the public of their legal rights. The Honorable Harry Weinberger of New York, for example, provided explanation and clarity about the extent of power that doctors from the Health Board could exert. Weinberger explains, "No laws are binding on the human subject which assault the body or violate the conscience. The right of personal security consists in a person's legal and uninterrupted enjoyment of his life, his limbs, and his reputation." (Weinberger, 1914, 393) He cites cases to illustrate how vaccination enforcement was enacted in the States of New York and Mas-sachusetts. "The only law in New York on the statute-books in reference to vaccination is that, in order to go to school—that is, public school—a child must be vaccinated." (Weinberger, 1914, 393) In Massachusetts, fines of five dollars or essentially a bribe to be vaccinated were charged to anyone refusing vaccination. Five dollars does not sound like a lot yet in 1914, this amount represented several days of labour.

The Public Health Boards succeeded in cultivating widespread fear among the general public. The fear of being convicted of not comply-ing with the Public Health Boards coincided with the also prevalent and general fear of contagious diseases. The fear of germs helped mold a population to default to compliance towards vaccination. Dr. Katz notes, "Never the belief in contagion has been so widespread as at the present time so that many people avoid, so much as possible, the contact with sick persons, in order to protect their own dear selves." (Katz, 1915, 428) Fear added, many early Naturopaths felt, to weakening the immune sys-tem and making people more susceptible. Echoing the concern of his naturopathic colleagues, Katz reiterates the counsel of Hippocrates, who "advised to be moderate in working, eating, drinking, sleeping and love, in such time, for a sober life gives the best protection against the so-called contagious diseases." (Katz, 1915, 428) Charles Zurmuhlen, MD cites

Hippocrates too, iterating in his writing and to his patients that living within the laws of Nature was essential for one to have a healthy immune system. Drugs and vaccines did not fit under the category of Nature or abide to natural laws, he felt.

Elsewhere, Charles Zurmuhlen, MD raises questions of the vaccines produced to prevent diphtheria. He ponders, "Why is the serum from the blood of horses suffering from natural diphtheria not a specific for diphtheria? Diphtheria is not a natural disease in horses; it must be produced by the artificial and unnatural method of injecting the bacillus of diphtheria into them." (Zurmuhlen, 1916, 537) Zurmuhlen next juxtaposes the flawed and irrational disease theory with the naturopathic adherence to natural laws. He warns that with the research efforts by the Rockefeller Institute on serums and vaccines, people may well come to disregard their habits of living. He concludes, "It teaches men that they can sin with perfect impunity for the serums manufactured under the methods of the Institute render men immune against disease." (Zurmuhlen, 1916, 541)

While the focus of regular medicine was on finding the next vaccine and serum, Naturopaths returned to the baseline of Nature. In "The Crime of the Century", Dr. E. D. Titus reminds readers that "the only way to prevent disease is to remove the cause through sanitary conditions, exercise and good wholesome food". (Titus, 1917, 130) He continues, "But these things the political doctor secretly fights." (Titus, 1917, 130) In the same article, he points out the value of fermented foods, "It has been demonstrated that bacterial milk will relieve pain and suffering in certain stomach and intestinal troubles where other known remedial agents have failed." (Titus, 1917, 131) Then, Titus concludes his article with a discussion of the political doctors who seemed to be in positions of control. He writes, "The only way for [the political doctor] to secure this control is to advocate government control of everything in sight." (Titus, 1917, 132) Titus is referring to the American Medical Associations and coined the term, "Medical Mafia" to describe the A.M.A.'s deliberate efforts to monopolize the practice of medicine by excluding any group who threatened their dominance. The historical record shows that the A.M.A.'s often brutal political ambitions spread to its research centers. The A.M.A.'s resolution to be the determining force for medicine in America corresponded to its public efforts to master the threat of disease.

In a lecture delivered at the 21st Annual Convention of the American Naturopathic Association held in New York City, William Bradshaw addresses the subject of "vivisection as a means of finding cures for diseases". (Bradshaw, 1917, 328) Vivisection was a practice employed by the Allopaths confining animals in laboratories for the experimentation in the pursuit of discovering new cures. As referenced earlier in this volume, the horrific truth of vivisection was as repulsive to Naturopaths as compulsory vaccination. The two were tangentially intertwined, though, and each of these triggered a public outcry. Bradshaw quotes Dr. Woglom of Columbia University, the head of a cancer research laboratory, who, in a lecture on the subject of Cancer and Experimental Research, stated that "over two million animals had been destroyed under circumstances of great cruelty, to find the cause and cure for cancer, but nothing of the kind had ever been discovered, and if anyone said that he had found a cure for cancer through animal experimentation, that man was a liar." (Bradshaw, 1917, 328)

One laboratory which caught the attention of Naturopaths was that of Dr. Simon Flexner, the director of the Rockefeller Institute and brother of the author of the Flexner Report which benchmarked medical schools in North America in the very early part of the last century. Simon Flexner was an avid vaccinationist and despised the Naturopaths for what he considered to be their lack of science. Flexner had developed a serum to fight infantile paralysis, making claims that his serum was 80% effective. In fact, his serum was a complete failure. Bradshaw recounts his encounters with Flexner and others bent on deluding the public about the real statistics and facts of serum failures. The concern was that those familiar with science learned to manipulate research data to produce the desired outcomes. This, the early Naturopaths and sympathetic Allopaths contended, was the way Flexner used science to cover his failures.

In any case, failure to achieve protective immunity with vaccination became a veritable battle cry of Naturopaths. As the debate and the record of problems accumulated, Lust wanted to address concerns of medical tyranny in the form of compulsory vaccination even more fully. He created a new column which he introduced in the *Herald of Health and Naturopath* called "Department of Medical Freedom" edited by Dr. Gilbert Bowman in the November/December issue in 1917. Bowman is irascible with rage and has left us with a factual and informative article on the subject of compulsory vaccination in the American military. Bowman writes,

> Let it be understood that, because of the absolute control of the military and naval affairs by the Medical Trust, every soldier, sailor, marine or airman, is required to submit to vaccination and to an injection of anti-typhus serum as soon as he enlists or is called to service, and as often thereafter as the medical officers may decree." (Bowman, 1917, 373)

He continues, "Should any soldier, sailor, airman or marine, refuse to submit to the treatment, he is promptly court-martialed for insubordination, the punishment for which is a prison term of probably one or two years." (Bowman, 1917, 373) Generally, it is thought that the most fit and healthy enlist into military duty. Indeed, Bowman reminds us to "keep in mind the fact that our army, navy and marine corps are made up of picked men; men who have been obliged to pass a rigid test of physical fitness before they could begin admittance to the service." (Bowman, 1917, 374) However, Bowman leaves a trail of statistics of mortality and morbidity that is dizzying to comprehend. The American military experienced a devastating toll of its soldiers and marines as a result of complications and adverse reactions to vaccinations. The failure of the smallpox vaccines was compounded by the emergence of new diseases in military populations, such as, tetanus, following a smallpox vaccination.

Oscar Beasley draws to our attention that tetanus naturally "exists in soil and in hay, and in the alimentary canal, the hair, and the manure of the calf. We can easily realize, therefore, that the very origin of vaccine virus is in an environment of tetanus." (Beasley, 1918, 70) The uncertainty of vaccination manufacturing and the diseases that accompanied smallpox vaccination left many to resist vaccination. Beasley comments, "Meanwhile, many hundreds of thousands of children had been inoculated with the vile stuff, and what disease is left in its train is not known." (Beasley, 1918, 72)

During WWI, 9 million people died. The Spanish Flu of 1918 brought WWI to the abrupt end in 1918, killing an estimated 35 to 50 million people worldwide. The Spanish Flu demonstrated that infectious diseases presented suddenly and were deadly and merciless. Significantly, the Spanish Flu presented early in America at Fort Riley, Kansas, at Camp Funston. A major troop staging and hospital camp in Etaples, France, it is alleged, became a major catalyst arena for this devastating pandemic. Back in America, the Allopaths used epidemics such as the Spanish Flu to foster fear and to promote their "Germ Theory". "Dover's powder, a preparation of ipecac and opium" (Havard, 1918, 865) was the golden standard of care by Allopaths and the thousands treated by this route became the horrible statistics that we associate with the Spanish Flu.

In an editorial, "Influenza, Immunization" written by William Freeman Havard at the zenith of the horrific and deadly Spanish Flu, we are exposed to alarming statistics. Allopaths lost patients and Naturopaths didn't. In fact, Naturopaths lost less than 1% and Allopaths as high as 80%. What differentiated their treatment protocols? Allopaths used drugs and experimented with serums and vaccines. The Naturopaths, on the other hand, administered baths, wet sheet wraps and fasted patients. And always lying at the core of naturopathic care is the belief that life style habits determined our health. Havard affirms,

> Natural immunity is with the individual who has a pure blood
> stream and such cannot be maintained or acquired on a diet of

animal foods, white bread, devitalized sugar, pastry, coffee, tea, alcohol and tobacco with bad air, overindulgence and lack of exercise as side partners of bad diet." (Havard, 1918, 867)

Havard, a student of Henry Lindlahr and Louis Kuhne, adhered to the doctrine that morbid matter accumulated over time would result in symptoms of disease. He adds,

Since the war we have had a splendid opportunity to study the action of serums for never before have they been administered in so many varieties and such great quantities. Procure this false immunity from one form of reaction and it takes another form. The serums themselves are an added encumbrance. (Havard, 1918, 867)

The various serums and vaccines that Havard alludes to spawned a rash of diseases and unexpected epidemics. E. H. Judkins, M.D. cites, "Recent epidemics of foot and mouth disease started from a vaccine virus. (Bureau Animal Industry, 147, *Farmer's Bulletin, No. 666*) Infantile Paralysis followed vaccination; and serums to cure that, as in one city hospital, caused 14 out of 15 deaths!" (Judkins, 1919, 201) Other diseases implicated with vaccination included the dreaded cancer. Judkins exclaims, "Besides pus cocci and bacteria of skin of cow, calf and horse are more or less mixed with all vaccine; and the cell of these animals grows nine times to one of human; hence, Drs. Snow and Bell show seven-tenths of all cancer and consumption is caused by vaccine serums, a 225 percent increase in cancer (New York) causing 80,000 deaths, and 2,500,000 consumptives in this country." (Judkins, 1919, 200) Perhaps Judkins is hyperbolic in his statements; even so, the fact of the matter is that in industrialized nations chronic diseases, obesity rates of over 60%, and cancer have not decreased with the advances made in medical science, including refinements in the production and dissemination of vaccines.

Per Nelson counsels us in his 1920 article: "Look around in any community and what will you find? You will find hundreds, yes, thousands of so-called incurables or chronics: men, women and children." (Nelson, 1920, 78) Nelson could be speaking of the 21st century but he is referring to a century ago. His article is poignant and masterful as he encapsulates in his article, "Naturopathy versus Medicine" many of the issues, strengths and weaknesses of Naturopathy and Allopathy. Henry Lindlahr had the gift of articulating with astute clarity the heart of Naturopathy. Nelson, also a gifted writer, had astounding insights that are enduring. These authors have left behind clinical pearls that deserve our attention.

Nelson was not convinced by the infallible arguments that medicine gave for their drugs and vaccines. Nelson challenges us to think, writing, "Germs are supposed to be equally dangerous to each and every one of us, and no matter how strong and healthy we are, if it should happen that they get into our systems, they will at once begin to raise 'cane' with us, especially so if we haven't had all of the 59 varieties of artificial anti-toxins injected into our blood." (Nelson, 1920, 78)

Per Nelson unravels the germ theory using scientific writings of his day to reveal the flaws and misinformation. He cites the work of a Canadian physician, John B. Fraser who showed that drinking a potion containing the Klebs-Loffler bacilli (diphtheria) did not have the expected results. Nelson recounts, "The first test was whether the Klebs-Loffler bacilli would cause diphtheria, and about 50,000 were swallowed without any result; later 100,000, 500,000, and a million more were swallowed and in no case did they cause any ill-effect." (Nelson, 1920, 134) His article is poignant and masterful as he encapsulates in his article many of the issues, and weaknesses of the germ theory that forms the foundation of allopathic medicine.

The issue of vaccination gave the Allopaths strong bidding powers in their efforts to mobilize and consolidate legislation to empower them with unilateral powers. Fear of disease was convincing and easy to convey to politicians that Allopaths were the only qualified doctors to contend with contagion and disease. In reaction, Naturopaths, Physical Culturists and other allied Drugless therapists rallied to take a position against the efforts of the Allopaths under the banner of *medical freedom*. One such person, Bernarr Macfadden was incensed that the A.M.A. had succeeded in championing seven bills in Washington. He called the drugless community together to take a stand, "If we do not defeat these bills we will deserve to die in the festering puss of the vaccination and serum poisons which these monopolistic doctors maintain is the accredited method of treating all disease." (Macfadden, 1920, 405)

Another prominent voice was Alfred Russel Wallace, referenced earlier for his work on the Royal Commission on vaccination in England, a scientist who embraced the task of understanding the dilemma of vaccinations. In his amusing yet brilliant article, "The 'Unvaccinated' Death Rate", Wallace examines the statistics in England to determine how vaccinations affected the death rate of smallpox. He cites once again the example of Leicester but also includes "Nelson and Northampton ... Loughborough, ... Kneighley, ... and Oldham all anti-vaccinationist centres [had] 645 cases of smallpox without a death". (Wallace, 1921, 137) Essentially he destroys the claims that medical doctors contend that unvaccinated people have higher mortality than those choosing vaccinations. He illuminates the scam,

> When we consider all the sources of error to which we have alluded we are led to conclude that the difference in fatality between the vaccinated and unvaccinated smallpox patients is not as great

as is sometimes contended, and that so far as it exists it cannot be merely to the effect of vaccination, while the fact that the fatality of all cases lumped together is practically the same now as it was in the unvaccinated of last century, when large numbers are taken for comparison, strongly suggests that of the inclusion of a large contingent of vaccinated persons has not exerted a mitigating effect on the average fatality of the whole. (Wallace, 1921, 138)

During this entire tumultuous period, Naturopaths, Allopaths and others continued to submit articles against vaccination to Lust's journals. In the early 1920s, Dr. Lust publishes segments of Dr. Louis Simon Katzoff, MD's views of vaccination. Katzoff writes "Vaccination never did prevent smallpox." He continues, "Upon observation and reflection I soon realized that smallpox is an illness which has its origin in filth that it follows closely upon flagrant violations of the laws of hygiene and sanitation." (Lust, 1922, 230) Katzoff recognized that without addressing hygiene, diseases would continue to be problems despite the advent of vaccines. Another statement from Katzoff is only too familiar: "The occurrences of *epidemics* or *scares* have coincided with periods of fatigue, anxiety and fear." (Lust, 1922, 230)

New vaccines came on the market and without delay reports of their entry and possible dangers were published. One such report comes from the London and Provincial Anti-Vivisection Society of England, disclosing the hidden dangers of the Schick Test for Diphtheria. The major fear was exposing "perfectly healthy persons ... to the dangers of successive inoculations for a disease which they may never contract." (London and Provincial Anti-Vivisection Society, 1923, 124) Several children died in Texas as a result of receiving this vaccine, details of which disaster were presented in the House of Commons in England to make a case against the use of this new vaccine.

The fear of the dangers that drugs and vaccines presented was indeed a recurring and incremental message from the early Naturopaths. Drugs and vaccines didn't heal disease, they insisted, and in their growing practices, Naturopaths certainly did not use them. Benedict Lust in the final article included in *Vaccination and Naturopathic Medicine*, wrote "Fallacy of Drugs". He states definitively that drugs are no substitute for abiding Nature's laws. Lust quotes Henry Lindlahr in this seminal piece: "Almost every virulent poison known to man is found in allopathic prescriptions." (Lust, 1923, 579) Vaccines and drugs hold out the promise of health and yet, that is not always the results. Lust continues to warn strongly about the dangers of drug therapies,

In view of what our foremost medical authorities say as to the worthlessness of drugs in the treatment of disease, how strange it is that any number of people will continue to believe that they can abuse their organs until they cease to function normally, and then when they are worn out make them over with drugs or have new ones to replace them. (Lust, 1923, 580)

Naturopathy as seen from the eyes of Benedict Lust did not include drugs or vaccines. Lust placed his faith in Nature. Nature and Naturopathy had much more in common that the roots of these word origins. Lust reminds us:

Health is the most precious heritage of man. It can be had by strict observance of and obedience to the law of his being, and in no other way. The body of man is governed by Natural Law, which is just as positive in its operation and requirement as the man-made law governing the mechanism of a watch. No man can violate this unfailing and unalterable law of Nature, which is older than the race itself, and expect to escape suffering the penalty by simply swallowing some poison drug. (Lust, 1923, 580)

Naturopathy began as a movement to restore people's understanding of the power of Nature to enhance and assure health. The early Naturopaths encouraged their patients always to live according to Nature's laws. What were these laws? Simply, as this early literature reminds us over and over again, to eat healthy food, drink pure water, breathe fresh air, exercise in Nature, sleep adequate hours, practice hygiene and choose a meaningful and moral life. The early Naturopaths treated infectious diseases with conviction and success, abiding by these principles. They restored patients to a wholesome diet; applied water applications; counseled patients to adopt sanitary practices, and witnessed their patients recover. Before the proliferation of poly-pharma and the monetizing of treatment around drugs, Naturopaths practiced with confidence and certitude. Their teachers, Priessnitz, Kneipp and Kuhne, laid a foundation for success which is as valuable today as a century ago.

What is most valuable is our recognizing in these voices from a century ago, *in their own words*, the familiar debates of today, attesting to how the fundamental issues surrounding vaccination theory and practice have not subsided. Notwithstanding contemporary claims about safety, efficacy and epidemiological data, the issue is very much with us still. Naturopathic principles and practice continue to be a powerful response to this persistent health dilemma.

Sussanna Czeranko, ND, BBE

1900

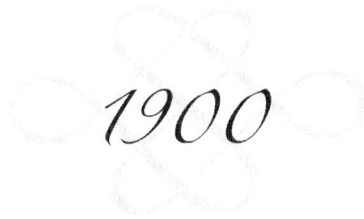

FOR THE LITTLE CHILDREN
BENEDICT LUST

CURE OF INFANTILE CHOLERA, IN ITS LAST STAGE
OTTO WAGNER

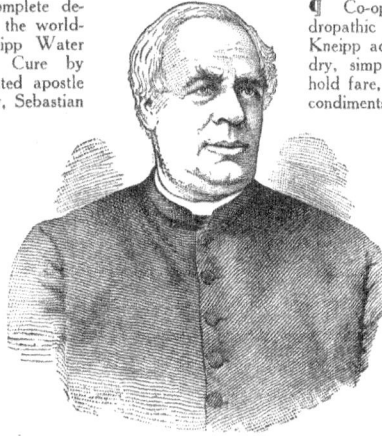

Father Sebastian Kneipp's methods of treatments formed the foundation for the early Naturopaths for the management and cure of infectious diseases.

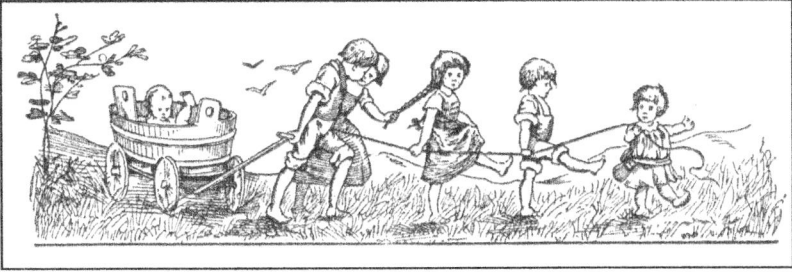

For The Little Children

by Benedict Lust

The Kneipp Water Cure Monthly, I (2), 28. (1900)

MEASLES AND SCARLET FEVER

Measles and scarlet fever commence like every other fever with a sudden decline of the physical strength of the little patient, loss of appetite, headache, chilly feeling and dry heat. The strength of the fever and the heat of the body increases. For years one was of the opinion that on account of the rash, cold water should not be applied. In thousands of cases Kneipp healed measles and scarlet fever by means of his water applications. If the chilly feeling [is] very strong at once make use of the hayflower shirt.

HAYFLOWER SHIRT

What are hay flowers? Hay flowers are the remains of hay, such as stalks, leaves, blossoms and seeds, which we find in every barn, where hay is stored. What is a hay flower-shirt? A shirt which is dipped into a decoction of hay flowers. To prepare the decoction take from 3 to 5 handfuls of hay flowers, pour boiling water over them, cover the vessel and let the whole mixture cool to the warmth of 88° to 90° F/31° to 32° C. It is of no consequence whether the hay flowers remain in the decoction or not; dip a shirt into the decoction, wring it out, put it on the child and leave it on for one hour. (See Kneipp's *My Water Cure*)

In cases of strong dry heat, a cold salt-water-shirt is used. What is a salt-water-shirt? A shirt dipped into cold salt-water. This shirt is also left on the child for one hour. To make the salt-water take a bucketful of water and put a handful of salt into it.

Very soon a rash will cover the body and with the appearance of the rash the battle is half won. Every hour thereafter the body is washed with cold water to produce wet heat and perspiration. By the perspiration all morbid matter is secreted.

All drugs which are prescribed in these cases cannot do much good or produce lasting results. They may stop the fever for some time, but very soon there will be other ailments and nature has to fight morbid matter again. Drugs could part the two fighters, but as soon as the influence of the drugs is gone, the fight is taken up again. The simple remedies of natural science are not satisfied with parting the fighting parties, nature and morbid matter, but force the fight to a finish; the weaker part, morbid matter, has to get out.

Drugs weaken the system while the water-applications refresh and strengthen the body.

DIPHTHERIA

Diphtheria is treated in the same way as measles and scarlet fever, but one may make good use of the half-bath, the upper-gush* and the sitting-bath in all three cases. In cases of diphtheria the upper-gush is of great advantage. The discharging of a lot of phlegm is a consequence of the application of the upper-gush. The half-bath is an even better remedy to remove the fever than the washing of the whole body. To produce a good effect, it is advisable to vary with the sitting-bath, upper-gush and washing of the whole body. The rash will appear in cases in which the water applications are effective. One does not need to feel frightened on account of it, for the rash is a natural consequence of the process of healing. Without it, there would be no cure, no secretion of morbid matter. To hasten on the appearance of the rash stout people may use one hay-flower-shirt or salt-water-shirt, one short package** (see under packages and their usefulness***) or these people may apply a shirt dipped into a fluid consisting of three quarter of water and one quarter of vinegar. Often the rash only appears on certain parts of the body, but nevertheless its appearance is a sure sign of nature's victory over morbid matter which is turned out in the form of a rash.

KNEIPP'S SHORT NOTES

Never give children a warm bath.

Harden the system of a child from the first months.†

Don't dress a child too heavy.

---

* Upper-gush is a specialized shower conceived by Father Sebastian Kneipp that is applied to the chest. —Ed

**Short pack or package refers to a cold compress that is applied around the body from the axilla extending to the calves. —Ed.

***Benedict Lust is making reference to a chapter in Sebastian Kneipp's book, My Water Cure. —Ed.

†Hardening was a key principle developed by Sebastian Kneipp to strengthen the constitution by using cold water applications. —Ed.

Allow children to walk barefooted as much as possible.

Fresh air and fresh water will always serve to make children healthy and well.

Improvements of health and strength have to be started by the mother.

Mothers should harden themselves, follow the rules of Kneipp's Water-cure and bring up their children accepting to these rules.

In every land good and healthy mothers are a guarantee of a happy future.

What are hay-flowers? Hay-flowers are the remains of hay, such as stalks, leaves, blossoms and seeds, which we find in every barn, where hay is stored. What is a hay-flower-shirt? A shirt which is dipped into a decoction of hay-flowers. In cases of strong dry heat a cold salt-water shirt is used.

The simple remedies of natural science are not satisfied with parting the fighting parties, nature and morbid matter, but force the fight to a finish; the weaker part, morbid matter has to get out.

One does not need to feel frightened on account of [the rash], for the rash is a natural consequence of the process of healing. Without it, there would be no cure, no secretion of morbid matter.

CURE OF INFANTILE CHOLERA, IN ITS LAST STAGE

by Otto Wagner, Director of the Bilz Sanatorium

The Kneipp Water Cure Monthly, I (3), 45-46. (1900)

On the 28th day of July, 1895, Herr Krebs, of M ... near Leipzig, a farmer, requested me to go with him to see his child, aged six months, who, he said, was very ill. During the drive to his house, Herr Krebs told me, that the above-named malady was prevalent in the neighborhood, and that a great number of children had died of it; that his child had been attacked by the malignant disease and been given up as beyond the reach of succor; that all the remedies employed had been ineffectual; that in the last week the child had been given laudanum* and a tablespoonful of brandy every day (to

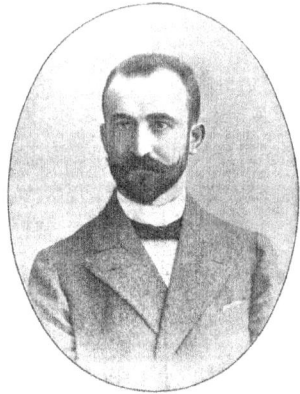

Otto Wagner

a child six months old!); and even that had failed to stop the diarrhoea. On my arrival the appearance of the little patient gave me the impression that my help had come too late. The body was a mere frame-work of bones covered with loose skin; the face was wrinkled and old-looking, the eyes dull and lusterless, half obscured. The whole body was cold to the touch, particularly the hands and feet; the pulse thin and thread-like, often scarcely perceptible; in short, the whole appearance was the reverse of reassuring. On enquiring what nourishment the child had had, I was informed that, besides pure milk, milk and water, and cream and water, trials had been made with almost all the artificial foods for infants, like Nestle's food, arrow-root, etc., but that not one of them had proved suitable.

I ordered: enemata, half a pint of water (90° F/32° C), to clear out the bowel of its contents, and to be given morning and evening; if the water returned, starch-water clysters, one table-spoonful (about 64° F/18° C), were to follow the enemata as a tonic for the bowels. A warm bath (97° F/36° C) lasting five minutes was to be given morning and evening, and followed immediately by an abdominal pack, and hot-water bottles applied to the feet—this pack to last from one and a half to two hours, and to be followed by a washing of the whole body with water of 77°

---

*Laudanum is an alcoholic solution containing morphine, prepared from opium and formerly used as a narcotic painkiller. —*Ed.*

F/25° C. The diet was to be oatmeal gruel without milk, and given a tea-spoonful at a time. On visiting the child two days afterwards I was very glad to find [the child] still alive. The vomiting had ceased, the diarrhoea diminished, the eyes were clearer—a sign that the vital power, supported by the proper means, had got the upper hand in the battle with disease. The only change I made in the directions was that only one cleansing enema was to be given daily, instead of two, and that rice water was to be the diet instead of oatmeal gruel. This agreed with the child very well. On my third visit, two days later, the child could be regarded as saved. There was no more vomiting; stools took place three or four times a day, still rather thin, but more paste-like in its consistency than before; sleep and appetite were good, appearance fresher. From that time the enemata were given up; a cool (82° F/28° C) washing of the whole body was ordered once a day, and an abdominal pack with calf packs of 77° F/25° C every night; the diet was more nourishing, consisting at first of oatmeal gruel with the addition of a few spoonfuls of new milk unboiled, and by degrees an increased quantity of milk till the proportion was reached of half milk to half gruel. This regimen suited the child exceedingly well; it thrived accordingly; at the end of a week it had thin whole-meal (wheat-meal) soup twice a day, and at the end of a month it had gained six pounds in weight.

The child was saved by the timely and correct application of the Natural Method of Healing*; while, in more cases than one, children in the same neighborhood were carried off by the disease under circumstances which included nourishment with artificial foods for infants and treatment with opium and cognac.

—Bilz, *The Natural Method of Healing*

The Natural Method of Healing was the title of Friedrich Eduard Bilz' encyclopedic work which was modelled upon Father Sebastian Kneipp's therapies. Those who followed the doctrines of Kneipp and Bilz used "Natural Method of Healing" as the phrase to denote Kneippian therapies. —Ed.

> *A warm bath (97° F/36° C) lasting five minutes was to be given morning and evening, and followed immediately by an abdominal pack, and hot-water bottles applied to the feet—this pack to last from one and a half to two hours, and to be followed by a washing of the whole body with water of 77° F/25° C.*

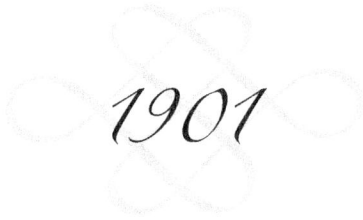

1901

VACCINATION
Frank D. Blue

ADDRESS TO THE PEOPLE OF ST. PAUL, MINNESOTA, ON VACCINATION
J. A. Clausen, M.D.

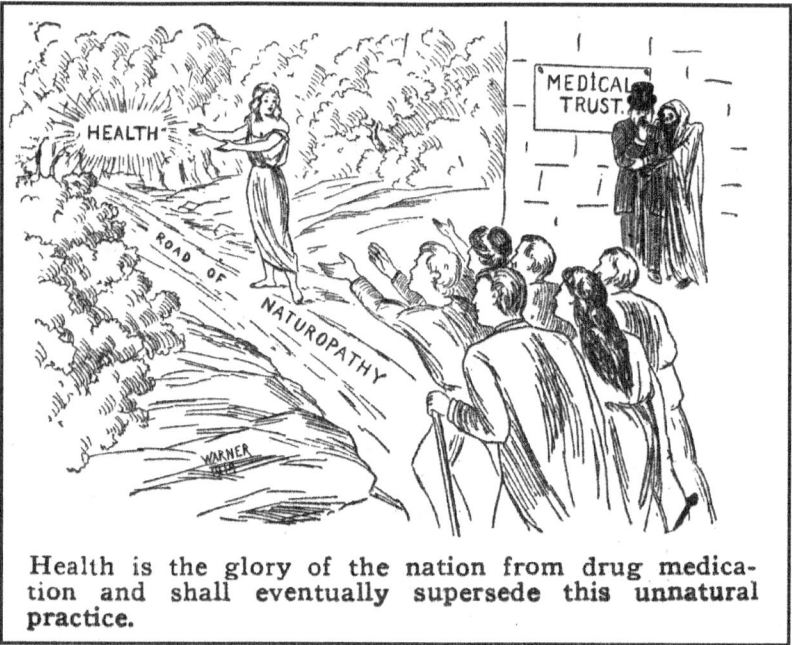

Health is the glory of the nation from drug medication and shall eventually supersede this unnatural practice.

VACCINATION

by Frank D. Blue

The Kneipp Water Cure Monthly, II (4), 116. (1901)

"Faith, fanatic faith, once wedded fast,
To some dear falsehood, hugs it to the last."

THE ANTI-VACCINATION SOCIETY OF AMERICA
OFFICERS:

L. H. Piehn, President...Nora Springs, Iowa
L. J. Weyprecht, Vice President...................226 2nd Ave., New York City
J. A. Clausen, M.D., Vice President.............................St. Ansgar, Iowa
M. R. Leverson, M.D., Vice President..............Ft. Hamilton, New York
C. Oscar Beasly, Counsel............................Fidelity Bldg. Philadelphia
Frank D. Blue, Secretary....................................Terre Haute, Indiana
E. C. Townsend, Assistant Secretary.........19 Broadway, New York City
E. B. Foote, Jr., M.D., Treasurer....................Box 788, New York City

CONSTITUTION, ARTICLE II

The object of this society shall be to oppose and prevent the enforcement of compulsory vaccination.

WHAT IS VACCINATION AND WHAT CAN I DO TO HELP ABOLISH IT?

Vaccination is the inoculation of a healthy person with pus poison, from a festering sore on a diseased animal, which may and often does cause most serious diseases and confers no certain immunity against smallpox. At this time the only way to attack this blunder, which is really worse than a crime, is by printing and circulating information in order to let the general public know just what a disease and death-producing agency vaccination is.

The Anti-Vaccination Society of America has been organized for this purpose. In order to accomplish its object it must have funds to pay for printing and postage; every additional member increases its influence, apart from its fee for membership. At present it has several hundred members, but it wants to have several thousand, and soon, too. Every cent given aids to the cause directly as all its officers serve without pay. The membership fee is but twenty-five cents, a nominal sum, and there are no dues; it being expected that all members will help as they are able. You should join our society at once and further aid this basic cause of humanity by inducing your friends to do likewise.

Also circulate our literature.

One great drawback to our cause is the fact that the public is generally not aware of the extent of the opposition to vaccination blood poisoning. Anti-vaccination is looked upon as simply a fad that will soon pass away; by others it is supposed to be confined to a few cranks and as of but little consequence anyway. The Anti-Vaccination Cause, already a power in the land, is greatly handicapped by the lack of good literature for circulation. By circulating good, neat, attractive literature, the solid basis of our movement is realized, and many who note these signs of its growth and stability will be led into our ranks to do battle with us, who now lack the courage to face popular prejudices. Never send out a letter without enclosing a tract [a pamphlet] at least.

VACCINATION

Issued monthly, for the Anti-Vaccination Society of America. Subscription 25 cents per year. Advertising rates on application.

Frank D. Blue, Editor
1328 N. 12th Street,
Terre Haute,
Indiana, U.S.A.

> *At this time the only way to attack this blunder, which is really worse than a crime, is by printing and circulating information in order to let the general public know just what a disease and death-producing agency vaccination is.*
>
> *One great drawback to our cause is the fact that the public is generally not aware of the extent of the opposition to vaccination blood poisoning.*

Address To The People Of St. Paul, Minneapolis, On Vaccination

by J. A. Clausen, M.D., St. Ansgar, Iowa
Second Vice President of the Anti-Vaccination Society of America
The Kneipp Water Cure Monthly, II (6), 158-160. (1901)

Mr. President, Members of the Anti-Vaccination Society of St. Paul and fellow citizens of the United States of America:
First of all, we will consider the individual's rights.

The right of man to his own body and the control and protection of his children's bodies are the most essential of all rights. And it is actually necessary at this time and date that the people of this country should call a halt upon the impositions of the tyrannical officialism which overrides their most essential right. It is a disgrace to all American citizens that more than one hundred and twenty-five years are required for them to fit themselves to accept the freedom secured for them by the Declaration of Independence and the Constitution of the United States of America.

It is enough to make a true American citizen black and blue with rage to see that a few bands of fanatics are high-handedly riding over a nation of 70,000,000 people in spite of all their constitutional rights. The toleration of the prohibition fanatics, the Sunday fanatics, the God in the Constitution fanatics is all a scandal to this nation, but worse than all of these is the toleration of the medical fanatics, who not only interfere with the people's constitutional rights to select whom they please to treat them when sick, but by force of arms, undertake to compel them to submit their bodies to the most deadly filth which these scheming criminals can study up as a means of creating sickness and good business for themselves. The demands of the medical fanatics of today are nothing less than the demand for absolute force to rule that the rest of the community may be their slaves! Before 1886, the medical profession used to be represented in the Iowa legislature by two or three physicians, but, after only fifteen years of medical monopoly, their representation has become so great that it is not deemed expedient to print the occupation of legislative members to learn that in fifteen years of medical monopoly, the medical fraternity has gained a representation of 900 percent. Sleep, dear people, sleep; in thirty years more all the members of the legislatures will be medical fanatics.

Judge Hord, when Attorney General of Indiana, rendered a notable decision bearing on this matter when he said: "The Health Board possesses no power of private espionage or unnecessary interference with the private rights of person or property. ... The Board cannot make regulations that are unreasonable, arbitrary and oppressive."

If there is anything a man owns, it is his own blood and just as a man has the unquestioned right to choose his political party, religion, physician, and to say whether or not a surgical operation shall be performed on his body, just so he has the right to reject vaccination.

THE COMMUNITIES RIGHTS

Col. Robert G. Ingersoll, in a lecture at Jersey City, gave utterance to these sentiments:

> This is my doctrine: Give every human being every right you claim for yourself, keep your mind open to the influence of nature. Receive new thoughts with hospitality. Let us advance. With every drop of my blood I hate and execrate every form of tyranny, every form of slavery. I hate dictation. I love liberty. I have given you my honest thought. Surely unresting action is better than unthinking faith. Surely reason is a better guide than fear. This world should be controlled by the living, not by the dead.

> How thoroughly now that fits the vaccination question!
> —*Newbury Daily News.*

The community's right over and against the individual's is on par with that of the individual over and against the community. In days gone by, when Minnesota was more civilized than it is today, this principle was recognized to the extent that cold-blooded judicial murder was not permitted.

The vaccinators know perfectly well that, if they should undergo to take from house to house and dose the people by force, they would speedily get themselves into trouble, and through frauds and political toadying they get the foolish or knavish lawmakers to assume the criminal part of the transaction, while they farm out the crime and spoils to the instigators of the crime.

Compulsory vaccination, direct or indirect, is a crime from both a theoretical and practical standpoint. While we could give you almost endless proof of this, we will simply call your attention to one instance right here close to home. In 1873, the Board of Health of Winona, Minnesota, made a vaccination order and furnished vaccine virus to the surgeons. P. Von Lackum, M.D., was appointed vaccinator for the third district. After the epidemic, he returned the virus furnished him and proved he had used pure cream instead. He showed his district did not have a single case of smallpox, and the general health was good, while in the other districts there were many cases of smallpox, and much sickness and many deaths, thus furnishing unquestionable proof that vaccination not only fails to prevent smallpox but that it is ruinous to the human race.

Dr. Von Lackum corroborates the statement made by Dr. C. Spinzir,

St. Louis, Missouri, in his *Variola, its causes, nature and prophylaxis*, page 7, St. Louis, 1878.

He says: "Vaccination is tantamount to inoculation and constitutes skeptical poisoning, a criminal offense to human health and life. It is statistically proved to afford no protection or mitigating power over smallpox; and, scientifically, in the nature of the case, it cannot possess any."

Also corroboration of the statement made in *Dungleson's Medical Dictionary* (See Vaccina, page 892, of 1856 edition; page 953 of 1860 edition; and page 1086 of 1874; that "smallpox occurs, at times, as an epidemic after vaccination."

We could cite evidence to fill a book. But it is generally known by the medical profession that vaccination nowadays is performed with smallpox virus, and in reality is the old practice of inoculation with smallpox virus, which is made a statutory crime by all civilized nations. The State Board of Health can start a smallpox epidemic at will, and they will every year from now on if the people will permit it.

The Civil Officer's Rights

The civil officer's right is to know that when he is sent to execute an order that such order is lawful. It is a scandal upon our judiciary to permit a superior official to go unpunished, when it is proved that such officer, through his own over-officiousness, caused the murder of an inferior officer.

The Health Officer of Albert Lea, Minnesota, is as guilty of the murder of Mr. Randall as if he had killed him with his own hands, and, in my opinion, all police officers in Minnesota should protect themselves from a similar fate by vigorous prosecution of the doctor who caused the murder of Mr. Randall. They should also be very careful in all executions coming from the Board of Health Department, inasmuch as such Boards have been proved to be irresponsible phantoms.

The Physician's Rights

Thousands of physicians understand the fraud of vaccination and it is their right to guard their friends against this foolish practice. To permit a law or ordinance which directly or indirectly practically overrules the constitutional rights between a physician and his patients, is a gross insult to the medical profession as a whole, and we dare say that 95 percent of the medical profession will candidly admit this statement to be correct, no matter what their opinion of vaccination may be. No one but the meanest and lowest in the medical profession would feel honored by being made a medical gallipot for a band of medical diplomat ward heelers calling themselves a Board of Health. Another thing, which should, or ought, to stir the pride of the profession is the practice of allowing medical men to become members of Health Boards; it smacks too much of fraud and a scheme to put in good work for selfish profit. There are plenty of men outside the medical profession who might better be trusted with the office than any professional man; both the medical profession and the public in general would be better served. Any sane man knows that the prosperity of the physician is in time of epidemics and much disease, and this alone is reason enough not to permit a physician to act as a member of a Board of Health nor to punish people or treating one another as we do now. There are many honest and upright men in the medical profession, but I believe that they also have a larger share of frauds than any other profession. Under the present protection laws, a scoundrel of a physician can play the confidence man with impunity for his own enrichment, and if his victims get tired of him and undertake to do what they can for themselves, he can retaliate by prosecuting them for practicing medicine. There is not one honest doctor who approves of such a state of things, and not one person outside of the profession ever approved it except through a misunderstanding caused by a misrepresentation of the facts, or else, a cash consideration, which is freely used in the lawmaking chambers by the class of physicians who expect to gain prosperity and prestige by such more than foolish acts. The respectable members of the profession are fast becoming ashamed of the scandal, and a little stir on their part and a little by the general public would, in a short time, burst this disgraceful bubble of the medical confidence men and stupid legislators.

THE CRIMINAL VACCINATOR

From where did he come? His home is in India, and he is not a physician but a priest, dealing out of the sacrament of the smallpox goddess whose name is *Matah*.

The Hindoos [sic] used to inoculate themselves with smallpox in order to appease the goddess, fancying that if they did so perhaps her majesty would kindly permit them to escape lightly. The Turkish court embraced this religion in 1721, and the English ambassador's wife, Lady Wortley Montague, of course, to be in the swim at court, found it an easy thing to embrace this, to her, new religion, and by her silly effort it was introduced into England, and as a result, smallpox epidemics became more common. This, in time, produced heretics who lost all faith in inoculation and looked for something better. The want was soon supplied by the smart alecks among the hustlers, who started the yarn that people who had once been affected by cowpox could never get the smallpox, and many people in the country embraced this new protestant religion of Matah faith. It is positively known that a farmer named Benjamin Jesty had administered this new protestant sacrament to two of his sons twenty years before (1796) when the Martin Luther (Jenner) permanently established this protestant religion in England, from whence it spread to the whole Caucasian race of man. As I have mentioned before, the protestant cowpox sacrament has in reality given place to the original smallpox sacrament of the mother faith. There are several reasons for this theological retrogression, which are as follows:

First of all, the cowpox is not as reliable to start a smallpox epidemic as the original sacrament smallpox. Second, cowpox inoculations have been found more dangerous as an infection than the smallpox inoculation, and in the next place, it is none of the people's business to know whether the Matah priests use the sacrament of his or that High Priest, as they are all standards.

And here you have them:

1. Jennerian equine (horse virus).
2. Sevine virus, with which Jenner inoculated his eldest son.
3. Horse virus, cow virus or horse grease (pus) passed through the cow.
4. The (said to be) spontaneous cow virus, the Gloucester brand.
5. Seely & Babcock's virus, the smallpox passed through the cow.
6. The Brangency virus.
7. The Passy virus.
8. Dr. Walomont's calf virus, supplied to the royal family in England, by which they were greatly injured.
9. The Sauroline virus, invented by Major W. G. Kind, and used in India and Burma.
10. Donkey virus, discovered by Surgeon O'Hare, used in India.
11. Buffalo virus, recommended in India.

To these must be added the viruses which have passed through numberless, more or less, diseased persons, which have been shown by high authorities to be capable of spreading leprosy, syphilis and other loathsome and incurable diseases.

Now, dear ladies, if you desire to be in the swim with the Asiatic Turks, and with the State Board of Heath Turks, you must do like Lady Montague, embrace the Matah religion, do penance, and have one of the mentioned sacraments administered to torture your body in honor of the goddess. Some of you may doubt the religious nature of vaccination, but let me tell you! The State Board of Health do not, and to prove this to you, I will give you a quotation from the pen of the Iowa State Board of Health Secretary, Dr. J. T. Kennedy, in the *Iowa State Board of Health Bul-*

letin, Vol. VIII, p. 52, where he says: "Nearly all well-regulated families, Jew and Gentile, felt it in their duty as parents to see that their offspring in early life had the protective influence of baptism, or circumcision, and vaccination. It would be well for Iowa parents to go and do likewise."

If you have the least little sense, you can plainly see that vaccination in the Matah religion is a sacrament equivalent to circumcision in the Jews and baptism in the Christian religion.

Now, then, when the State makes any religion in the State religion and compels its inhabitants to accept that religion under penalty, it is performing an unconstitutional act.

The Proper Way To Prevent And Treat Smallpox

We will now take a look at the means scientific men make use of to prevent and cure smallpox. Dr. George Dutton says: "Smallpox is a zymotic disease. It originated in decomposition and is powerless against cleanliness, within and without. Zymosis implies fermentation and fermentation is one of the earlier stages of decomposition. Dr. Carl Spinzig, in a paper read before the St. Louis Medical Society, Jan. 15, 1881, states that the eruptive character of smallpox is the outward manifestation of a process of decomposition of the blood produced by an excess of urea.

> Urea is the product of waste in the tissues of the body and is usually eliminated by the kidneys. Normal human blood contains about two percent of urea, while variolous (smallpox) blood has about eight percent. Smallpox, scarlatina, and measles generally occur in the early winter, when the cutaneous elimination is checked, and an increased burden of eliminating waste is thrown upon the kidneys. Accordingly, we find more eliminated by the kidneys in winter than in summer, when perspiration is freer. In tropical regions, it is observed, that smallpox is more generally confirmed to the higher elevations, where the temperature is lower than on the plains.

Knowing these facts, the preventative and curative means are simple. To prevent smallpox, we eliminate the urea by sweating and mild diuretics, and when these preventatives have been neglected longer than twenty-four hours after the beginning of the fever, all we can do is to aid nature to eliminate the urea in her own curative way, and this has been done many times with the most favorable results, even in the worst form of the disease. In one case among many others, the patient had been declared lost by the attending physicians and she had been unable to speak for several days, but the free use of Black Cohosh tea brought back her speech in a few hours, and she recovered rapidly, notwithstanding her old age. Many ordinary cases are on record where this line of treatment was found to be of great success, even two families who had been inoculated by small-pox according to law, and were treated with this Cohosh tea, while the court held the physicians under arrest to await the outcome of these cases; fortunate for the physicians, they succeeded in preventing the inoculation from taking effect, and consequently were released without further punishment.

But let it be remembered that our Materia Medica is brim full of remedies which will prevent smallpox. But even if this was not the case, we can fight smallpox successfully with water alone. Kneipp has proved this to the world beyond a doubt; and the time has come, when the people of this world must arise in their might and throw off one more detestable yoke of arrogant oppressive tyranny inherited from the dark ages of man.

Before 1886, the medical profession used to be represented in the Iowa legislature by two or three physicians, but, after only fifteen years of medical monopoly, their representation has become so great that it is not deemed expedient to print the occupation of legislative members to learn that in fifteen years of medical monopoly, the medical fraternity has gained a representation of 900 percent.

If there is anything a man owns, it is his own blood and just as a man has the unquestioned right to choose his political party, religion, physician, and to say whether or not a surgical operation shall be performed on his body, just so he has the right to reject vaccination.

The State Board of Health can start a smallpox epidemic at will, and they will every year from now on if the people will permit it.

Smallpox is a zymotic disease. It originated in decomposition and is powerless against cleanliness, within and without. Zymosis implies fermentation and fermentation is one of the earlier stages of decomposition.

1902

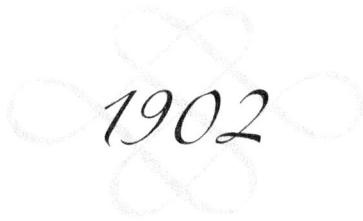

Influence Of Water On Health And Longevity
A. L. Wood, M.D.

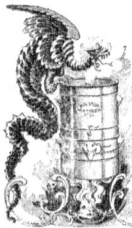
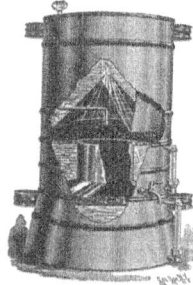
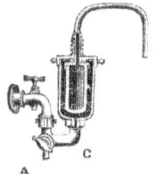
Distilled water was considered to be the safest and purest water to consume.

Influence Of Water On Health And Longevity

by A. L. Wood, M.D.

The Naturopath and Herald of Health, III (3), 127-132. (1902)

Read before the 100 Year Club at Hotel Majestic, 72nd St and Central Park West, New York, Nov 26, 1901.

Diarrhoea And Dysentery From Impure Water

Prof. William T. Sedgewick, of the Massachusetts Institute of Technology and Biologist of the Massachusetts State Board of Health, in the *Journal of N.E. Water Works Association* for March, 1896, gives an interesting account of the city water supply of Burlington, Vermont, and its effect upon the public health which is very instructive and from which the following information has been gathered. The natural conditions, location and surroundings of Burlington are exceptionally favorable to health. From 1870 to 1894, a period of twenty-four years, there existed a *mild epidemic of diarrhoea* gradually growing worse, year after year, until 1894. The same was true in a lesser degree of dysentery, and, while the deaths from typhoid fever were not considered excessive, they far exceeded what they should have been.

This long continued and excessive prevalence of diarrhoea and dysenteric diseases was attributed to organic impurities in the water supply which was taken from Lake Champlain, into which the sewage of the city was discharged.

In 1894 the intake pipe of the water supply was extended three miles from the sewer outlet into the lake with the result that, to use Prof. Sedgewick's own words: "The peculiar diarrhoeal disturbances that had so long prevailed in Burlington have, since the extension of the in-take pipe, wholly ceased; and the physicians are enthusiastic in their recognition of the salutary change, which they attribute entirely to the improved water supply."

This was written in 1896. In answer to my recent letter of inquiry, I have received the following reply from Dr. Watkins, the present Health Officer of Burlington:

Dr. A. L. Wood,   Nov 21, 1901.
Burlington, Vermont,
Brooklyn, New York

Dear Sir:

In reply to your letter of inquiry relative to the diarrhoeal disturbances which at one time prevailed in Burlington, will say that the conditions which followed the change of the in-take of water from the lake have continued to the present time. Burlington is very free from such troubles.

Sincerely yours,

H. R. Watkins, Health Officer.

Thus it will be seen that the remarkable, and for a long time unaccounted for, 24 years reign of diarrhoeal disorders, from 1870 to 1894, ceased suddenly and absolutely upon the change for the better in the city water supply. Not only this, but for seven years past the same freedom from these intestinal diseases has continued.

Does not this conclusively prove that this large class of diseases which causes the death of nearly 50,000 people a year in the United States, in addition to the 35,000 killed by typhoid fever, is caused by the use of impure water?

City Water Supplies Unsafe

The question naturally arises, what water shall we drink? What water shall we use in the preparation of the various articles of food and the different liquids, other than simple water, which we introduce into our stomachs to nourish the body, or for other reasons? I will say here that there are thousands of intelligent people who would not think of drinking our impure city water who allow their cooks to use it in the preparation of all their food, tea, coffee, etc., without once thinking that it is more important to use pure water for cooking than for drinking. But more of this later.

Where shall we obtain pure water? Certainly not from the city water supplies. They are rendered impure and dangerous to life and health by the drainage from cultivated fields where the rains wash the fertilizers, both animal and commercial, into the streams, and by pollution from shops, factories and other sources as will be shown further on. That such conditions exist can be seen by anyone who will take the time to investigate as I have done.

The Ridgewood water of Brooklyn contains an immense number of bacteria and animalculae. At one time, a few years since, there were as many as six million of a kind of vegetable starfish named asterionella in one glass of this water. This is all the more interesting from the fact that each one of these bacteria contains a minute globule of oil. (There would have been a good opening for the Standard Oil Company.) The decomposition of these bodies naturally produced a decidedly unpleasant taste and smell. There are more or less of these microorganisms present at all times.

What a vegetable garden the Ridgewood reservoir must have been when a single glass of its water contained six million of vegetable organisms. This asterionella, be it remembered, is but one of over 200 different forms of animal and vegetable life contained in our city waters. They are all fully illustrated by George Chandler Whipple, the present biologist of Brooklyn's Water Supply, in his recent book, *The Microscopy of Drinking Water.* Five minutes spent in examination of these illustrations ought to be sufficient to cure any one of the desire to eat or drink Ridgewood water whether its inhabitants are living or dead.

I would refer any one desiring to investigate the condition of the city water to an article in the May, 1901 number of the *Brooklyn Medical Journal,* by Dr. Hibbert Hills, now Director of Bacteriological Laboratory of the Boston Board of Health, but who, a few years since, was Chief Biologist of the Brooklyn Health Department, with Sanitary Supervision of the water shed; also to the *Annual Report of the New York State Board of Health* for 1898, which contains definite statements of the condition of hundreds of farms, residences, shops and other places bordering the streams and ponds of Brooklyn watershed, where the drainage from horse and cow stables, barnyards, pig pens, hen houses and yards, rabbit pens, duck yards and ponds, stagnant and filthy water pools, piles of manure, ashes, garbage and all kinds of animal and vegetable refuse, together with actual sewage from houses, shops, sinks, cesspools, urinals, privies and water closets, empty into, and form a part of, the delicious Ridgewood water which the people of Brooklyn have been accustomed to brag about and drink in its natural state or in the form of mineral waters, ginger ale, soda water, tea, coffee, etc., and to eat in all kinds of food prepared from it, in their bread, cake, pies, puddings, cooked fruits and vegetables, soups, fruit ices, etc., etc.

Anyone who can drink the city water from any beverage made from it, or eat anything cooked in it, or prepared with it, after reading these articles, must have an exceedingly strong stomach.

These articles, be it remembered, refer to the Brooklyn water, which in the past, has enjoyed the reputation of being one of the purest city waters.

For the delectation of the inhabitants of Manhattan Island, I will say that their Croton water is much more impure and unwholesome than Brooklyn's Ridgewood. I think it is superfluous to say anything more about Croton water.

The only way to avoid this pollution is to keep the watersheds which gather the water used, entirely in a state of Nature, free from cultivation and population. This may possibly come in the next generation, but probably not in this.

Many people, who realize the danger of using the impure city water, boil it and feel happy; others filter it and rest secure. Let us see if they have remedied the trouble.

BOILED WATER

Boiling impure water, aside from the destruction of the life of *some* of the disease germs, the elimination of some of the gases, and the deposit of a portion of the carbonate of lime, *always makes it more impure.* Boil a gallon of water until there is but a quart left and the quart will contain all the impurities of the gallon except as above stated, and be nearly four times as impure as before. Continue the boiling and all the impurities, animal, vegetable and mineral, except the gases thrown off, will be reduced to one solid mass. The water which is evaporated and passes off as steam is pure. But, you will say, it kills the dangerous germs. We will suppose it does, but their remains furnish material for bacterial life to feed upon. Do you relish the idea of eating in food, or drinking their dead and decomposing bodies which poison the water by their decomposition? The fact is scientific investigation has proved that boiling only kills the *feeblest*, the least injurious germs.

Prof. Percy Frankland, Ph.D., F.R.S., the noted English scientist and a recognized authority on water, says: "The germs which propagate epidemic or zymotic diseases may be boiled three hours and yet not be destroyed."

Try a simple experiment. Put unboiled city water in one bottle and the same that has been boiled for half an hour, or more, in another; cork tight and keep in the sun or in a warm place for a week or longer and note the difference. The unboiled water will show a marked depreciation in looks, taste and smell, but that which has been boiled will be so much worse in these respects that no one would think of using it. In comparison with these, you can submit a properly sealed bottle of pure distilled water to the same conditions and at the end of a year, it will be found to be as pure, sweet, and perfect as when first bottled.

FILTERED WATER

The domestic filter is a dangerous article of the worst description. People rely upon the fancied security while in 99 cases out of every 100 the water is more dangerous to health and life after passing through it than before. All soluble mineral salts and all impurities of every description, including the deadly poisons from disease and germs, which are held in solution, pass through the very best filter at all times, as freely as the water itself, and unless the filter is cleaned and sterilized several times a day, which is rarely, if ever done, the germs of typhoid fever and other diseases multiply with great rapidity within the filter itself and pass through with the water. Many eminent chemists and scientists have testified to the truth of these statements.

Cause Of Old Age—How To Retard It

Water laden with the germs of disease and the poisonous substances called toxines [sic] produced by them, and decomposing animal and vegetable matters poison the system and produce typhoid and other fevers and many acute intestinal and other diseases and cause the sudden death of thousands. The mineral elements contained in the water we drink and in that which is used in preparing our food are far more disastrous to health and life, but, being much slower in their action, are consequently unrecognized and unthought of.*

A French Physiologist has truly said: "A man is as old as his arteries."

Please remember this, for it is very important, "A man is as old as his arteries." What makes our arteries old? Young, healthy blood vessels are very elastic and allow the blood to circulate freely through them. In old age they become hard and unyielding, their capacity is diminished, and the blood stream becomes smaller and moves with less rapidity. These changes are caused by the deposit within the walls of the blood vessels, of fibrous and gelatinous substances, and of lime and other earthly compounds contained in the water taken into the system in food and drink. This deposit is liable to take place in the dense structures of any of the joints, in the tendons and muscles, in short, wherever the blood circulates, which, of course, is in every organ and tissue of the body, in the heart, the lungs, the digestive system, &c., [etc.] producing various diseased conditions, impairing the action of one and all and hastening the time when the human machine will cease to act and the spirit take its departure.

The following from Dr. C. W. De Lacy Evans, the noted author, physician and surgeon of London, states the case truly and forcibly.

> The combinations of lime held in solution in the water we drink, when taken into the stomach, are soon distributed throughout the system and deposited in all the tissues, exactly as they are precipitated and form incrustations on the bottoms of kettles in which water is boiled. The result is general induration, partial, and often in some organs and tissues, complete ossification. The bones become brittle; the joints and muscles stiff and rheumatic; gravel and stones form in the bladder; the kidneys, liver, heart, nerves and brain become indurated and sluggish in their action; all the bodily functions are impaired; the nerves weaken; the mind loses its vigor; the memory fails and senility and death creep on.

The evil influence of hard and mineral waters is, therefore, a chief producing cause of the conditions that constitute old age as well as many of the more serious diseases of mankind, and demands the earnest consideration of everyone who desires health, activity and length of days.

---

*This statement was made at a time when biochemistry was in its infancy. We now know mineral water has therapeutic properties. —Ed.

It is a common idea among the people that the minerals contained in spring and other waters are necessary to properly nourish the body, but chemists and physiologists know that inorganic minerals, such as contained in water, cannot be assimilated and used, but must be removed from the body or remain to obstruct and impair vital action. A volume could be filled with scientific testimony as to the truth of these statements in regard to minerals in water.

Our food contains in organized forms suitable for immediate use, all the minerals necessary for the needs of the body.

All city supply waters, and all spring and well waters, necessarily and inevitably contain more or less of these inorganic minerals and earthy matters in solution, and are objectionable in proportion to the quantity present. The purest are the best, but the purest are not good enough. The purest spring waters, and the most popular ones, are those which come nearest in analysis to distilled water.

Some of the so-called spring waters sold in this city are nothing but city water which has been passed through ordinary, improperly cared for filters. This I personally know to be a fact.

The presence of organic and inorganic impurities in the spring waters sold in this and other cities is a matter which demands the serious consideration of the Boards of Health of such cities. In the last *Annual Report of the Connecticut Agricultural Experiment Station*, the result of the analysis of 24 spring waters sold in the State and elsewhere, showed that 14 of them were unsafe and unfit for use on account of organic contaminations alone. The report of the Massachusetts State Board of Health gives the analysis of 45 spring waters sold in that State, which showed that 34 of them contained the waste organic products of human or animal contamination, or, in other words, filtered sewage. The spring waters of Massachusetts and Connecticut are probably no worse than those of other States.

No dependence whatever can be placed upon the quality of spring waters. They may be comparatively good at one time, and very bad at another. The amount of organic and mineral matter which they contain varies with the season of the year, with the amount of rain fall, and many other changing conditions.

Distilled Water The Purest And Best

The purest and best and the only absolutely safe water to use for drinking and the preparation of all foods and artificial drinks, is that produced by distillation. There are many processes of distillation, but the most imperfect one produces a water far superior in purity and healthfulness to the very best spring waters under their most favorable conditions. The nearest approach to it in purity is rain water, which is distilled water of Nature's own production, when collected on clean surfaces, in uninhabited sections, where the air is pure and uncontaminated by smoke, dust, city factory gases etc. I wish to correct a quite natural impression that boiled water and distilled water are practically the same. In boiling, the steam, the pure part, passes into the air and is lost, while all the impurities are left behind and condensed into liquid form again, giving a pure and wholesome water.

But some will say distilled water has a flat, insipid, disagreeable taste. This is true of distilled water produced by the old processes of distillation which do not get rid of the ammonia and other gases which in boiling pass off in the steam.

The most modern and perfect process of distillation not only eliminates these gases, but, to assure a perfect product, *re-distills* the distilled and purified water, giving *double distillation* and an absolutely pure and palatable water for drinking, cooking and many other uses in the household, and in the arts and manufactures. Unlike all spring and city waters, double distilled water is always uniform in quality and always pure.

Pure water is colorless and odorless. Any water, be it distilled or not, that has the slightest disagreeable taste, color or smell, is more or less impure and unsafe to use.

Distilled Water A Great Solvent

The great value of distilled water aside from its purity and palatableness is its great solvent powers, and the property of absorbing any impurities with which it comes in contact. *The Century Dictionary* says: "Of all liquids, distilled water is the most powerful and generally solvent."

Nature's distilled water in the form of rain percolates through the earth and in its course dissolves and absorbs various organic and inorganic substances with which it comes into contact, thus rendering it impure. In the same way distilled water taken into the body in food or as drink, circulates through the minutest parts of the system and dissolves, absorbs and carries with it out of the body, the unused and waste organic and mineral matters that poison and injure the system. In this way it purifies the blood and tissues, washing away the weak uric acid and other poisons that produce rheumatism, gout, congestion of the liver, kidneys and other organs.

Dr. De Lacy Evans, before quoted, says:

> Distilled water, used as a drink, is absorbed directly into the blood; the solvent properties of which it increases to an extent that it will keep salts already existing in the blood in solution, prevent their undue deposition in the various organs and structures, and favor their elimination by the different *excretae*. If the same be taken in large quantities, or if it be the only liquid taken into the system, either as a drink or as a medium for the ordinary decoctions of tea, coffee, etc., it will in time tend to remove those earthly compounds which have accumulated in the system, the

effects of which usually become manifest as the age of forty or fifty years is attained.

The daily use of distilled water facilitates the removal of deleterious compounds from the body by means of the excretae, and therefore tends to the prolongation of existence. The use of distilled water may be especially recommended after the age of thirty-five or forty years is attained; it will of itself prevent many diseases to which mankind is especially subject after this age; and were it generally used, gravel, stone in the bladder, and other diseases due to the formation of calculi in different parts of the system, would be much more uncommon.

The presence of organic and mineral substances in water destroys this solvent power in proportion to the quantity present, and, while not removing from the body as much as it should, it also leaves some of its own impurities in the system.

A German chemist, who evidently knows nothing about physiology and the laws of life and health, has stated that distilled water is absolutely poisonous, and that it is dangerous to use it because it dissolves the earthy salts and removes them from the system. This is one of its most valuable properties, for it only dissolves the *excess* of these salts, which are deposited throughout the system as foreign substances, and thus frees the body from their health-impairing and age-producing effects. It has no such an effect upon the living tissues of the body. If distilled water is a poison, then God is poisoning his children every day of their lives, for He distills every drop of water on the earth over and over again continually.

Do you relish the idea of eating in food, or drinking their dead and decomposing bodies which poison the water by their decomposition? The fact is scientific investigation has proved that boiling only kills the feeblest, the least injurious germs.

The nearest approach to it in purity is rain water, which is distilled water of Nature's own production, when collected on clean surfaces, in uninhabited sections, where the air is pure and uncontaminated by smoke, dust, city factory gasses etc.

I wish to correct a quite natural impression that boiled water and distilled water are practically the same. In boiling, the steam, the pure part, passes into the air and is lost, while all the impurities are left behind and condensed into liquid form again, giving a pure and wholesome water.

1903

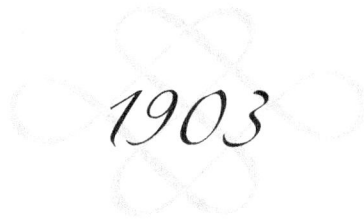

Compulsory Vaccination
Benedict Lust, N.D.

Children's Diseases
Sebastian Kneipp

This advertisement appeared in *The Naturopath and Herald of Health* in 1902 indicating that Benedict and Louisa Lust had three venues to promote Naturopathy. The New York Naturopathic Institute and College located at 135 E 58th Street would have different names throughout Lust's lifetime. The Health Store was one street away on 111 E. 59th St., and the Bellevue Sanitarium was open during the summer and located 30 miles from New York City in Butler, New Jersey. Benedict and Louisa Stroebelle were married July 11, 1901, and shortly after, the Bellevue Sanitarium was renamed the Naturopathic Health Home Yungborn.

COMPULSORY VACCINATION

by Benedict Lust, N.D.

The Naturopath and Herald of Health, IV (5), 127. (1903)

The readers of *Naturopath* were reasonably cautioned in regard to Stewart bill, No. 235, in the New York Assembly, because it contained five lines to provide for compulsory vaccination.

At the meeting of the Naturopathic Society of America, held February 13th, strong resolutions were presented by Dr. E. B. Foote, Jr., with a few brief remarks, and were unanimously adopted. Copies were mailed to the press and the committee in charge of the bill. Dr. Foote also appeared in person at a hearing on the bill before the Assembly Committee of Public Health, and found the State Commissioner, Dr. Lewis, there to address the Committee in favor of the whole bill. It was therefore evidently a sort of *official* or administration bureau bill, and one likely to pass, but we are now glad to be able to report that the Committee conceded the one point asked for by the opposition, by cutting out the lines making compulsory vaccination possible at the dictation of the State Health Department, so that the great State is saved the shame of legal enforcement of disease by its health officers, and so far as the bill now stands, it simply facilitates this department in the performance of its proper sanitary functions, while it may also bestow some new primers of the kind known as *political graft*. Possibly the Health Department feared it might lose all (including new access to the public purse) if the compulsory vaccination clause were retained, for the *Press-Knickerbocker*, one of Albany's wide awake dailies, was administering frequent hard knocks on this account. At least we may congratulate ourselves that the vigilance of a few has protected the many from a very imminent danger of the worst sort of compulsory vaccination law, and let us hope for continued immunity from such infliction.

Children's Diseases

by Sebastian Kneipp

The Naturopath and Herald of Health, IV (8), 237. (1903)

Scarlatina, Measles

Scarlatina demands every year a large number of victims among our children; it is generally prevalent in the spring and summer and on account of its great infection spreads very quickly. Even among grown people some few cases occur.

The symptoms are languor and apathy, dullness in the head, indifference to play, etc. Soon a few red spots appear on the body and fever sets in accompanied by great thirst. These outward symptoms are as a rule last from 5 to 8 days. Immediate recourse to the water cure never fails to give prompt relief and speedy cure.

The child should be dressed with a salt-shirt, i.e., a night shirt dipped into cold salt water and then wrung out; then it should be well covered all around with a woolen blanket, but not too tightly. Let the child remain thus quietly for about an hour and then the shirt can be removed and replaced by a dry one. Afterwards, give the child a quick ablution of the entire body and keep [the child] in bed. A cold half-bath, of about two seconds, may occasionally be applied and this treatment is continued until the fever has disappeared and all danger has passed. Should the fever return, apply again an ablution of the whole body with cold water, as before.

Diet during the time of illness must be as plain as possible; give small portions at a time and rather repeat them often.

Scarlatina and measles are caused by insufficient exhalation of the body during the winter. The diseased matter, not having been excreted, has gradually settled under the skin, and makes its appearance in these two forms with the change of air in early spring. This is a tangible proof of the good effects of fresh air.

Measles differ from scarlatina only by greater discharges of fluid matter. The diseased matter manifests itself by small pustules which appear on the surface of the body, and the best remedy for their extirpation is certainly water, which in two or three days' time will eliminate all signs of the disease.

In a case of measles the throat and palate are also covered with pustules which cause irritation and a tendency to cough. For their dissolution, the best remedy to be applied is a teaspoonful of *Foenum-graecum* decoction, to be taken every fifteen minutes. Take a little on the end of a knife to half a pint of water.

Tea of shavegrass* or oak bark, in similar doses, have a somewhat

---

*Shavegrass is Equisetum. —*Ed.*

stronger effect. It would be well for children if every two years they would have an attack of measles or scarlatina, as this would cleanse the system most effectively of all impurities. It is a well-known fact that children who have recovered from either of these two diseases, are much healthier and feel much better than those who have not had them.

The temperature in the sick-room must be kept low—lower than 70° F/21° C degrees, which is too much even for healthy people. Care should also be taken to keep the apartment well ventilated, but all draft must be avoided.

There is some danger of contagion from scarlatina, for children as well as grown persons, but only when the scarlet spots are visible on the surface of the body of the patient.

The child should be dressed with a salt-shirt, i.e., a night shirt dipped into cold salt water and then wrung out; then it should be well covered all around with a woolen blanket, but not too tightly. Let the child remain thus quietly for about an hour and then the shirt can be removed and replaced by a dry one.

Scarlatina and measles are caused by insufficient exhalation of the body during the winter. The diseased matter, not having been excreted, has gradually settled under the skin, and makes its appearance in these two forms with the change of air in early spring. This is a tangible proof of the good effects of fresh air.

Measles differ from scarlatina only by greater discharges of fluid matter. The diseased matter manifests itself by small pustules which appear on the surface of the body, and the best remedy for their extirpation is certainly water, which in two or three days' time will eliminate all signs of the disease.

For [pustule] dissolution, the best remedy to be applied is a teasponful of Foenum-graceum *[Fenugreek] decoction, to be taken every fifteen minutes.*

1904

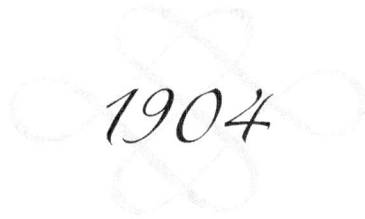

ON THE MECHANISM OF PROTECTION IN OUR BODY

CARL STRUEH, M.D.

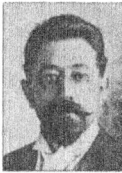

Carl Strueh, M.D., an outspoken practitioner of Naturopathy, practiced in Chicago and had a health sanitarium at McHenry, Illinois. For many years, Strueh placed regular monthly advertisements in Benedict Lust's journals.

On The Mechanism Of Protection In Our Body

by Carl Strueh, M.D.

The Naturopath and Herald of Health, V (4), 81-83. (1904)

Man, like every living being and every living plant is, during the entire time of his existence, subject to injurious influences—influences which are antagonistic to the conditions essential to living, and which would be powerful enough in themselves to put an end to his life were the body not endowed with a mechanism capable of preventing the effects of these influences or of neutralizing them. Life is an unceasing struggle of the organism for existence, an everlasting battle between influences detrimental to health and the mechanism of protection and resistance of the body. Are the latter unequal to the task of

Dr. Carl Strueh

warding off the noxious influences [or] our organism will succumb; i.e., it will sicken and finally perish. The marvelous manner in which our body protects itself against all the different noxiousness's may be observed in an endless line of processes going on in our organism. When we run a dirty sliver of wood into the finger, the body at once calls forth an inflammation and suppuration in order—if at all possible—to coax the sliver of wood in the finger, as it were, to expel it together with the noxious substances attached to it, and in this way to prevent blood-poisoning. When we choke, i.e., when some substance finds its way into the respiratory organs, a violent coughing fit at once sets in for the purpose of expelling the foreign substance and of preventing its remaining and thus causing a fatal illness. In some cases of paralysis it not infrequently happens that the patient owing to the insensibility of the respective nerves is not aware of the swallowing in consequence thereof the swallowed substances remain in the respiratory tubes and cause a fatal pneumonia.

Sneezing after taking a pinch of snuff is a part of the mechanism of prevention in our body, and only after the nerves of the nose, by repeated and persistent use of snuff have become insensible, reflex sneezing ceases. When we partake of unsavory things our body generally rids itself of them by vomiting or diarrhoea. The hardening of the skin against influences of cold; all those manifold processes are observed during disease: fever, pain,

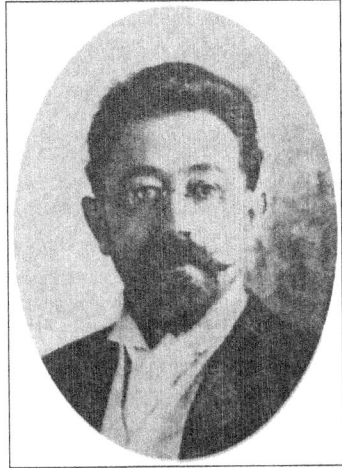

perspiration, coughing, cutaneous eruptions, etc.; all these represent the mechanism of protection and prevention in our body. Hence, we commit the most flagrant error in repressing instead of assisting these curative efforts of Nature. Again, the enlargement of the heart-muscle in irregular circulation, the enlargement of one of the kidneys in affections of the other, the augmentation of the sense of touch in blindness, the compensatory enhancement of the activity of one organ in case of suspended function of another serving the same purposes, the feeling of fatigue impelling rest, the want of appetite which induces us not to burden our body with needless nourishment, the feeling of hunger and thirst, telling how much and what kind of nourishment and how much liquid our body is in need of for the time being, the numberless states of inflammation, the most varied hemorrhages, as, for instance, bleeding piles. All these symptoms are not independent irregularities, but necessary consequences. They belong to the mechanism of protection and prevention by which our organism is rendered capable of maintaining its existence as long as it is possible under the circumstances.

Only when all these curative means which Nature employs are insufficient, which is especially the case with the lasting effect of the causally disturbing influences, does our organism succumb. Bacilli also belong to the mechanism of protection and must not be considered as causes, but as effects of physical disturbances. We are not sick because of the presence of bacilli, but bacilli are present because of our sickness. Bacilli were not created to make us ill, but to restore our health. From unphilosophical minds only could emanate the absurd idea that Nature created these low beings with the express and evil intent to impair our health. Nature destroys us only after we have become unsuitable for further existence and proper propagation by our wrong mode of living. The metabolic process must have been disturbed before bacilli can make their appearance to remove the dead substances created by the disturbances in the metabolic process and to restore our health in this way; and only in case of the continuance of the casual disturbances will continue the formation of dead substances and presence of the bacilli until we succumb.

Bacilli by themselves are never the cause of illness; they are everywhere in Nature; they are always swarming about us, but they never settle in our organism and multiply if there be nothing to do for them, i.e., if they do not find any dead material on which they can subsist. One man's meat is another man's poison. That we find in different diseases different bacilli is explained by the fact that the cells decaying in different diseases are composed of different elements, and that these different elements furnish the subsistence for the different species of bacilli. The same conditions [apply to] lice. We distinguish head-lice, body-lice and clothes lice. A head-louse does not thrive in clothes, a clothes louse does not thrive on the head, and the body-louse thrives only in the region of the genitals. Why? Because the conditions of existence and subsistence are different for the different species; the head-louse finds favorable conditions on the head only, the clothes-louse in the clothes only, and the body-louse only about the private parts. Exactly the same is the case with the different species of bacteria. The bacillus tuberculosis, for instance, is found only where there is the material necessary for its subsistence, and not where conditions are favorable to the existence of the bacillus of diphtheria or smallpox.

In this way, then, we must explain the attempts at vaccination. If ten persons are inoculated with a certain bacillus it must not be presumed that every one of the ten will be attacked by the same disease, but perhaps only five or but three, because only five or three had the requisite material, the necessary food for the particular bacillus. A goat does not eat lobster-pie, nor does a cat eat cabbage, and thus different bacilli presumable have different predilections. A so-called infection always requires, besides the bacillus, a so-called predisposition, which means the presence of decayed substances furnishing the conditions of existence to the bacilli. The decomposition and removal of this material proceeds in the nature of an acute feverish illness, which latter must not, on that account, be considered as disease per se, but as the process of reaction and healing, and hence must not be repressed. The acute illness being permitted to run its course, complete recovery will take place in almost all cases ending favorably because the system has been freed from all decayed matter and thoroughly cleansed. An incomplete recovery is most always the result of an interference with the process of reaction and healing by incorrect treatment, especially by improper diet and absorption of chemical remedies. By so-called preventive vaccination (immunization) the disease, i.e., the predisposition, i.e., the morbid material in our system is preserved. The serum employed in these inoculations alter the nature of the fluid elements of our body in such a manner as not to meet the taste and requirements of the bacilli; so that these cannot develop and execute their healing work as long as the more or less preventive agency of the inoculation endures, i.e., as long as the fluid is altered by the inoculated serum so as not to meet the requirements of the bacilli.

This alteration of the fluid gone, the system again becomes susceptible, i.e., bacilli will reappear to free the system of all latent decayed substances and thus cure us. Vaccination, then, must be condemned for the very reason that it preserves the disease, because it prevents the acute feverish reaction, i.e., the self-delivery of the system of any pathological metabolic products. The effect of vaccination is attributable to the fact that it causes such a change in the chemical composition of the elements of the body as not to meet the requirements of the particular bacteria preventing these to take root and propagate. We can, indeed, render the choicest soup unpalatable by undue seasoning; and there are leeches and fleas that will not touch certain persons because the blood of the latter, for some unknown reason, is not to the liking of the former. Again, just as well in such a case the change in the blood renders the latter unsuitable for food of leeches and fleas, it may be presumed that by the absorption of a particular serum the chemical composition of the blood is changed to such a degree that it ceases to offer the conditions necessary for the subsistence and development of bacilli, thus preventing the reactive process of healing, which we call acute illness.

Bacilli were not created to make us ill, but to restore our health.

Bacilli by themselves are never the cause of illness; they are everywhere in Nature; they are always swarming about us, but they never settle in our organism and multiply if there be nothing to do for them, i.e., if they do not find any dead material on which they can subsist.

The bacillus tuberculosis, for instance, is found only where there is the material necessary for its subsistence, and not where conditions are favorable to the existence of the bacillus of diphtheria or smallpox.

The acute illness being permitted to run its course complete recovery will take place in almost all cases ending favorably, because the system has been freed from all decayed matter and thoroughly cleansed.

1905

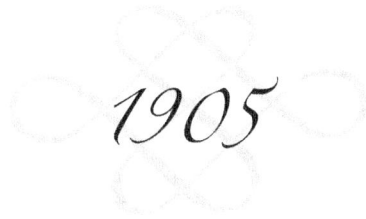

DIPHTHERIA
BENEDICT LUST, N.D.

DIPHTHERIA AND ANTITOXIN
DR. SCHULZE

An advertisement appearing in 1900 in *The Kneipp Water Cure Monthly* for books on health and hygiene.

DIPHTHERIA

by Benedict Lust, N.D.

The Naturopath and Herald of Health, VI (1), 12-15. (1905)

Diphtheria is one of the most dreaded diseases and claims a great many victims. According to Professor Rose of Berlin, there have been in one single hospital in the infirmary Bethanien, one of the best conducted hospitals, in one single year no less than three hundred and forty cases of diphtheria in which two hundred and forty-one operations became necessary, and in which five-sixths of the patients died. With the natural method of healing, the cure of this disease requires only a few days, and operations become therefore unnecessary; cases of death, alas, are also here recorded, but not by far at the same rate as with medical treatment.

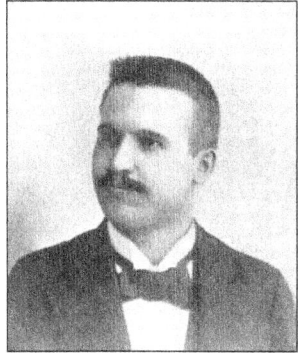

Benedict Lust, N.D.

This disease greatly resembles croup, but diphtheria is contagious and croup is not; the diphtheritic coating bears characteristics of decay; in croup, however, a real membrane forms. People of any age are subject to the former, children only to croup; in the former swelling and suppuration of the sub-maxillary glands, but not in the latter. Thus various differences exist which are described in a more detailed manner in the following.

This disease is, as already mentioned, very much like croup; also like thrush aphthae, and catarrhal inflammation of the throat. To be perfectly clear, we will give a concise and yet somewhat more circumstantial account of the respective distinguishing characteristics:

DIPHTHERIA OF THE PHARYNX, [VINCENT'S] ANGINA

The exudation (membranous exudation), which is white or greyish white, is located in the mucous membrane, is therefore firmly attached and can be removed only with difficulty. The cure is affected with loss of substance and the formation of scars and putrid smell.

CROUP

The excretion has a pale yellow color, clings very fast to the mucous membrane and is difficult to place [identify]. Cure takes place without loss of any substance. Barking cough, commences suddenly and generally at night.

CATARRHAL INFLAMMATION OF THE THROAT

White or yellowish point-like prominences, easily squeezed out and wiped off, frequently form on the tonsils.

APHTHAE

Aphthae are principally found on the edges and the undersurface at the point of the tongue, where croup never touches.

THRUSH

The odium* is white, easily wiped away with a handkerchief, and makes its appearance in the whole of the throat.

SYMPTOMS OF DIPHTHERIA

General feeling of illness, depression, indifference, loss of appetite, followed by occasional vomiting, headache, delirium, high fever, shivering, heat, thirst, heaviness in the limbs, and pressure in the pit of the stomach. Next, pains in the throat when swallowing, inflammation and swelling of the tonsils and the gullet, and the appearance of a grey or whitish grey fungus-like coating. Sometimes also brownish spots on the tonsils or the uvula spreading rapidly behind, above and below. If removed, the mucous membrane beneath it is seen to be an open, bloody or ulcerous place. Further a peculiar unpleasant gangrenous smell, fetid discharge from the nose, dry, barking cough, etc. This disease appears independently or accompanied by other diseases, such as scarlatina, smallpox, etc. It affects principally children of from five to two years old, and appears more rarely in later years.

CAUSES

Indigestible food and faulty diet, and consequent weakness in the digestive organs and of the nerves, spoiling children and effeminizing them, and thus causing them to forfeit all the strength which should go towards resisting injurious and morbid influences. Next, unhealthy, damp, dark dwelling places, often kept dirty, which are never aired, and overcrowded with people; and next too little exercise in the open air. Vaccination also from arm to arm, whereby the blood and the humors of healthy children are tainted or permanently poisoned, and the systems of the little ones thus rendered susceptible to diseases of that description is one of the causes of diphtheria. Lastly, infection, etc.

----

*Odium albicans is the organism that settles chiefly in the mouths of newborns whose general condition is in some way below par. —Ed.

TREATMENT

Separation of the affected from the healthy. The room must be cool and airy and therefore the windows constantly open and sometimes also the door. At a temperature of 46° F/8° C, there need not be a fire in the room. A patient, with a fever upon him, cannot easily catch cold; therefore, he must be slightly covered; best a blanket because it allows the morbid exhalations to pass through, while feather beds [down duvet] rather retain the morbid matters. This blanket, or better two of them, must daily be hung up in the open air several times, if possible in the sun; the floor of the room must be cleaned every day, but not be carpeted. The following simple but wonderfully effective treatment must, above all, be adopted.

Full steam-bath in bed* and cool neck-compress. For the latter a medium-sized towel is usually taken for children, dipped into (54° to 66° F/12° to 19° C) water and wrung out moderately dry—but it must be as wide as possible, so as to reach up to the ears and be put around the whole neck. The upper half of this wet compress is left without any woolen covering. Therefore the compress must not be too thin, and be kept on all the time the patient is in the pack. When he is not in his steam-bath (66° to 72° F/19° to 22° C) cool neck-compresses are constantly applied and changed when getting warm. With peevish children, three-quarter steam-bath in bed and shoulder pack (duration of the bath three-quarters of an hour to one hour). Should the patient become restless the pack must be removed. If needful this pack must be repeated two or three times within twenty-four hours. After it, a lukewarm (72° to 86° F/22° to 30° C) full washing to be given. The higher the fever, the thicker and wetter the sheet for the steam-bath in bed. Moreover trunk and foot packs are to be given. Both packs to be changed in high fever, i.e., when they get hot—which a little child soon shows by its restlessness—according to requirement; when the fever is only moderate, about every two hours. Water should be taken into the mouth to absorb and loosen the exudations in the inflamed mucous membranes, etc. The patient must gargle several times during the hour, and with little children, injections made into the nose and throat with lukewarm (77° F/25° C) water, which may be acidulated advantageously with lemon juice, one-fifth of a lemon to a glass of water. If there is no ball-syringe, a well cleaned common syringe must be used, but it must be applied with a mild pressure. Besides fresh water, mixed with plenty of lemon juice, must be drunk freely because firstly, it helps to quench the thirst, and, secondly, it soothes the heat and pain in the throat; the suppurating places are cleansed of their corrosive poisonous excretions, and, thirdly, the inward fever heat is mitigated, and

---

*A full description of the steam bath in the bed will be found in a future volume of the Hevert Collection, *Hydrotherapy in Naturopathic Medicine.* —*Ed.*

the injurious substances removed from the blood. Nourishment is only given the patient when he asks for it. Non-stimulating, cool, semi-liquid food, buttermilk, apple-jam or other boiled and raw fruit. Egg-flip with sugar, oat or barley—gruel and similar decoctions. For constipation and for derivative purposes: cool (64° to 66° F/18° to 19° C) enemata. In the evening a lukewarm half-bath (88° to 92° F/31° to 33° C) for ten minutes. If the diphtheria is of a croup-like character, and the coating begins to cover the larynx, it is advisable, when a choking fit takes place, to put the child into a tub containing warm water about five inches high, and to give affusions with cold water from the neck over the back. I have seen many a child saved by this heroic treatment. Also, the hip-baths combined with wet rubbing mentioned by Kuhne and continual lavations of the abdomen are effective.

That injury may be done by physical application is proved by the following illustration: A homeopathic doctor applied inhalations of steam in diphtheria by causing the patient to inhale the steam of boiling water from a tub, which process is generally fatal to life. The inhaled vapor is, by reason of its moist warmth, the very thing to promote the growth of fungi and effects only considerably aggravated respiration. The consequence of it is mostly aggravation of the croup and poisoning of the blood with carbonic acid (choking fits).

A Second Treatment

According to the patient's strength, a lukewarm (80° F/27° C) soothing three-quarter pack, morning and evening (if needful with a hot-water bottle, wrapped in a wet cloth, at the feet) and neck-compresses containing plenty of moisture, as above, to be kept on for an hour and a quarter, and followed by a lukewarm (90° F/32° C) bath. For the rest, continual tepid (72° F/22° C) stimulating calf-packs to be kept on about an hour and a half, and combined with (66° to 72°F/19° to 22° C) cooling neck-compresses (duration half an hour) and tepid (68° F/20° C) gargling or injections into the gums (also for half an hour). If there is fever, there are to be added (88° F/31° C) soothing trunk or abdominal packs (duration one hour). This treatment must be continued through one or two nights, as it is just then, whilst the patient sleeps, that an aggravation of the disease takes place. Non-stimulating light food, lemonade (the juices of fruit, especially of lemon). Tepid (72° F/22° C) enemata twice daily contents eight to ten spoonfuls of water. When the disease has been overcome, it is advisable to give the patient a wet rubbing of the whole body every day for about a week, and a full pack or steam-bath in bed every other day.

Treatment By Massage

The swollen glands and muscles of the throat must be rubbed gently from the beginning in spite of the patient's great pain and the resistance offered to it by him, but with more pressure gradually in a downward direction for from two to four minutes with the fingers dipped previously in oil and water. At first this treatment is not applied to the swollen parts but to their neighborhood, and the manipulation of the affected places is gradually entered upon and to be repeated every half hour. The treatment by massage is always to be combined with the above applications of water.

This treatment by massage in diphtheria has been characterized by many as absolutely injurious because the friction of the tonsils, auricular salivary glands, muscles of the throat, and glands at the shoulders, all of them swollen and exceedingly painful, causes the poison to be rubbed farther into the system. On the other hand, experience has taught over and over again that it is just these threatening swellings, which massage combined with the applications of water calculated to stimulate excretion (as steam-baths, succeeded by packs, enemata, etc.) has caused to disappear in surprisingly short time. Notwithstanding this explanation, I do not advise treatment by massage in diphtheria to be undertaken without professional advice or, if applied, to be used only in the mildest manner possible, especially as the above applications of water are quite sufficient of themselves to cure the disease.

At the beginning of the disease, when the throat and the tonsils begin to get inflamed and the first diphtheritic coating is discernible, frequently changed cool (59° to 66° F/15° to 19° C) throat compresses are of excellent effect, and must not be done without. But it is not necessary to put the compress right round the whole neck, and thus to trouble the child at every renewal of the compress to raise its head, which would be every ten to fifteen minutes or oftener, because it takes that time in the beginning for the compress to get hot. I chose for this purpose a large pocket handkerchief, folded lengthways in four, to be placed behind the neck of the child, and have besides two compresses made, folded in eight, about three fingers wide and composed of old soft, white linen, long enough to cover the whole forepart of the neck and the tonsils (in other words: reaching from ear to ear, measured under the chin). A wash-hand basin or other basin with cool water is placed by the side of the bed, and both these compresses are dipped into it; they are wrung out, not too dry, and one of them is applied to the child's throat, so as to cover it, whilst its two ends are turned up at both sides of the tonsils, towards the ears, and then pinned together loosely with the dry cloth behind the neck. After some time, when it feels warm to the touch, it is unpinned and exchanged for the other compress lying ready in the basin, the dry cloth clapped over it as before and its ends tucked under the shirt. This process is continued till the compresses do not any longer get warm so quickly, which happens simultaneously with the decrease of fever and inflammation. When that is the case, i. e., when the compresses take longer to get warm, a wet pocket-handkerchief, folded in four, is put round the child's whole neck in such a way that the ends reach in front up to the ears beyond the part where the tonsils are situated, and on which the diphtheric coating forms, so that the damp warmth may tell effectively upon the detachment of the coating and the excretionary process of the respective part of the skin, for which reason this compress is left on till it has become quite hot and begins to dry, which is within four or five hours or more. By this contrivance one has the advantage that the child is not obliged to raise its head every time a compress is put on. Let me emphasize once more only at the outset, where there is considerable fever and violent inflammation of the throat and tonsils, are the wet cold compresses to be changed frequently for the purpose of reducing and limiting the inflammation and the formation of the fungus-like covering. If these exudations, however, producing the diphtheric coating are embedded already in the mucous membranes of the throat to any considerable extent, or if fever and inflammation are moderated and entirely reduced, then frequently changed throat compresses are absolutely injurious, because nothing else than damp warmth (stimulating compresses) is necessary to dissolve the mucus and effect a cure. This is an undoubted fact, and one of which any physician who has the opportunity of treating patients affected with diphtheria cannot help being convinced. It is always preferable in this disease to ask the advice of an efficient Naturopath.

The higher the fever, the thicker and wetter the sheet for the steam-bath in bed. Moreover trunk and foot packs are to be given.

The patient must gargle several times during the hour, and with little children, injections made into the nose and throat with lukewarm (77° F/25° C) water, which may be acidulated advantageously with lemon-juice, one-fifth of a lemon to a glass of water.

According to the patient's strength, a lukewarm (80° F/27° C) soothing three-quarter pack, morning and evening (if needful with a hot-water bottle, wrapped in a wet cloth, at the feet) and neck-compresses containing plenty of moisture, as above, to be kept on for an hour and a quarter, and followed by a lukewarm (90° F/32° C) bath.

Diphtheria And Antitoxine

by Dr. Schulze

The Naturopath and Herald of Health, VI (I), 16-18. (1905)

No age has been so rich in inventions and discoveries as ours, and it is worthwhile to investigate the causes of this phenomenon. I fear that the source of most discoveries has not been altogether an unsullied one, and that they have arisen in great measure from mere ambition, or, worse still, from desire of gain. Or shall we, on the other hand, designate the guiding motive by the well-sounding term "Love of Truth"?

During the last two decades an irresistible tendency has asserted itself in medical science, constantly to seek out new remedies, many of which enjoy only a brief existence and are again replaced by newer ones. The progress which has been made in chemistry, physiology, and especially in microscopic research, has given rise to a host of new ideas, resulting in a new system of therapeutics, based on the hypothesis that diseases are caused by organisms and the *modus operandi* of which consists in the introduction into the circulation of the new remedies by means of inoculation and injections. It is a question, however, how far these so-called remedies have stood the test of experience and proved really serviceable to humanity or even to the animal world. I would remind the reader of the system of inoculation against hydrophobia, introduced by Professor Pasteur in France, the success of which has been doubted by his own countrymen, and which has met with no favor in this country. Also of the claim of the same man to have discovered a remedy for anthrax in inoculation, a claim which was examined and rejected by a commission appointed by the Prussian Government, in the district of Mansfeld, where the disease was epidemic. I would refer once more to the pernicious tuberculin injections of Koch, which have resulted in a complete fiasco, in spite of the manner in which they were lauded to the skies and trumpeted forth to the world, but which continue to be employed by credulous fanatics, and are still puffed in medical periodicals. I admit that sufferers from the dry cough, which forms the earliest stage of tuberculosis of the lungs, have recovered after inoculations with tuberculin; but are we justified in drawing the conclusion that these patients owe their recovery to the inoculations, in view of the fact that equally favorably results have been obtained by a strictly regulated manner of life, by the removal of the patient to a healthier house and bed-room, and by breathing exercises carried out in pure and mild air?

And now a new discovery has lately been brought to light, viz., the cure of diphtheria by injecting the serum of animals rendered immune to the disease (i.e., protected from contracting it) by inoculation with the lymph of other animals which have been attacked by it.

There has been no little jubilation in the newspapers over this discovery, and the high-sounding title of Antitoxine has been applied to the remedy, though men are by no means convinced as yet that the virtues which have been attributed to it will be confirmed by further experience. Since, however, according to the discoverer, the remedy is only effective in the early stages of the disease; the question arises whether all the cases which have been announced as cured were really of diphtheritic character. I am very frequently sent for by anxious parents who have noticed grayish-white patches on their children's tonsils, and in most cases I have been able to comfort them with the assurance that there were no symptoms of diphtheria. I have even known cases which have been diagnosed by physicians as diphtheritic, and notified as such to the police, which, however, were not cases of diphtheria at all.

While on this subject I must mention a fact which, I am sorry to say, does not redound to the credit of the medical profession, viz., that it has been the custom of late, at any rate among young doctors, to exaggerate the gravity of the disease when speaking to the patient's family, a custom which I cannot approve of, and can only account for as the result of the desire on the part of tyros to establish for themselves a reputation as saviors of life.

In the reports of experiments with antitoxine it is stated that the remedy is effective only at the beginning of the disease. What, however, is meant by the beginning of diphtheria? No other disease approaches so treacherously and breaks out so suddenly in its fully characteristic developed form, before the least suspicion has been entertained of the presence of the danger. How often are we not informed by parents that their children are at one moment playing gaily, and then suddenly lose all inclination for play, and complain of indisposition and pain in the throat, and that then for the first time they observe patches on the tonsils and gums of the children. But since the patches were observed as soon as the children complained of feeling ill, the disease must already have been developed. Is this moment then to be considered the beginning of the disease, or have other phenomena been discovered on the apparently healthy individuals indicating the commencement of diphtheria?

It is now more than half a year since I first heard of the alleged curative virtues of antitoxine in cases of diphtheria, and yet we are still in the experimental stage. It might have been supposed that, diphtheria being a disease of frequent occurrence, especially in Berlin, some definitive conclusion would long since have been arrived at, for this continual experimenting tends to produce a feeling of skepticism in regard to the *beneficent discovery*.

Among the criers of the new system must be included the committee formed for the object of making antitoxine accessible to the poor.

In their appeal attention is drawn to the high price of the remedy, the necessary dose costing seven marks, which sum has even been demanded from doctors by an enterprising apothecary in a circular. I would suggest to the benevolent committee that they should apply direct to the laboratory, which, I am informed on sound authority, makes a handsome profit by selling the remedy for two marks, whereas the apothecary is not satisfied with less than 200% profit in addition.

A Case Of Death

A case of death through antitoxine which at the time was reported in all the papers, and which shows how dangerous the administration of serum may be in many cases, may find a place here:

The *Vossische Zeitung* had the following announcement in its issue of the 9th of April:

> Our dear son Ernest, aged one year and a half, died yesterday evening at six o'clock, in the midst of perfect health, from the effects of an injection of Behring's antitoxine, administered for the purpose of procuring immunity from diphtheria.
>
> The undersigned request silent sympathy.
>
> Dr. med Langerhans,
> Mrs. Langerhans

It need hardly be said that the above deeply affecting case, in which the child of a well-known medical man, in the midst of perfect health, fell a victim to an injection of antitoxine, will afford food for reflection to sensible people, especially in regard to the administration of antitoxine as a preservative [preventative].

The *Berliner Lokal Anzeriger* writes as follows concerning this case:

> Dr. Robert Langerhans, Professor at the Moabit Hospital, son of the Chairman of the Town Council, Dr. Langerhans, has just been visited by a terrible calamity. He has lost his little boy, aged one and three-quarter years, who died immediately after an injection of Behring's antitoxine. The circumstances, as far as we have ascertained them, are as follows: The Professor's cook was suddenly seized with violent pains in the throat, and was sent to the diphtheritic department of the Moabit Hospital. On the advice of his colleagues, Prof. Langerhans, who had lost two of his children the year before, determined to secure his little boy against infection by an injection of antitoxine on the following day. Having procured a supply of antitoxine from the apothecary at the hospital, he administered the injection towards evening. In an instant the boy was a corpse. A sudden failure of the heart put

an end to his life. Dr. Max Asch, of Charlottenburg, made the following remarks: "Are we to see in the tragic fate which has befallen the family of Professor Langerhans only an exceptionally unfortunate accident, or are there reasons for supposing that a causal connection exists between the death of the child and the previous injection of Behring's antitoxine? Are there other cases within our knowledge tending to show that injections of antitoxine are dangerous to life?"

An article in the February number of the *Monthly Therapeutical Journal*, edited by Prof. Liebreich, setting down simply and dispassionately the results of the experience gained up to the present affords us some instructive information on this point. In the first place we find a list of cases in which the administration of antitoxine has been followed by severe illness, often lasting for weeks and months. The most notorious of these cases is one reported by Dr. Pistor in Berlin, and which happened to his own daughter. The latter, a girl of seven, was treated, on account of inflammation of the throat, which it was afterwards proved was not diphtheritic at all, with one injection of antitoxine, and this was speedily followed by severe and protracted illness, confining her to her room for three months. Dr. Variot, of Paris, who has perhaps had the widest experience in this matter, expressly raises a warning against the administration of the antitoxine for preventative purposes, the danger attending such administration being too great. Not only, however, has disease been known to result from the injections in question, but there have been cases in which their administration to healthy children for preventative purposes has been followed by death within a few days.

The experiences here brought to light ought to be sufficient to refute the assertion, so constantly and publicly repeated in interested quarters (by interested parties) the application of antitoxine is unattended with danger. On the contrary, it must be emphatically pointed out that there are few remedies out of the vast number known to medical science the use of which has so often led to disastrous results as this much vaunted antitoxine.

Referring once more to the case of Dr. Langerhans' little boy, who I will add a few words of my wife's, who, though not possessing the advantage of a university education like physicians and professors, nevertheless has plenty of common sense. She says: "One feels tempted to regard this case as a dispensation of Providence intended to show clearly to the believers in inoculation that these and all other inoculations are unnatural and presumptuous errors of the age, especially as Professor Langerhans has shortly before been questioned by a Government Commission as to his opinion of the value or non-value of vaccination, and had spoken warmly in favor of it. In consequence of this, compulsory vaccination, against which thousands of petitions had been for many years sent to the Reichstag, remained in force."

However much our over-clever atheists may make merry over the idea of messages from the above, the matter cannot be disposed of in this easy fashion. I would remind such people that there are more things in Heaven and Earth than are dreamed of in their philosophy.

— *Journal of Popular Hygiene*

During the last two decades an irresistible tendency has assert-ed itself in medical science, constantly to seek out new reme-dies, many of which enjoy only a brief existence and are again replaced by newer ones.

I would refer once more to the pernicious tuberculin injec-tions of Koch, which have resulted in a complete fiasco, in spite of the manner in which they were lauded to the skies and trumpeted forth to the world, but which continue to be employed by credulous fanatics, and are still puffed in medical periodicals.

What, however, is meant by the beginning of diphtheria? No other disease approaches so treacherously and breaks out so suddenly in its fully characteristic developed form, before the least suspicion has been entertained of the presence of the dan-ger.

Not only, however, has disease been known to result from the injections in question, but there have been cases in which their administration to healthy children for preventative purposes has been followed by death within a few days.

1906

Vegetarians Safe. Are They?
Ellen Goodell Smith, M.D.

Vaccination: Should It Be Enforced By Law
Montague R. Leverson, M.D., Ph.D., M.A.

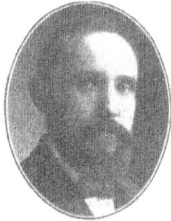

Although raw vegan diets are the rage today, a century ago George J. Drews, author of *Unfired Foods And Tropho-Therapy,* caused a surge of interest in a new wave of vegetarianism that endorsed raw and vegan foods. Benedict Lust began publishing a column dedicated exclusively to Apyrotrophy for his readers in 1913.

Vegetarians Safe. Are They?

by Ellen Goodell Smith, M.D., Amherst, Massachusetts

The Naturopath and Herald of Health, VII (4), 159-160. (1906)

An excellent article by A. S. Hunter in September *Naturopath* has keenly interested me. I quite agree with her that vaccination, the custom that causes as much disaster and death, should be abolished. But the fact that we are vegetarians does not protect us from all illness, neither renders us immune to all contagious diseases.

The larger and broader the outlook we bestow upon the world of so-called vegetarians, the more surprises will we meet, or such has been my experience. I once thought a vegetarian need not have any disease that was going the rounds of a community, and that rheumatism and gout were unknown. But later, when I found both to exist, it was quite a setback.

Now with regard to the smallpox, I can give you a personal experience. In my youth I was twice vaccinated, at intervals of a year or more, but it refused *to take*. In 1885, I became a hygienist and a vegetarian, and decided that I would not be vaccinated again, but would take my chances with smallpox if ever it came my way. In 1861, I graduated from Dr. Trall's college in New York. I had been appointed to make a presentation speech and read my thesis on graduation day. At that time the smallpox was in the city. I was not accustomed to having a cold, but for several days previous to that last day, I was contending with what was supposed to be a very severe cold in head and lungs. Although I had eaten but a trifle during the time, I could hardly speak and was flushed with fever, I determined that no one else should do my work and overcame all physical conditions, and performed my part as though in perfect health, making such a success of it that students said "you will be on the public platform someday".

The rosy cheeks and brilliant eyes doubtless impressed them favorably. I started for home the next day and spent four days in visits on the way. The morning after reaching home I noticed a few pimples on my face and thought I might be having a second edition of the measles. I had a three-mile sleigh ride that day and the next day visitors in the afternoon. Three more days passed, the eruption getting more profuse each day; then on a bright morning when I awoke there was the unmistakable smallpox. The family physician was summoned. He was well equipped with common sense and wisdom enough to let Nature have her way when she had such a fine start. "Yes," said he, "your first case is one of genuine smallpox in the distinct form. You could not have done better for yourself had you been aware of exposure to it. Your baths and packs and fasting could not have been improved and you do not need a drop of my medicine." A room upstairs was soon unfurnished except the bare necessities. I walked up to it and remained two weeks as a prisoner in a quarantined house, that the doctor said was so thoroughly sanitary no one would take the disease if they came in.

My mother had the care of me. She had not been vaccinated since a young child, and at this time there appeared a slight eruption on her hands.

All the treatment I had during those two weeks was plenty of fresh air, all the sun I could bear, and a tepid water-towel bath when I felt the need of it, my face protected with well-oiled linen cloths. I had none of the skin irritation as common with this disease.

At the doctor's next visit I would neither see nor speak. He said I must eat or I would go into a typhoid condition. My drinks were cold water and lemonade, but I ate nothing until hungry, and at his third and last visit, he remarked upon the wonderful recovery and said: "I begin to believe that medicine is hardly needed in acute sickness." My first meal was one tablespoonful of fine corn meal gruel, cooked three hours. The next day: two spoonfuls of the gruel. Then into fresh gruel a beaten egg was stirred and the ration increased as Nature dictated. Before I was out of bed, I detected the odor of a boiling dinner (minus flesh) and insisted upon having what the family had. The cook said "it will be the death of her", and under protest sent me a small plate of vegetables and bread, and I assure you that meal was a repast fit for the gods. Not one of the twenty or more people I met during the ten days after graduation, when I first detected the true disease, caught it, although terribly frightened if they had a headache.

One member of the family who had a deep vaccination scar an inch or more in diameter, and was much out of health at this time, looked into a room as I was passing through it, and in just two weeks he was in bed with the "confluent" form of smallpox. I assisted in nursing him, but his resisting power was so deficient, he passed away at the end of the week.

Until five years of age I was a healthy specimen of child life. I then had scarlet [fever], and became a target for experiment. The doctor told mother (after he had saved my life) that he "gave me calomel enough to kill thirteen men"! From that day until I was twenty-two years old I was a stranger to health, and never free from suffering in some form. I was exposed to all the ills of childhood, and during these years of lowered vitality, was living as others did and dosing with something constantly. But repeated exposure to mumps and measles never touched me.

Some months after my restoration to health in *water cure* (where I passed through a very serious crisis, a week's salvation included) I had the mumps, supposedly taken from another person.

The next year, while in college, I had a severe attack of measles, and several other students were thus afflicted. The next year the smallpox came my way, and in the way of some others of the class.

Can anyone explain why I had these diseases when in excellent health, with a faithful record of six years of vegetarian and hygienic living, and not have them with unhygienic living, flesh eating and drug taking were the rule.*

Please explain. We may have theories on various matters, but we are after truthful statements, that may be best learned from experience.

---

*As the writer reveals in the previous page, that she had received enough calomel to kill thirteen men speaks volumes. Calomel, a mercury derivative, is an extremely toxic drug that would have adverse effects for a lifetime. —*Ed.*

VACCINATION: SHOULD IT BE ENFORCED BY LAW?

by Montague R. Leverson, M.D., Ph.D., M.A., Brooklyn, New York
The Naturopath and Herald of Health, XII (7), 260-261. (1906)

That in any one of these United States it should be necessary to discuss the question as to whether any medical dogma or practice should be forced upon its citizens by law, illustrates in a striking degree how very little TRUE LIBERTY is understood or respected among us, and that while we are wont to mouth the Declaration of Independence on every recurring 4th of July, and even teach it in parrot-fashion to the children in our schools, the principles of that noble instrument are strangers, alike to the conscience and to the intellect of our people.

Even if vaccination were all that Jenner alleged it to be, it would yet be the most infamous of tyrannies to force it upon those, who or whose lawful guardians are unwilling to receive it. It is usurpation precisely like that of enforcing a religious dogma. It is no more within the proper function of law to enforce a surgical operation than a religious creed; to insist that a person shall be vaccinated than that he shall take the communion. To allege that a healthy person is, or can be a *focus of infection* is as absurdly false as to allege that free thinkers or persons who deny the thirty-nine articles of the English church are foci of moral pestilence; the right to kill, burn, maim or imprison the latter is just as well founded as is that to enforce conformity with medical dogma, and the legislatures which have yielded to solicitations of medical coteries, and endeavored to enforce a medical creed upon the people, deserve to be branded with shame as much as they would be if in obedience to a coterie of priests they had passed laws to inflict penalties upon those who might refuse to go to church on Sunday.

Such would be the case even if vaccination were what it was pretended to be when the thin edge of the wedge of persecution for medical heresy was first inserted into our laws.

The pretext that compulsory vaccination is necessary to protect the community from infection is logically absurd as well as a violation of the most sacred rights of family and personal liberty.

Vaccination either protects the vaccinated from smallpox or mitigates it when it is taken, or does neither. If it neither protects nor mitigates, then, it is useless and even its present warmest advocates must admit that it ought not to be enforced by law. If it only mitigates, then since the mildest attack is confessedly as contagious as the most severe, vaccinated smallpox is no less dangerous to the community than un-vaccinated, and there can be no pretext of public utility to warrant its imposition. But if it really does protect from smallpox, then those who are vaccinated are protected and can incur no danger from the unvaccinated; and here too there can be no pretext of the safety of the vaccinated to warrant compulsion upon those who do not believe in its efficacy.

Now while the foregoing considerations are sufficient to condemn the enforcement of this medical creed in the minds of all who are not wanting in even the smallest modicum of a sense of justice and of a love of equal rights, even if the operation were a harmless one and prophylactic against smallpox, the truth is that it is neither.

Of all the innumerable fads which have beset the medical profession, I know of none more hideous than this of *thrusting into the blood of healthy human beings the putrefying matter of a beast's disease!* And mark you well, gentlemen of the Medico-Legal Society,* there never has been the smallest evidence deserving the attention of a rational being, that vaccination does prevent or ever has prevented an attack of smallpox, *except by killing the patient before smallpox reached him.*

I know, gentlemen, this assertion will seem strange to you. I should have hesitated to believe it myself three years ago; like the rest of my professional brethren, I remained in a state of sleepy acquiescence until aroused to investigation, and then I soon found the truth.

One among the commonest errors of the vaccinationists has been that of magnifying the evils of smallpox. It is really marvelous how, in the face of facts, official doctors, aided by pseudo-historians, such as Macaulay, have succeeded in scaring the world about smallpox. Until the doctors got in their fads, first of inoculation and then of vaccination, smallpox was but one of the diseases which expressed the filth and gluttony of our ancestors, and was really one of the mildest of the lot.

----

* Brief extract from a paper read before the Medico-Legal Society.

Even if vaccination were all that Jenner alleged it to be, it would yet be the most infamous of tyrannies to force it upon those, who or whose lawful guardians are unwilling to receive it.

Vaccination either protects the vaccinated from smallpox or mitigates it when it is taken, or does neither.

Of all the innumerable fads which have beset the medical profession, I know of none more hideous than this of thrusting into the blood of healthy human beings the putrefying matter of a beast's disease!

Until the doctors got in their fads, first of inoculation and then of vaccination, smallpox was but one of the diseases which expressed the filth and gluttony of our ancestors, and was really one of the mildest of the lot.

1907

Vaccination Wholly Empirical
C. S. Carr, M.D.

Whooping Cough
Benedict Lust, N.D.

The Columbus Medical Journal was published by Dr. C. S. Carr who shared many of the same views as the Naturopaths.

Vaccination Wholly Empirical

by C. S. Carr, M.D., Columbus, Ohio

The Naturopath and Herald of Health, XIII (7), 220-222. (1907)

I have for many years been oppos- ing vaccination and inoculation of all sorts for the cure of disease. Twenty-five years ago I was connected with a bacte- riological laboratory and was therefore acquainted with this science in its earliest infancy. At that time I made myself rea- sonably certain that the production of an artificial immunity from any disease was a practical impossibility, and would at least be always attended with great uncertainty and risk.

But since that time many things have happened. I have been busily engaged with other matters and must confess that I have not watched the progress made by

C. S. Carr, M.D.

the science of bacteriology very closely. To be sure, I have read the articles that occur in the leading medical journals, and have a cursory knowledge of what has been going on. But I did not pretend to be a strict student of the science of bacteriology for at least fifteen years.

Yet I have continued my opposition to the whole thing on general principles, believing that if any new or especially convincing evidence had arisen since my connection with that sort of work I should have learned of it.

In order to make quite sure that my opposition to vaccination had not been too sweeping or uncompromising, I began several months ago to look about me as to the best authority upon the recent developments on this subject, promising myself that I should read some good, solid work on the subject carefully, from end to end.

After making some inquiries from men who are posted on the litera- ture of this subject, I fixed upon the book entitled *Immunity in Infective Diseases*, by Elie Metchnikoff, foreign member of the Royal Society of London, professor at the Pasteur Institute, Paris. This book was translat- ed from the French by Francis G. Binnie, of the Pathological Department of the University of Cambridge, and was issued in 1905.

Perhaps no other book can lay claim to greater authority on the sub- ject and surely no book of so great worth has been issued later. Any one reading this book may feel practically certain that he is reading the

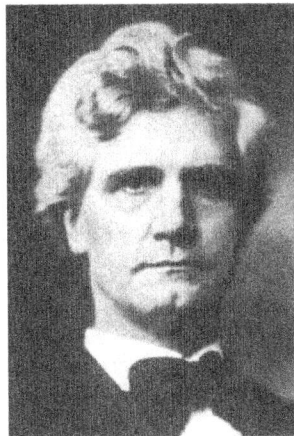

last word which the advocates of artificial immunity have to say upon the subject.

But I shall not have the space to dwell on many details, however interesting they are. The purpose for which I read the book was mainly to discover what, if any, support the practice of vaccination has found in these laboratory researches. Can the author of the book which I am reviewing throw any light on the practice of cowpox vaccination to prevent smallpox?

He does not attempt to make any such claim. He squarely confesses that he knows nothing whatever about smallpox. Neither he nor any of his colleagues have been able to discover the micro-organism of cowpox. In other words, they do not know what smallpox is, and they do not know what vaccine virus is. After all this flurry and flutter, expense and array of laboratory apparatus, these savants are obliged to confess that they have been able to do nothing to sustain the promoters of vaccination. Dr. Metchnikoff, like all the rest of us, was obliged to go back to one Jenner, of London, and his supposed discovery of cowpox.

This Jenner was a London barber, who lived at the time when everybody was inoculated with smallpox virus. It was deemed necessary, in those days, that everyone should have smallpox who could possibly be made to take it. Thus it was that instead of trying to prevent the people from getting smallpox, instead of keeping the people who were afflicted with smallpox separate from those who had not taken it, they did everything they could possibly invent to produce smallpox. It was in those days that Jenner lived. It was in those days that every third person met on the streets of London was pitted on face and hands with the scars of smallpox. The wonder is that any one escaped at all.

It was in those days that Jenner made the astounding discovery that the pastoral people of Scotland did not have smallpox as much as the people in pestiferous London. He is reported to have gone to Scotland to study into the reason why. He found them milking diseased cows; cows whose udders and teats were covered with sores exuding serum.

Filled with the notion that everybody must be inoculated with something or other, Jenner imagined that the serum exuding from the cows' teats inoculated the milkers, which fortified them against smallpox. Therefore he thought he would try some of the stuff on other people. Having collected an abundance of the cow serum, he began to vaccinate people, instead of inoculating them with the smallpox.

This, of course, led to good results. Having ceased peddling smallpox and begun in its stead to peddle another animal poison not quite so vicious, a great gain was experienced.

On this experience depends the whole theory of smallpox vaccination, and not one scintilla of scientific truth has been added to the above inference. Everybody is in the dark concerning the nature of smallpox, and in gross darkness concerning the nature of vaccine virus.

In times past I have offered again and again $50 to any physician who would tell me what vaccine virus is. I had no idea, however, that the task was such an impossible one. I really supposed that there were manufacturers of vaccine virus, or perhaps laboratory experts, who could tell me what vaccine virus was. But, according to this book, no one knows, not even the manufacturer.

All the doctor knows about vaccine virus is how to make the stuff. He takes a healthy heifer, shaves the hair off the lower part of the belly, and then punctures into the flesh of the heifer some of the serum which he has obtained from other sores made in the same way. This serum poisons the system of the heifer, causing her belly to break out with large sores containing quantities of serum.

This serum is carefully extracted from the sores and put into glass tubes and conveyed through the trade to the physician, who punctures it into the flesh of the people.

The manufacturer does not know what this virus is. He simply knows how to make it. He does not know whether it contains micro-organisms of a specific character or not. He has never seen such organisms. He has never seen anyone else who has seen them. He rests his whole case on statistics.

The doctors, who take this vaccine virus and puncture it into the flesh of the people, say that it protects them from smallpox. Health Boards repeat this assertion, and thus it is that those people only who are interested in the spread of vaccination are the witnesses of its efficacy.

It is certainly pitiful that in the midst of such uncertainty the scientific investigator cannot come to our rescue one way or the other. I had hoped that in reading this book I should get some glimpse of scientific authority for the practice of vaccination. I really hoped that I had overlooked something, and that I was about to discover something that would place me in the rank and file of doctors who believe in vaccination. It is much more pleasant to belong to the comfortable majority than to the despised minority. It is much easier to be in the swim, float down the stream, than to be constantly beating against the current in an effort to go in a contrary direction. Therefore, I had secretly wished that I should discover something among the annals of the various bacteriological laboratories that would shed one ray of light on the practice of vaccination.

But Dr. Metchnikoff, after all his array of sagacity, patience, skill and scientific information, when he reaches the subject of vaccination, lays down all his paraphernalia of science, turns his back on his laboratory, and proceeds to quote the fables of smallpox statistics. He did not gather any statistics himself. He simply took those gathered by other people.

I wish Dr. Metchnikoff could realize how these statistics are gathered, and what a farce the whole thing is.

In this city, several years ago, there was an epidemic of smallpox, so called. Many people were vaccinated. In the reports kept by the Health Boards over one hundred people who had this so-called smallpox were classed as "never vaccinated".

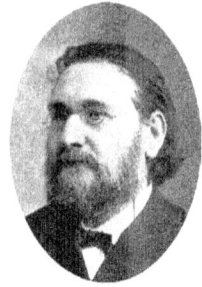

Elie Metchnikoff

Anxious to know the truth of the matter, I obtained a list of those people that were alleged to have never been vaccinated, and upon investigation, I found, to my astonishment that the great majority of them had been vaccinated.

Instead of apologizing for this discrepancy, the principle of it was defended. It was frankly stated by the health officer in charge that if these people had been successfully vaccinated, they would not have had smallpox. Therefore, he felt entirely justified in classifying them as never vaccinated.

This exactly illustrates how smallpox statistics are gathered, and it is to such trash as this that the renowned Dr. Metchnikoff subscribes his name when he stoops to quote statistics as a basis for his belief in vaccination.

Not a single thing has been discovered in the laboratory, up to date, that justifies the use of vaccine virus to prevent smallpox. Not a single thing has been discovered in the laboratory to justify the use of anti-diphtheritic toxine to prevent diphtheria. Not a single thing. The whole thing is empirical, based on statistics. Not a single thing has been discovered in the laboratory to furnish any scientific basis for the use of serums to prevent tetanus. Its use is wholly empirical.

The apparatus proof of the usefulness of these treatments is explained by the peculiar nature of the disease involved.

A thousand cases of sore throat occur where one proves to be diphtheria. And it is in these thousand cases of innocent sore throats that the statistician finds his material to prove the efficacy of anti-diphtheritic toxine.

A hundred people are injured in such a way as might produce tetanus, and yet not have tetanus. The diseased people who escape by natural immunity have furnished the supposition that something has been done to prevent tetanus.

The same may be said of rabies. The institutes where patients are treated who have been bitten by dogs suspected to be mad are supported by the peculiar uncertainty that attends this terrible malady. In the first place, it is very uncertain whether any supposed mad dog is really afflicted with rabies. But even when this detail has been made certain it is again very uncertain whether the person bitten by such a dog will acquire rabies. It is upon these uncertainties that institutions to prevent rabies find their support.

It is with regret that I turn from this elaborate attempt to uphold the modern practice of vaccines and antitoxines and inoculations. It is with regret that I turn from this book without having gained a particle of confidence in the desperate effort now being made by the medical profession to produce artificial immunity against disease.

It may be that sometime in the future the laboratory will be whipped into line and made to render some support to the practice of vaccinations and inoculations, but up to date its voice is silent. After all his assertions and speculations, the vaccinating physician has received no support from that source, and the whole trend of bacteriological science seems to me to be in the opposite direction.

After carefully reading the latest word that bacteriology has to say, I find that the laboratory lends little if any support to the practice of vaccination, inoculation and the use of serums and antitoxines. Whenever these practices are referred to, the author deals with them kindly, but presents no evidence, further than the statistics furnished by those who practice them. So far as the human family is concerned, acquired immunity from disease rests wholly on empirical grounds, and finds little or no support from the investigations of the laboratory. Natural immunity has been uncovered with wonderful accuracy and entrancing detail by the bacteriologist, but up to date this indefatigable worker has not been able to offer any practical assistance to that class of doctors who practice the arts of artificial immunity.

> *Thus it was that instead of trying to prevent the people from getting smallpox, instead of keeping the people who were afflicted with smallpox separate from those who had not taken it, they did everything they could possibly invent to produce smallpox.*
>
> *This exactly illustrates how smallpox statistics are gathered, and it is to such trash as this that the renowned Dr. Metchnikoff subscribes his name when he stoops to quote statistics as a basis for his belief in vaccination.*
>
> *Not a single thing has been discovered in the laboratory to justify the use of anti-diphtheritic toxine to prevent diphtheria. Not a single thing. The whole thing is empirical, based on statistics.*

The Whooping Cough

by Benedict Lust, N. D.

The Naturopath and Herald of Health, VIII (12), 355-356. (1907)

A bugbear for the mother, a torture for the little ones is the horrid whooping cough which demands its victims almost at all seasons of the year. Up to this time opinions differed about its cause: some authorities supposed it to be a catarrh of the mucous membrane of the larynx and the bronchi and stated that the catarrhal secretion irritates the larynx and the bronchial nerves and thus causes the violent spasmodic coughs. Through the *Deutsche med. Wochenschriit* we learn that two professors in Koenigsberg, Messrs. E. Czaplewski, M.D., and P. Hensel, M.D., have succeeded in discovering the real exciters of the whooping cough in small bacteria which they found in the sputum.

The bacilli are there and that they can be very viscous is proven by the fact, that Dr. Czaplewski while experimenting was not only seized by a violent coughing fit, but also fell sick.

Children between three and ten years are mostly seized by the whooping cough in spring, fall and winter. It lasts, though not without interruption, from six to ten weeks; it then stops for a time and appears again until the whole process is run off, if not stopped by some remedy.

The whooping cough begins with long-drawn whistling and panting; then follows violent spasmodic coughing, agitating the whole body, interrupted by a whistling, painful respiration until, finally, a tough, gluey transparent phlegm will be thrown out. This attack is preceded by restlessness and anxiety; the little patient complains of scratching and tickling in the throat and tries to suppress the outbreak. During this coughing the patient becomes blue, even blue-black in the face; the eye-balls protrude and the poor sufferer is the very personification of anxiety and horror— for the tender-hearted mother a most painful sight. The carbonic acid in the blood, having been accumulated, stops the respiration and causes the discoloration, while the violent agitation of the diaphragm will bring on vomiting, involuntary secretion of the urine and excrements; often blood will rush out the ear and nose; though exciting these phenomena for the poor mother may be, they do not imply any danger for the child.

The attack over, the child is greatly exhausted and tired; it will complain of pains in the stomach and now and again will cry—but that is passing; soon [the child] will be composed.

There are three stages in pronounced whooping cough. In the first stage the children are photophobic; they begin to cough and have fever—this is the moment the mother has to stop its further development. The second stage is the real attack; the third stage is the throwing out of the tough cathartic phlegm. By and bye, these attacks diminish until they altogether cease.

Taken all in all, the whooping cough belongs to the non-malignant disease; it becomes only dangerous if another sickness appears. Now it is the mother's duty to be most careful; lest inguinal hernia, umbilical hernia, pneumonia, emphysema of the lungs, dyspnoea appear by which the breaking out of the sickness will be impeded.

The treatment of this sickness by the Allopaths, as they themselves will frankly admit, is in no ways satisfactory. Their only remedies are the following ones: belladonna, hydrocyanic acid, inhalations of the nitrate of silver and bromide of potash, infections of morphia and so forth. Such treatment is real nonsense and is not only without any affect at all, but often enough accompanied by baneful consequences.

Kneipp's treatment, on the contrary, is very simple and always successful. As soon as the first symptoms, as mentioned above appear, as photophobia, fever, coughing, the mother has to put a shirt, dipped in a decoction of hayflower, on the child, wrap it* airtight into a woolen blanket and let it rest for an hour; then she gives the child a cold wash and puts him/her to bed. As long as the child's body is warm, these washes have to be repeated two or three times during the day. If the whooping cough is fully developed, the child gets three times a day a thyme-bath at 98° F/37° C, in which it remains submerged to the throat for ten or twelve minutes. On taking the child out it has to be washed quickly with cold water at 70° F/21° C lightly wrapped up and put to bed. During the day light warm linen handkerchiefs dipped in hot water and covered with flannel, have to be put on the sufferer's breast for ten or fifteen minutes; plus, cold washes, three times a day, will be of great benefit. If the cough is spasmodic, a thorough wash, and wrapping up in a shawl, will bring relief. As well, the child has to be given warm fennel or silverweed tea and twice a day from 6 to 9 drops of fennel oil. As soon as the child begins to recover, usually after the first day fewer applications have to be made.

It is a matter of course that the food has to be light and not stimulating and care has to be taken that the child does not catch cold. In order to prevent a hernia, a body-belt of stiff linen has to be put around the child; the air in the room has to be perfectly pure and not too dry. During a coughing attack the child's head has to be softly pillowed; the best is to put the child to bed and give the child fennel tea.

Such a patient has to be kept apart from other children, the whooping cough being contagious. The sputum has to be burned. By this kind of treatment the whooping cough can be overcome within a week.

---

*Benedict Lust's use of the pronoun 'it' to refer to a child is reflective of how children were called a century ago. —Ed.

Kneipp's treatment, on the contrary, is very simple and always successful. As soon as the first symptoms, as mentioned above appear, as photophobia, fever, coughing, the mother has to put a shirt, dipped in a decoction of hayflower, on the child, wrap it airtight into a woolen blanket and let it rest for an hour; then she gives the child a cold wash and puts him/her to bed.

If the whooping cough is fully developed, the child gets three times a day a thyme-bath at 98° F/37° C, in which [the child] remains submerged to the throat for ten or twelve minutes. On taking the child out it has to be washed quickly with cold water at 70° F/21° C lightly wrapped up and put to bed.

In order to prevent a hernia, a body-belt of stiff linen has to be put around the child; the air in the room has to be perfectly pure and not too dry.

_1908_

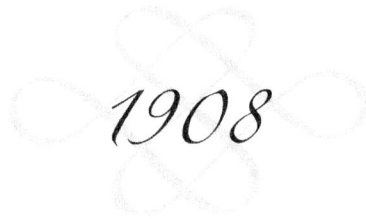

Anti-Compulsory Vaccination
Walter E. Elfrink, M.D.

This ad appeared in 1905 in *The Naturopath and Herald of Health*. The interest in hygienic measures to achieve health standards was top of mind for the early Naturopaths.

Anti-Compulsory Vaccination

by Walter E. Elfrink

The Naturopath and Herald of Health, XI (3), 95. (1908)

Chicago, Dec. 24, 1907
Dr. Benedict Lust,
124 E. 59th St., New York.

My Dear Doctor,

I am sure that you will be interested in the anti-vaccination fight which we are making here in Chicago. This movement grew out of the expulsion of Louise Jenkins from the public schools because she was not vaccinated in accordance with the ideas of the medical inspector. Mr. Jenkins, her father, does not believe in vaccination, and has refused to have the operation performed. The result is that his little girl is out of school and is being educated at home.

An application has been made in the courts for a *writ of mandamus* to compel her admission into the schools. This we regard as something of a test case and we are confident that we will win.

We also have another case in court in which we are asking for damages because of the forcible expulsion from the schools of an unvaccinated child. We expect both of these cases to come up for trial very soon.

We are distributing thousands of circulars and collecting the names of hundreds of people who are opposed to vaccination. Although this work has only been in existence about six weeks we already have over one thousand names on our list.

The authorities have been very arrogant. One mother came to us with her little boy, who had been vaccinated four times, but as he was strong and healthy it would not take, consequently the doctor said that he must stay at home and be re-vaccinated until it would take. Think of putting this vile poison into a healthy body until its resistance is broken down to a point where this kind of infection is possible.

In another case a mother reported that although both of her children had had smallpox, yet they were refused admission into schools without vaccination.

Another mother reported that her little child in the kindergarten department had been vaccinated without even consulting her.

The Health Department refuses to accept the certificates of physicians in good standing, and insists that every pupil must exhibit a typical scar not smaller than a ten-cent piece before he can be admitted to the schools. They insist that they will push this thing and enforce it if it requires a dozen operations on each child.

Dr. WALTER E. ELFRINK,

Osteopathic Physician,

Instructor in Chemistry, Dietetics and Hydrotherapy,
in the American College of Osteopathy,
Medicine and Surgery.

OFFICE: RESIDENCE:
Suite 507 Burton Building   6056 Monroe Avenue,
39 State Street, Chicago,   Corner 61st Street.
9 A. M. to 12 M.   Tues. Thur. Sat. 3 to 6 P. M.
Telephone, Central 3670.   Tel. HydePark 5784

The authorities have been very discourteous to practically all who have protested against their tyrannical conduct.

This society was organized on a permanent basis; has been incorporated and will fight this thing, if necessary, in the courts and legislature, and by educating the people to the facts in the case until such time as our rights are established.

The Supreme Court of this State has decided several times that compulsory vaccination is not warranted by the State laws, but in the city of Chicago, under cover of an ordinance which, with its drastic provisions, would do credit to the fourteenth century, they have submitted the people of Chicago to tyrannous acts and insulting treatment in thousands of instances. We feel that you, as an editor of a liberal health magazine, could do much to help us, and we shall be glad if you will give this work as much publicity as your interest and space will permit.

With best wishes, I am yours fraternally,
Walter E. Elfrink, Secretary.

One mother came to us with her little boy, who had been vaccinated four times, but as he was strong and healthy it would not take, consequently the doctor said that he must stay at home and be re-vaccinated until it would take. Think of putting this vile poison into a healthy body until its resistance is broken down to a point where this kind of infection is possible.

The Health Department refuses to accept the certificates of physicians in good standing, and insists that every pupil must exhibit a typical scar not smaller than a ten-cent piece before he can be admitted to the schools.

This society was organized on a permanent basis; has been incorporated and will fight this thing, if necessary, in the courts and legislature, and by educating the people to the facts in the case until such time as our rights are established.

1909

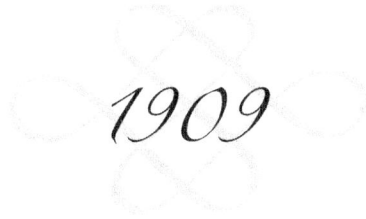

A System Of Autocracies
J. T. Robinson, M.D.

The Plague
Hereward Carrington

Brief, Regarding Vaccination
William D. Gentry, M.D.

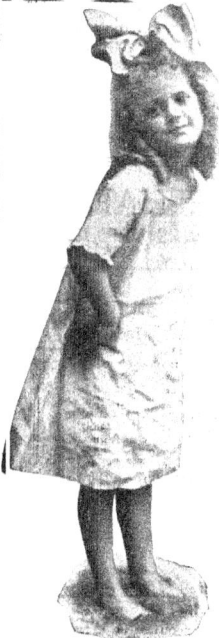

The issue of compulsory vaccination ignited public outrage and consequently prompted the organization of the International Health Society with a mandate to put an end to medical tyranny. The early Naturopaths recognized the importance of medical freedom and believed ardently that every American citizen had the right to choose their doctor and the kind of medicine to ail their ills.

A System Of Autocracies

by J. T. Robinson, M.D.

The Naturopath and Herald of Health, XIV (2), 116-120. (1909)

The greatest evil that confronts the American people today is the monopoly evil. We hear much of the Standard Oil trust, the political trust, but the worst that was ever inaugurated in this country or in the old world is the trust upon human life. There is a trust upon the medical colleges. There is a trust upon the practice of medicine; the practitioner who does not hold credentials from one of the trust or monopoly colleges is not allowed to practice medicine or heal the sick; it is no longer a question of ability to relieve suffering humanity, but a question of authority and prestige. It should ever be our wish and most ardent desire to know all that is worth to be known. It should not be a question of method or system as the regulars would have us believe, but the ability to heal the sick. The great trust and monster evil now at work organizing every State of the Union and employing lobbyists in every legislature to pass selfish monopolistic medical bills is better known as the American Medical Association.

The purpose of this association is to control or monopolize the healing art in every State of our Union. These medical trust pirates pretend that their object is to protect the people against the imposition of quacks and impostors, judging from the size of the medical fees and the wholesale butcheries in our hospitals infirmaries, the people will not appreciate such protection. These would-be humanitarians are flattering the public on the one hand and picking their pockets on the other hand. They are invading the homes and inserting poison virus into the bodies of children which in many instances produces death. They are enforcing surgical operations against the consent of parents and friends; nine times out of ten these operations prove fatal; they are cultivating a practice and bringing on a mania for butchery in so-called appendicitis. The future historian will record thousands and millions of butcheries and murders by the members of the American Medical Association. Why not pass a law prohibiting anyone from practicing who injures his patient; a law that allows everybody to practice so long as they do no harm.

The members of this medical trust make it a crime for irregulars to cure patients and a virtue for the regulars to poison and kill. The old regular Allopath would rather see death on the pale horse and pagan Rome with a red sword than to see a just law passed which provides that every doctor shall be punished who injures his patients or administers poison to the sick. When a father has a son and he does not know what to make of him, he has not piety enough to make a preacher, intelligence enough to make him a lawyer, or industry or ingenuity enough to make a mechanic or farmer, he makes an allopathic or regular doctor. We have a great many of these who are doctors only in name. These are the doctors who are asking for medical laws to protect them against the real, genuine physician who is in possession of too much gray matter for them; they cannot stand the competition of quacks and impostors. After a four-year's course in the monopoly college of medical wisdom and learning, they begin to bawl for protection against men who never saw one of these colleges; these medical imbeciles continue to bawl for State and National medical poorhouses.

The brainy men of the medical art have never asked for medical laws, neither will they accept a position on one of the Board of Health or examining boards. It is always the small incompetent fellow who wants a fee and political position to bring him into notice; they are the doctors who cannot stand on their own merits, and like John Bunyan's tub they should be rolled down the hill. It is a confession of incompetency and weakness to ask for medical laws. Dr. Senn, who is acknowledged to be one of the most noted surgeons in the United States, gives a fearful statement of affairs. He states that victims by the thousands from the flower of American womanhood are falling thick and fast around us, and yet we have called attention to a small portion of the murderous work being done by the graduates of monopoly medical colleges whose infamous quackery is only possible because the American Medical Association, medical monopoly colleges and the various so-called State Boards of Health, have by their united efforts smuggled the most infamous laws through the legislatures of nearly all the States.

It is pretended that the object of said laws is to protect the people. Just how the people are protected can be seen by the very nature of these medical trust laws. The people are not only unprotected, but they are deprived of their most sacred rights. So cunningly have the word combinations of laws we have referred to been in some States, that they succeed in prosecuting, fining and imprisoning those who save life, whereas [the medical doctors] only make the patient worse. Think of it, how common highway robbers and murderers are treated, the jails and penitentiaries await them; but this combination composed of allopathic medical college professors, State Boards of Health, and members of the American Medical Association, can meet and calmly discuss such outrages but do little or nothing to terminate them and actually form insurance companies to protect these infamous murderers who perform these outrageous and death-producing operations. Should we succeed in helping to instruct and arouse the public to the great danger of this legalized robbery and death dealing practice we will be well paid.

In 1836 the American people became so disgusted with medical laws that they went to the ballot box and voted every medical law out of existence, from that time until after the Civil War there was not a monopoly medical law on the statutes in any of the States of the Union.* More advance and real progress were made during that period than was ever made before or since that period of time.

Remember, that members of the medical trusts have ever fought medical progress; all the great discoveries in the art have been made by those on the outside of this so-called profession. We condemn a system that enables one set of men to enslave another set of men; we condemn a system whose most prominent effect is to create more reverence for authority than for truth. We condemn the spirit which in effect binds men to a blind, unreasoning routine practice and forbids advance in intelligent thought. We condemn a system which makes medical heterodoxy a social crime; we condemn a system which is the principal hindrance to the development of the noblest, most humane, most useful of all arts.

We denounce this heterogeneous combination of trust, the steel trust, the Standard Oil trust, the railroad trust, the commercial trust, the medical college trust, the doctors' trust, the drug trust, the trust upon all the necessaries of life, the trust upon human life itself formed by this infamous system of autocracies—a wheel within a wheel, a system within a system—that knows no bounds, that knows no mercy, that is as heartless as a hyena, who rapacious maws swallow all the wealth of this world and is deaf to the cries of orphans, and sees not the tears of widows and feels no sympathy for the sick distressed. We condemn this gigantic system of autocratic tyrants as the most diabolical and villainous in all the annals of history. It is on behalf of the weak, the defenseless, the distressed and the outraged people of the United States of America that we make this appeal and it is to you the noble souls who are in the everlasting struggle of the human race for liberty, justice and life that we step in the fore front of the battle without rest or furlough in the most deadly conflict that has ever been recorded upon all the blood-stained pages of history, liberty, home and heavens.

The most priceless jewels in the diadem of honor, the most exacting rulers that beguile the brain and soul of man. She, the proud bird of freedom, the American eagle, will have nothing of him who will not give her all. She knows that the pretended love of her enemy serves but to betray. But when once the fierce heat of her quenchless, lustrous eyes has burned into the victim's heart, he will know no other smile but hers. Liberty! Float not from us in the far horizon, but come and take up thy abode in our hearts, in our homes, and perch up on the dome of our capitol. Liberty! Let us have none but the great, devoted and glorious souls

---

*A meeting held in Philadelphia in 1847 and attended by 200 medical doctors inaugurated the American Medical Association.

who have promises and boundless hopes and infinite charms that lures these victims over the hard and stormy ways of life. We have a desperate enemy to fight, and enemy that will not meet us in the open and give steel for steel—an enemy who is controlling Congress, the Senate, the Supreme Court, the legislatures, the church, the press and the entire world.

To the politico-medical, commercial oligarchy, and system within a system of autocracies, we ask you, did you ever place your important skillful combination outside the field of contest long enough to see what nature can do and is doing? Do you fully understand that your feeble efforts are simply what nature has done thousands of times before medical Solomons came into existence? Did you ever watch nature perform an amputation, a version, plane off a mass of granulations, tie off a tumor, drain a lung abscess, or a hopeless case of appendicitis? She may bring safety after all hope has been abandoned; nevertheless you political medical sharks get the credit of cures. Do you realize that the wild, false theories of bugology and the mania for surgical operations constitute a pathway which leads to an ignominious medical oblivion? Are you so blinded in your own conceit that the medical laws for which you are bawling is simply a confession of your weakness? It is the last struggle for existence. God pity the medical imbeciles and commercial pirates who unite their forces to rob and murder the American people.

Twenty-five years ago the most infamous trust that ever disgraced a civilized people was organized; it originated among physicians known as Allopaths or Regulars. These doctors are easily recognized, as they are the most frequently seen as they are—the self-appointed leaders of this medical trust and have absorbed a large number of homeopathic and eclectic physicians on condition that they have agreed to become regulars. In the District of Columbia this medical trust has obtained the passage of laws through Congress which absolutely prohibit any person from practicing medicine or healing the sick who is not a member of this medical trust. The doctor must also be a graduate of one of the medical trust colleges. They have established a scale of fees, none may charge less, but may charge as much more as each individual member may desire, and if any of the poor people, employing a member of the trust, are unable to pay the enormous fees they are put upon what is termed a black list, and thereafter no member will treat such a family.

The members of this medical trust can trace their origin to the dark ages and with but little improvement since the year A.D. 425, when the world lost its true Christianity and confidence in the All Mighty. Sickness was at a time previous to the above date considered a disgrace because of its origin in ignorance. No longer than one hundred and fifty years ago the blood of black cats and white puppies, earthworms, snakes, toads, lice, burnt owl feathers, powdered human skulls, priest-craft, the spittle of a king and many other disgusting things too numerous to mention were used to cure the sick. How much better is it today? Let us see. Vaccination, the great smallpox cure and preventive is nothing but rotten, diseased pus taken from an ulcer from the body of a cow or calf. Rotten, stinking pus, the vilest poison on earth, from a diseased animal that lives only a few years; this poison is injected into the bodies of children who should live to the age of one hundred years. Antitoxine is rotten, poisoned pus from diseased horses. This vile stuff is injected into little children to cure diphtheria. Tuberculin is a rotten poison pus taken from a consumptive cow. This is the great cure for consumption. This is what the members of the medical trust term the science of medicine.

The history of vaccination has been appalling. The inventor, Jenner, was considered a quack and imposter, but after he had succeeded in fooling the King of England out of a fortune, he got a compulsory vaccination law passed. The doctors saw they had a bonanza, and every one of them, old sore heads, were ready to carry Jenner on their backs. The arm to arm vaccination was in practice for fifty years, and then the parliament of England abolished it, making it a crime to inject this syphilitic poison into healthy bodies. During the fifty years almost the entire white race was poisoned with syphilis (see *Encyclopedia Britannica*). Then comes the cow pock vaccination in its place. We have had fifty years more of syphilis and a few years ago a few members of this great medical octopus met and decided that consumption came from the cow and now we have no more vaccination from the cow; but they use calves as calves are not cows. So now we get the virus of cow pox from the sucking calf, preserve it in glycerine. The name of the vaccine is glycerinated calf lymph; it sounds very scientific you know. Now they wish to impose this same old, rotten pus in a new dress on the people fifty years more, but they can't do it unless they get odious laws to protect them. Vaccination killed more American soldiers in the late Spanish American War than the bullet and all other causes combined.

There is a drug trust in the United States with over forty million invested, with a membership of over sixty-five thousand—the American Medical Association.* These two terrible curses are deceiving and robbing the people in every hand. They have kept the fire of smallpox and syphilis burning for more than one hundred years; some patient who has been vaccinated several times starts an epidemic of smallpox, measles, syphilis, mumps, la grippe and many other diseases, which keeps the medical trust doctors at work night and day until another epidemic is worked up. Should they find the practice running short it is an easy matter to

---

*In 2015, the number of medical practitioners in USA is approaching one million doctors and in addition 170,000 Osteopaths and over 190,000 Nurse Practitioners. —*Ed.*

produce another scare by administering iodide of potassium and mercury for a short time, which will produce a rash all over the body that makes a doubtful case of smallpox. Then another vaccination epidemic and the same thing over and over from Jenner's time to the present. When the people absolutely refuse to have their children poisoned with this rotten pus, one-half of all human ailments will disappear from the earth. They are becoming aroused everywhere and are no longer deceived by the medical trust who claim that their infamous medical laws are to protect the dear people.

The old regular medical trust pirates have stolen everything they failed to throttle in way of discoveries in the healing art. Now they are trying to steal Osteopathy and Christian Science, calling one only massage and the other simply suggestion. In order to find out what is the matter with them, the Allopath doctor feels every inch of the body of this patient; he must go through an indelicate examination with the ladies; it is immodest, indecent, uncalled for, a base shame, infamous, diabolical and contemptible practice that should be condemned by all decent people. The medical men as a rule have become so corrupt, have proven themselves so dishonest, so unreliable, their treatment of the sick so unsuccessful, it has placed the art in disrepute to such an extent that the title of doctor has become a stench in the nostrils of decent, intelligent people. When we go upon the tower of observation and gaze upon the great battlefield of medical practice, medical butchery miscalled surgical operations, when we count the millions of mutilated and bleeding human forms we exclaim with emotion too high for utterance; this is by awful odds the horror of the world.

The words of these members of corporations and trusts are accepted as law—law greater than any contained in the statutes of any of the States of the Union. The well-paid leaders are the potentates of the nation. This insidious influence invades the sacred precincts of hallowed homes, and is wafting its deadly breath and malicious thought against all intelligent, decent people while cravenly and cowardly masquerading under the cloak of deception and claiming to protect the people. There are over one hundred and fifty thousand unfortunate insane people in the United States in the many asylums who are being treated the same old way that was in use two thousand years ago, yet these old, ignorant regulars or Allopaths have the cheek and unmitigated gall to ask for a monopoly on their old, mossback methods. There is no law to force the unfortunate insane to be associated in the same building and same wards which any intelligent person knows is injurious and detrimental in many ways. These patients should be separated and kept at home as much as possible.

We could multiply instances of nations that have been overwhelmed with bitter disaster through the vicious practices and diabolism of the political and medical leaders. And Babylon, the glory of kingdoms, the beauty of the Chaldees' Excellency, shall be as when God overthrew Sodom and Gomorrah. It shall never be inhabited, neither shall it be dwelt in from generation to generation; neither shall Arabian pitch there; neither shall shepherds make their fold there, but wild beasts of the desert shall lie there, and there houses shall be full of doleful creatures; and owls shall dwell there and satyrs shall dance there. And wild beasts of the island shall cry in their desolate houses, and dragons in their pleasant palaces. How to avoid or overcome this strange curse, which is a form of black magic and travels in vibrating waves and injects its mental poison in the mentality of innocent people? We are in possession of the key to this vibrating treatment, which has proven itself to be an absolute defense against the wiles of black magic, no matter what name whether malicious magnetism or mental malpractice or any evil or impure thought, it is a barrier strong and effective.

J. T. Robinson, M.D., specialist in cancer and chronic disease. San Antonia, Texas

The purpose of this association is to control or monopolize the healing art in every State of our Union. These medical trust pirates pretend that their object is to protect the people against the imposition of quacks and impostors, judging from the size of the medical fees and the wholesale butcheries in our hospitals infirmaries, the people will not appreciate such protection.

Antitoxine is rotten, poisoned pus from diseased horses. This vile stuff is injected into little children to cure diphtheria. Tuberculin is a rotten poison pus taken from a consumptive cow. This is the great cure for consumption. This is what the members of the medical trust term the science of medicine.

We have had fifty years more of syphilis and a few years ago a few members of this great medical octopus met and decided that consumption came from the cow and now we have no more vaccination from the cow; but they use calves as calves are not cows.

THE PLAGUE

by Hereward Carrington*

The Naturopath and Herald of Health, XIV (6), 353-358. (1909)

CONSIDERATIONS ON THAT MOST FATAL AND LITTLE KNOWN DISEASE

From the earliest times there seems to have been constantly present, in one part of the world or another, diseases of a more or less malignant type— prominent among which is one that has come down to us under the term **plague**. Biblical accounts of such visitations are numerous, and Josephus, in his *Antiquities of the Jews*, refers to certain diseases and symptoms which seem to indicate that the scourge was none other than the plague of modern times. "Emerods of the secret parts" are probably equivalent to our inguinal buboes; vomiting is mentioned, also hemorrhages; "they died of the dysentery and flux". The connection of rats with the more ancient disease is a suggestive fact, when we remember that they have been found to be great spreaders of the disease, when the causes have been closely studied.

VITALITY, FASTING
AND
NUTRITION

A PHYSIOLOGICAL STUDY OF THE CURATIVE
POWER OF FASTING, TOGETHER WITH A
NEW THEORY OF THE RELATION OF
FOOD TO HUMAN VITALITY

BY

HEREWARD CARRINGTON
Member of the Council of the American Institute for Scientific Research;
Member of the Society for Psychical Research, London; Author
of "The Physical Phenomena of Spiritualism," etc.

NEW YORK
REBMAN COMPANY
1123 BROADWAY

The terrible epidemics of the Middle Ages are probably familiar to all. Prominent among these is the Black Death of 14th century—perhaps the most fatal epidemic on record, but which is held by some writers to have been a different disease from the plague of our time. It seems improbable that this should be so, but, in the absence of fuller knowledge, this point is likely to remain an unsettled one—as our knowledge of the old epidemics is very incomplete and uncertain. There are certain marks of difference between the old and the newer diseases; but there are also many points of agreement. The blue and purple spots, so frequently mentioned by the old writers, as appearing suddenly in various parts of the body, is comparatively rare phenomenon now-a-days, but hemorrhages, bleeding from the nose, vomiting, spitting of blood, weakness and malaise are all characteristic symptoms of the modern disease. The offensive breath indi-

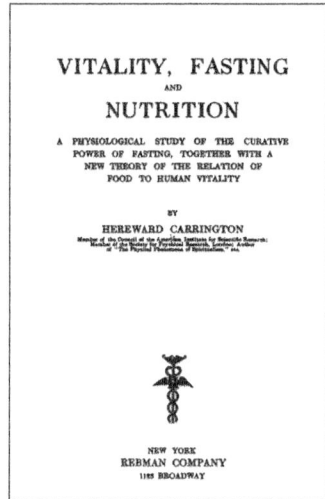

---

*Hereward Carrington was the past member of the Council of the American Society for Scientific Research; Author of *Vitality, Fasting and Nutrition* and other books.

cating gangrenous inflammation of the lungs is seldom associated with the pneumonic variety of plague now-a-days. Diarrhoea is seldom seen.

The mortality from plague in some of the older epidemics was enormous. It is stated, e.g. that in London, over 50,000 corpses were disposed of in one burial ground alone. In one week (that ending September 19th, 1665) more than 10,000 persons are reported to have succumbed to the plague alone. Many of the graveyards could not hold their dead, and wholesale burials were resorted to. Defoe, in his *Plague of London*, draws us a vivid and fascinating picture of the times—the frightful panic of the populace; the helplessness of the authorities—medical and civil; the shocking prevalence of crime; the doleful passage through the streets, at night, of the driver of a huge cart, ringing a bell and crying out the customary, "Bring out your dead! Bring out your dead!" The presence of quackery and charlatanism among venders of quack medicines—exactly paralleling the quacks of our own day—all is dwelt upon a masterly fashion—holding our attention, while it repels us at the same time. Nor is such a state of affairs past and gone from our history—a page to be forgotten. In India, and in a lesser degree, in other Oriental countries, the plague still continues to claim its victims by the hundred; it is a disease with which medical men who reside in the East must cope; and it will consequently be of interest to us to review here, briefly, the symptoms and treatment of this ill-understood disease; and see how far the current theories explain the facts, and to what extent the regular treatment may be said to be rational.

Plague has been defined as "a specific contagious and infectious febrile disorder, characterized by extreme mental and physical depression, generally attended by hemorrhages in different parts, bubonic swellings in one or more of the glandular regions, and occasionally, by involvement of one or more of the other systems (especially of the respiratory, central nervous, and cutaneous); a disease, though reputed to be endemic in some areas, occurring generally at long intervals, in epidemic or pandemic form".

The general tendency of modern scientific medicine is to regard this disease as due to the presence of a specific infective agent—in short, a germ. These bacilli have been found, isolated and studied. I need not enter into the details of this part of the subject, which would probably be of small interest to readers of this magazine. Suffice it to say that they have been found to be present in this disease, and that they have considerable vitality. Experiments have shown that the materials composing the floors of the majority of native houses afford ample pabulum for their growth and development. I shall come to this again in a minute. Just now I shall only remark, *en passant*, that almost the only animals susceptible to the plague (except man) are rats, mice, squirrels and monkeys; and if kept in close confinement, cats, rabbits and guinea pigs. It will be seen from this that the plague is very similar, in many respects, to other blood-diseases with which we are more familiar.

Let us now turn, for a moment, to the **symptoms** of this peculiar or deadly disease. The period of its incubation is short—from two to five days, as a rule. It is acknowledged, however, that although the oncoming of the acute symptoms are so sudden, there is generally present, for several days before such symptoms, a general feeling of depression or malaise, and frequently soft pulses, nausea, headaches, diarrhea, impairment of mental functioning, etc. All seeming to indicate that the attack was not nearly so *sudden* as had been imagined, and that there was a previous condition of the body, at least predisposing it to become diseased in this direction.

Vomiting is one of the earliest symptoms to appear. It is generally followed by intense thirst. The face wears a grave, anxious expression; the memory and thoughts become confused, and the patient soon assumes the look of one entirely helpless. Insomnia is frequently noted; the tongue becomes swollen and thickly furred. The temperature invariably rises, and remains abnormal throughout the disease; the respiration becomes rapid; the pulse also rises greatly; the gait becomes staggering, and the patient weak. In fatal cases, the temperature suddenly falls to below normal, and the face assumes a dusky hue. When the patient happens to recover, it is always a matter of weeks, and during that period any sudden or violent exertion is apt to result in cardiac failure and fatal syncope.

It will thus be seen what a fatal and terrible malady this is, and why it should be so dreaded by all black and white alike, who live in those districts where plague is common. It is apparently exceedingly infectious, and may be contracted by merely sleeping in an infected house, or coming in contact with an infected person. At the same time **all** persons do not contract the plague, and it yet remains to be explained, satisfactorily, **why** certain persons contract the disease and others do not, though they may both have been exposed to the same influences. That seems to be a crucial point of difficulty, with the medical investigators, though it should be, at least in part, clear enough.

Taking the *pests* of our own country—smallpox, e.g., we know very well the only rational reason why some persons escape and others do not. It is simply because the body of the first man is clean and pure, and the body of the second man is foul and impure; in other words *susceptible*. This rule holds well in all diseases of this type—though many medical men would dispute the fact. It is true, nevertheless. Were it not true that only healthy men can resist disease, and that only the predisposed *catch* it, there would be no sense or science in hygiene, in health or morality; there would be no object in preserving the body and in keeping well; in truth, there would be no health in us. But the fact is that these influences do play a part in all contagious and all other diseases that we know, and it is only natural to think that similar conditions should play at least some part, if not a highly important part, in withstanding the plague. Let us see if this factor is considered important, or even considered at all, by medical authorities who have written upon this subject.

It is claimed that "among the agencies which exert a deleterious influence upon the organism (the plague bacillus) are heat, circumstances which favor desiccation, light, efficient ventilation and chemical disinfectants". It is to be presumed that this means when the bacillus is without the human organism, as health is not even mentioned in this list!

But let us take some standard book upon the subject, and see what its author has to say upon the relation of health to the possibility of infection, and the proportionate value he attributes to it. I have before me e.g., *A Manual of Plague*, by William Ernest Jennings, M.B., C.M., Chief Medical Officer for Plague Operations in the Bombay Presidency, etc., and stated by Surgeon-General Bainbridge to be an "accurate exposition of our present knowledge of plague". This we may expect, therefore, to be a fair presentation of the subject.

Now our author has a whole chapter devoted to the "Etiology of the Plague". After showing that this disease is apparently spread by more or less direct infection—from clothes, beds, merchandise, etc., the author takes up the "circumstances affecting the liability of the individual". Age, sex, race, occupation, temperament, heredity, etc., are discussed at the usual length, and the usual opinions arrived at. These conclusions are only those which a fair knowledge of the laws of hygiene, and a fair amount of common-sense, would render obvious—that those who breathe foul, vitiated air, and lead a sedentary life are more disposed to *take* the disease than others who have an opposite and more favorable environment, etc. Climate, locality, and general hygienic conditions are also enumerated; the general conclusions being that the first two play but an insignificant role while the third is, naturally, very important. So important, in fact, that the author evidently considers it all important and ends his discussion of predisposing causes with it. Personal health, personal hygiene, personal cleanliness, are not even mentioned; they are unworthy of recognition! They occupy no part in the modern scheme of medical science, which recognizes germs, and serums and viruses and antitoxins as all important, and the vital element as insignificant by comparison; not even worthy of mention in the list of predisposing causes! What is one to do with such a *science* as this?

The exciting causes of the plague are of course considered to be the germs, which find entrance into the body, generally through the skin, respiratory passages, or other mucous surfaces. I am not going to question the fact that germs do, in some sense, cause this extraordinary and fatal disease; but I think there are other ways of looking at the facts which enable us to see that they (the germs) do not cause the disease in the simple and sure way that it is generally supposed they do. Let us consider some of the facts from another than the usual standpoint.

I have long contended that, merely because germs were found to be present in certain diseases, it by no means proved that they **caused** those diseases. The mere coincidence did not prove any casual agency one way or the other. In fact, there is a good deal to be said for the *other* side, that the diseased state *caused* the germ rather than the germ the diseased state. There is a story of an old Irishman who, when returning home one day, discovered by the wayside, that *rara airs*—a dead donkey. He looked at it for some time, endeavoring to puzzle over what had killed it, or how it had died, but went away still puzzled in his mind. A few days later, his curiosity being still unsatisfied, he determined to revisit the donkey, to see whether further investigation would throw any further light on the cause of the donkey's death. He found the carcass very much alive, as can well be imagined—since the body had lain for some days in the hot sun. At once the mystery of the animal's death was plain to him! "Ah, sure," he said to himself, "no wander th' poor b'ast died! He was being eaten aloive by those vermin!"

To return to the serious side of this question, it will be seen that the above way of looking at the facts clearly reverses their order of cogency, and, in fact, placed the cart before the horse. It is the same in many of the orthodox medical views about germs. These do not always **cause** diseases, but may in fact **result** from them: their presence in the organism proves nothing more than the mere coincidence, and does not for one moment say which is the producer and which the produced. Orthodox medical science contends that the germs cause the disease; many nature-curists contend, equally firmly, that the foul conditions of the disease rendered possible the presence of the germ. Doubtless there is much truth in both of these views. They act and inter-act, and my own view of the matter is that they are both produced or rendered possible, in the vast majority of cases, by causes and conditions operative within the body which produced or rendered possible, both. This third thing is equally the cause of the disease and of the germ (roughly speaking) and is generally an excess of mal assimilated food material floating at large within the organism. I have elaborated all of these points at considerable length, in my *Vitality, Fasting and Nutrition,* and cannot stop to consider them at greater length here. The point of view is all that is required.

Now, when we come to the plague, there can be no doubt, it seems to me, that this question of the state of the individual's health is relegated to a very unimportant and subsidiary position, when it should hold a very

---

*For authority for this statement, see *Report of the Indian Plague Commission,* p. 320; p. 273; p. 280-1; p. 319, etc.

important, if not preeminent one. Various antitoxines have been tried, but the results have been absolutely inconclusive, so far, to say the least of it, and raise no hope whatever that any definite and beneficial results will ever be obtained in this manner, or by this treatment.*

In many cases it was found that the antitoxines did actually fatal harm; and the results never had the chance of being balanced against a number of cases cured or treated along the general hygienic plan. Local treatment was found of little or no avail; in most cases, actually undesirable. Medicines were found to be practically useless and worthless, "In many cases they are entirely contraindicated, and tepid or cold sponging, or the wet-pack have to be relied upon for the reduction of the temperature. In cases in which it is considered advisable and safe to use them, they should be combined with agents which counteract their depressing effect by stimulating the nervous system and strengthening the circulation." (Jennings: *The Plague*, p. 125) It will thus be seen that medicines are only *safe* in rare cases, and doubtfully beneficial at all. Wet-sheet packs and other simple devices after all have to be relied on! Why not try them in the first place, instead of first depressing the circulation with drugs, and then elevating it again with stimulants? If the real medical men understood the real nature of the action of the drugs and stimulants, they would be both ashamed and unable to write such rubbish. At all events, we find that drugs and drug treatment is totally worthless in this disease, as in all others.

We are driven, then, to the only two remaining plans of treatment— the general Hygienic and the Dietetic. Under the first of these we find, as essential, rest, good ventilation, plenty of light and pure water, all of which the hygienist has been in the habit of insisting upon from time immemorial. It is only a recognition of nature's power of self-restoration, and willingness to conform to her dictates in this question. They have found nothing new; they have merely rediscovered an old truth; and the only part of the current treatment that will ultimately prove of any value is these very agencies, so long despised!

But when it comes to the dietetic part of the regular treatment, it is much to be regretted that the common-sense aspect of the case is lost sight of, and that the prevalent errors are observed here, as elsewhere. Thus: "In order to support the powers, food should be administered in small quantities at frequent intervals!" When will the medical man learn that food, in time of sickness, does not *support the powers*, but on the contrary detracts from them? That it cannot nourish the body and that the body has no need for nourishment; that it is, in fact, over-nourished already? Fancy attempting to force food *at frequent intervals* into a patient suffering from the plague! I cannot conceive anything more preposterous or opposed to all true common sense. The principles of the fasting cure and of hygiene generally are so ill-understood by the medical profession that it will take many years, probably, before they fully appreciate their value, and not until then can we expect any real progress in the treatment of the plague or any other infectious or epidemic disease. If, instead of devoting years of time and millions of money to inspection of railway trains, vessels, traffic, bundles, etc., the authorities devoted their energies—or a part of them—to instructing the populace how to keep their houses sweet and clean, and their bodies in a thoroughly pure, properly balanced and internally antiseptic condition, they would be doing far more service, not only to the existing, but to all future generations. It is to be hoped that time is not so far distant as some of the more pessimistic are in the habit of thinking.

The mortality from plague in some of the older epidemics was enormous. It is stated, e.g. that in London, over 50,000 corpses were disposed of in one burial ground alone.

At the same time all persons do not contract the plague, and it yet remains to be explained, satisfactorily, why certain persons contract the disease and others do not, though they may both have been exposed to the same influences. That seems to be a crucial point of difficulty, with the medical investigators, though it should be, at least in part, clear enough.

I am not going to question the fact that germs do, in some sense, cause this extraordinary and fatal disease; but I think there are other ways of looking at the facts which enable us to see that they (the germs) do not cause the disease in the simple and sure way that it is generally supposed they do.

Now, when we come to the plague, there can be no doubt, it seems to me, that this question of the state of the individual's health is relegated to a very unimportant and subsidiary position, when it should hold a very important, if not preeminent one.

Brief, Regarding Vaccination

by William D. Gentry, M.D.
Author of *The Concordance of Materia Medica*
The Naturopath and Herald of Health, XIV (10), 633-635. (1909)

For The Consideration Of The Committee On Education Of The House Of Representatives Of The Illinois Legislature

Mr. Chairman and Members of the Committee: I greet you as Representatives of Education, in the House of Representatives, of the great State of Illinois, and as such you are evidently educated and learned men; but if you are like others of intelligence and education, you are still seeking to learn all you can. Speaking for myself in regard to this thought, although I am seventy-three years of age, have practiced medicine for quarter of a century, an author of medical books in daily use by leading physicians of the Homeopathic School, and now, having been a minister of the Gospel for thirteen years, I am still a learner, and thankful to learn something and advance in knowledge every day, and I presume each of you are seeking all the information and knowledge possible on the subject before you, which is that of Vaccination, referred to in the House Bill Number 23, entitled:

> A Bill to provide for the vaccination of children and for the vaccination and revaccination of all inhabitants of towns or cities, the vaccination of the inmates of almshouses, reform and industrial schools, hospitals, prisons, jails or houses of correction, or any institution which is supported or aided by the State, and for the exclusion of unvaccinated children from the public schools.

As a friend of humanity and especially of children, I wish to speak to you regarding the subject of this Bill and to protest most earnestly against it becoming a law.

I appeal to you, Gentlemen, of this honorable committee, to consider well this most important matter; for if you do, I feel sure that you will not recommend the passage of this Bill.

You have been told, and doubtless know, that vaccination originated in the early part of the past century, by a physician by the name of Jenner, who discovered during an epidemic of smallpox, that those who milked cows having cowpox or vesicular eruptions on the udder, and having lacerations or cuts on their hands and thereby becoming inoculated with the virus from the vesicles on the udders of the cows they milked, would either escape having smallpox, or have a light attack of what Dr. Jenner was pleased to call varioloid, or a mongrel disease.

As a physician I was led to investigate the whole subject of smallpox, cowpox, variola and vaccination, and as one who passed through three epidemics of smallpox, having treated many cases successfully, I feel myself competent to instruct you learned men on this subject.

When a person is vaccinated, the virus or unclean, loathsome matter, which in some cases (on account of the diseased condition of the cow) is only pus, is introduced through the skin into the arm or part of the person subjected to the operation. In three days a process of fermentation and inflammation takes place, which results in about seven days in the formation of a scab or crust over the wound, under which is either cowpox matter or pus, which being absorbed into the blood causes a fever, with chilly sensations creeping over the body, attended by more or less lassitude, with painful or uneasy feeling.

If the person is not perfectly healthy, or has been using stimulation, such as alcoholic drinks, tobacco, coffee, tea or other drugs to excess; or if the person has inherited or acquired some weakness in one or more of the organs of the body, the combination of the poison produced by the fermentation, with that already existing in the circulation, will frequently produce a life-long morbid condition, if not a fatal disease.

Frequently, on account of the ignorance regarding constitutional conditions, characteristics and liabilities to results attending and following vaccination on the part of the physician or other inexperienced person performing the act, persons are vaccinated who are already diseased, owing to weakness of some vital organ. In such cases vaccination positively subjects such persons to death or permanent injury.

Besides this, the virus from cowpox, or worse still, vaccination with virus mixed with pus, or from the vesicles produced from the inoculation of cattle with matter from true smallpox pustules, which I am told, dealers are now supplying, is nothing but the act of impregnating the system of a little innocent child, or even a pure and healthy adult, with a loathsome disease-producing matter, which will, ever after, cause such person to be unhealthy and suffer.

A great amount of money is being made by men and women in the business of producing virus of various degrees of effectiveness in producing disease, and in vaccinating, whose business and income will be greatly increased by having this Bill become a law.* These are the individuals who are using every influence in their power to persuade you to approve and recommend this Bill for passage. It certainly is not the people; for on inquiry in different sections of the State, I find that people are kept in ignorance of the fact that even such a vitally important and dangerous enactment is proposed. The people have not been informed and know absolutely nothing of this Bill.

---

*The American vaccine manufacturers generate revenues in the billions. In 2011, the US federal government awarded 6 pharmaceutical companies $5.7 billion dollars to produce vaccines for children alone. —Ed.

The honorable gentleman who introduced the Bill was careful to state, he only introduced it at the request of others; and on inquiry it was found that the authors of the Bill are two prominent doctors, holding political offices by appointment in the State, who will probably be financially benefitted, more than any others.

I know as a fact and which has been repeatedly proven in my practice, that there is a more efficient and preventive against smallpox than cowpox virus or vaccination. It costs but a trifle and will make no person sick. It is simply fumes of pure apple vinegar, or acetic acid, produced by saturating a towel or apron with the vinegar and hanging it in the room of the house inhabited by people subjected to contagion.* If this is done, no one inhaling such fumes can take smallpox. This has been thoroughly tested by me in homes of families where there was a single case of confluent smallpox. Not another member of the family took the disease, though exposed daily.

This is done only on truly scientific principles, as I will now show. The eruption and other concomitant symptoms produced in a case of smallpox is not the disease. The disease causing the symptoms is invisible. It may be called a spirit. It is not certainly a germ. One susceptible to smallpox does not have to come in touch with or breathe the breath of one having the disease in order to take it. All they have to do is to come within ten or twenty feet of the individual who has the disease. Nothing visible or material passes, but only a spiritual unseen something, and in seven or eleven days the disease is reproduced.

It is found that the peculiar spirit in the fluid, known as vinegar, communicated in the evaporation an unseen power, which totally destroys or makes null and void the spirit producing smallpox.

The virus of cowpox only produces another disease, which reduces the virulence of smallpox. The danger and the almost universal injury to any person who has been vaccinated, should cause intelligent people everywhere in this enlightened age to strenuously oppose vaccination and the enactment of any law to enforce it.

Human beings are divided into, at least, twelve different families or species, just as apples or potatoes are divided. Each one of these families are subject to some peculiar disease, or family of diseases, so that a wise and competent physician may, by knowing which family of human beings is subject only to some kindred or similar diseases, can by exclusion of all other diseases, determine the character of any sickness in the individual he is called upon to treat. It has become known that only about one-twelfth of the whole human family is subject to smallpox. It has also become

---

*Vinegar mixed with water and boiled to steam in the living quarters occupied by infectious patients was a common and effective practice used by the Chinese to strengthen the Wei Qi and improve immunity during times of infections. I have used steamed vinegar as a standard prophylactic with patients in times of flus with astounding success. —Ed.

known that whenever any person belonging to one, at least, of the other families, perhaps three, is forced to have, by compulsory vaccination or otherwise, the disease produced by cowpox virus, will be permanently injured in some way.

Smallpox is not a fatal or dangerous disease except to those who have symptoms weakened by syphilitic or scrofulous infection, or have weakness of vital organs caused by the use of stimulants or harmful, unhealthy foods or habits. A perfectly healthy, clean person will not be greatly affected by smallpox any more than by any other disease. They will soon recover, and ever afterwards be immune from nearly every disease in the catalogue.

Most conscientiously and earnestly, on behalf of the ignorant and innocent children and adults of our commonwealth, I protest against the proposed Bill becoming a law.

A Bill to provide for the vaccination of children and for the vaccination and revaccination of all inhabitants of towns or cities, the vaccination of the inmates of almshouses, reform and industrial schools, hospitals, prisons, jails or houses of correction, or any institution which is supported or aided by the State, and for the exclusion of unvaccinated children from the public schools.

If the person is not perfectly healthy, or has been using stimulation, such as alcoholic drinks, tobacco, coffee, tea or other drugs to excess; or if the person has inherited or acquired some weakness in one or more of the organs of the body, the combination of the poison produced by the fermentation [from being vaccinated], with that already existing in the circulation, will frequently produce a life-long morbid condition, if not a fatal disease.

A great amount of money is being made by men and women in the business of producing virus of various degrees of effectiveness in producing disease, and in vaccinating, whose business and income will be greatly increased by having this Bill become a law. These are the individuals who are using every influence in their power to persuade you to approve and recommend this Bill for passage.

Smallpox is not a fatal or dangerous disease except to those who have symptoms weakened by syphilitic or scrofulous infection, or have weakness of vital organs caused by the use of stimulants or harmful, unhealthy foods or habits.

1910

BULLETIN

OF

The Anti-Vaccination League of America

517-518 Crozer Building, 1420 Chestnut Street, Philadelphia, Pennsylvania

February 1, 1916   No. 2   Price, Five Cents

CHILD VICTIMS OF A DEADLY RITE

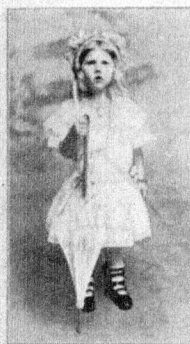

MARGARET A. GRAHAM
Age 4 years, daughter of Edward J. Graham, 6337 Paschall Ave., Philadelphia, Pa. Vaccinated October 27, 1910. Died November 13, 1910, from tetanus.

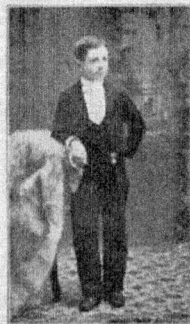

CHARLES WARE
Age 9 years, son of C. M. Ware, 601 High Street, Millville, N. J. Vaccinated about October 20, 1910. Died October 26, 1910, from tetanus. Charles in the box wearing a white sweater, standing on the extreme right, at the top.

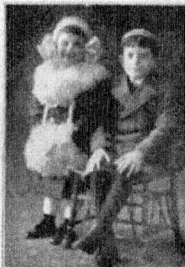

JAMES MOCK, JR.
Age 4 years and 3 months, son of James Mock, 2336 East Allegheny Avenue, Philadelphia, Pa. Vaccinated August 28, 1912. Died September 3, 1912, from internal abscesses.

WILLIAM PLUMRIDGE
Age 6 years, son of Frederick W. Plumridge, 6631 Vine St., rear of 236 North Robinson St., Philadelphia, Pa. Vaccinated September, 1909. Died October 18, 1909, from tetanus.

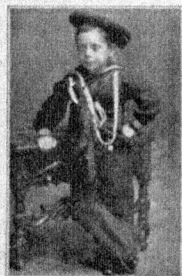

CATHERINE AICHER
Age 5 years and 10 months, daughter of Mrs. Elizabeth Aicher, 215 Chambers St., Phillipsburg, N. J. Vaccinated August 20, 1912. Died September 13, 1912, from meningitis and lockjaw.

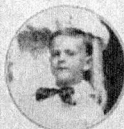

JOSEPH GOLDIE
Age 11 years and 7 months, grandson of Captain Francis Campbell, 312 North Fifth St., Camden, N. J. Vaccinated in Bristol, Pa., October, 1901. Died November 11, 1901, from blood poisoning and tetanus.

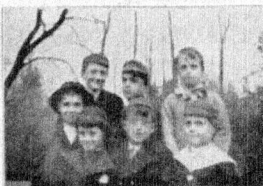

FRANK HIGHAM, JR.
Age 8 years and 9 months, son of Frank Higham, 466h Hawthorne St., Philadelphia, Pa. Vaccinated September 3, 1912. Died September 17, 1912, from tetanus.

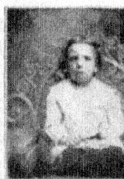

ALBERT R. THOMPSON
Age 6 years, son of Edward F. Thompson, 2425 Ogden St., Philadelphia, Pa. Vaccinated about August 24, 1909. Died September 16, 1909, from tetanus.

The first Anti-Vaccination League of America was founded by two doctors, Drs. Robert A. Gunn and Alexander Wilder in 1879 to counter the compulsory vaccination laws. In 1902, Frank D. Blue of Terre Haute, Indiana, succeeded as president and launched a publicized campaign to increase public awareness in *The Naturopath and Herald of Health*. To make their position clear, the Anti-Vaccination League of America published a Bulletin with images of children who died as a result of compulsory vaccination.

Tuberculosis and Vaccination

by John W. Hodge, M.D.

The Naturopath and Herald of Health, XV (2), 75-77. (1910)

The following article appearing in the *Niagara Falls Gazette* in Jan. 22 is reprinted here by request:

Tuberculosis exhibitions [prevalence] are now the order of the day all over the country. While the combined efforts of doctors and laymen in combating this great scourge of humanity are commendable it is a notable fact that one of the most prolific agents in the probable causation of this disease has been almost entirely overlooked by the medical profession. For the past two years I have been reading the reports of the transactions of tuberculosis' congresses which have convened in various parts of the world and have failed to find in all these voluminous reports a single reference to vaccinations as a probable factor in the spread of tuberculosis. It is universally conceded that the bovine race is peculiarly liable to tubercular diseases, and the distinguishing pathologist, Cohnheim, declares this conviction that so-called "vaccine lymph used for the purposes of vaccination is tuberculosic [sic] in its nature".

Within the last few years a number of pathologists of world-wide renown have expressed the suspicion that so-called *pure calf-lymph* may be a prolific source of the tuberculosis which has been so affrightingly on the increase in all jennerized countries.*

In Germany where vaccination is rigidly compulsory, tuberculosis has become so formidable in its ravages that the death rate from that disease has more than doubled within the last two decades, while in England where vaccination is not compulsory, the death rate from this disease has diminished by one-half during this same period. In many jennerized countries where tuberculosis was practically unknown prior to the introduction of vaccination, the *great white plague* is now a veritable scourge. According to Dr. Perron, a distinguished member of the French Legion of Honor, "Tuberculosis which was at one time an exceptional disease in France, has in the last hundred years been steadily extending its ravages, in spite of the general advancement in hygiene, till it has attained the rank of a pestilence." Dr. Perron tells us that he finds himself compelled to the conviction that the causal connection is with vaccination which has advanced step by step with tuberculosis. Herein Dr. Perron finds explanation of the extraordinary devastation of wrought by tuberculosis in the European armies (especially in the first and second years after enlistment) where re-vaccination is the order of the day in spite of the great care

---

*'Jennerized countries' refers to countries who adopted the vaccination practice that was introduced by Edward Jenner in late 18th century. —*Ed.*

otherwise lavished upon the soldiers' physical welfare. With this clue we may find significance in the official figures recently published showing the deaths from tuberculosis in Germany (where vaccination is so much at home) as thrice more numerous than in England where vaccination is much neglected. That there is a causal relation between vaccination and tuberculosis cannot be seriously doubted by any observer who has given attention to the subject.

The inoculation experiments conducted by M. Toussaint, in France leave no room for reasonable doubt that tuberculosis can be communicated from a tuberculous cow to a healthy human subject. Toussaint vaccinated a tubercular cow with lymph from a vaccine vesicle raised on a previously healthy child. Then, in turn with the lymph from the pocks on the cow, he vaccinated four rabbits and a pig. The rabbits were killed two months afterwards, autopsied and found to be infected with tubercular disease at the points inoculated; in the glands and in the lungs. The vaccinated pig also developed tuberculosis, both local and general. These results have been corroborated by other experimenters.

Here we are confronted with a fact of grave significance. These inoculation experiments prove conclusively that tuberculosis is communicable through vaccination; and as cows are peculiarly subject to tuberculosis, both in its latent and active forms we can never be certain that the so-called calf-lymph used by vaccinators is free from the subtle and insidious foe: tuberculosis.

To the members of the medical profession who are sincerely interested in the extirpation of *the great white plague* I earnestly recommend a careful perusal of the following pithy paragraph which I quote from a recent number of *Life*:

> Several doctors appeared before our Tammany Mayor the other day asking for money to fight tuberculosis. Life hopes they will get it. But if these benevolent doctors really wish to conquer tuberculosis—or any other disease—why persist in injecting other people's diseases into healthy bodies? There is a rather solid belief in this country—all wool and a yard wide—that tuberculosis will continue to consume us so long as Dr. Vaccine Virus is allowed to pour petroleum on the flames.

Doctor, do you see the point? Think it over.

Jan. 22, 1910.
Niagara Falls, N. Y.

For the past two years I have been reading the reports of the transactions of tuberculosis' congresses which have convened in various parts of the world and have failed to find in all these voluminous reports a single reference to vaccinations as a probable factor in the spread of tuberculosis.

In many jennerized countries where tuberculosis was practically unknown prior to the introduction of vaccination, the great white plague *is now a veritable scourge.*

These inoculation experiments prove conclusively that tuberculosis is communicable through vaccination; and as cows are peculiarly subject to tuberculosis, both in its latent and active forms we can never be certain that the so-called calf-lymph *used by vaccinators is free from the subtle and insidious foe: tuberculosis.*

But if these benevolent doctors really wish to conquer tuberculosis—or any other disease—why persist in injecting other people's diseases into healthy bodies?

THE ANTI-VACCINATION CRUSADE I

by Henry Lindlahr, M.D.

Copyright by The Nature Cure Publishing Co., Chicago

The Naturopath and Herald of Health XV (3), 129-132. (1910)

To vaccinate or not to vaccinate", that is the question of the day in Chicago.

In order to solve this much discussed problem intelligently and rationally, it becomes necessary to understand the true nature of acute and chronic diseases.

Modern *regular* medical science is built on the germ theory of disease. The microscope discloses to the astonished eye of science the wonders of the world of micro-organisms. Many forms of disease are found to be accompanied by the production of certain kinds of germs, bacteria, and parasites.

In malarial diseases we find in the blood in great numbers of the *plasmodium malariae*; in cholera, the cholera bacillus; in

Henry Lindlahr, M.D.

consumption, the tubercle bacillus, etc., and forthwith scientists argue that these germs are the true causes of disease. As a natural corollary to this assumption they further conclude that in order to cure the disease they must kill the germs.

From these premises have evolved our modern theory and practice of medicine and surgery, culminating in the lymph, serum, vaccine, and antitoxin therapy.*

Kill the bug and cure the disease, that sounds possible—but is it true?

Only a few years ago the world was all aglow with excitement over Dr. Koch's wonderful discovery, and he was heralded as one of the great figures of humanity. He claimed that the tubercle bacillus was the cause of consumption, and that his tuberculin, a decoction of tubercle bacilli, was certain death to the bacilli and a sure cure for consumption. The German Parliament, in the first excitement over the wonderful discovery, presented to him in the name of the nation a vote of thanks, and the sum of 100,000 marks.

From all parts of the world consumptives and those who were in dread of becoming such came to try the new treatment. But, alas, today

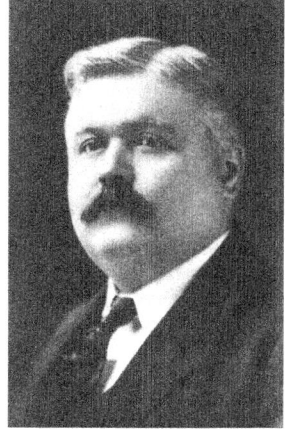

---

*There were two common spellings of antitoxin and antitoxine used by the early Naturopaths. Antitoxin refers to the vaccine developed for diphtheria. —*Ed.*

tuberculin is almost forgotten. Only here and there a lone fakir poses as the original Dr. Koch from Berlin, and sells to poor deluded sufferers the wonderful tuberculin as a sure cure for consumption, and in Berlin people show you *Koch's graveyard*, where lie buried thousands of victims of tuberculin.

Like the tuberculin and like many other *ignis fatuus* [deceptive] of medical science, every other form of lymph, serum, vaccine, and antitoxin will also in time sink into merited oblivion. Health can never be created by putting viral poisons into the human body.

Naturopathy holds that germs, bacteria and parasites are products of disease rather than its cause. The sugar solution may create yeast germs, but yeast germs cannot create a sugar solution. Disease matter in the body, as we shall see, corresponds to the sugar in a fermenting fluid.

Which is the more probable, that foul air, filth, and dirt create fungi and vermin in a house, or that the fungi and vermin create the foul air, dirt, and filth? Is it not evident that medical science has put the cart before the horse?

What would the learned professor of bacteriology say if some day he found his trusted Bridget going through the house with a carbolic acid sprinkler trying to extirpate dirt and microbes, instead of using a good supply of soap, water, fresh air and sunlight?

Cleanliness inside and out, in the body, the home, the street and the alley, is the only rational preventative and cure of infectious, bacterial and parasitic diseases.

Naturopathy claims that germs of themselves alone cannot create disease—if they could, humanity would soon be extinct. Disease germs are present everywhere: on the food we eat, and the water we drink, and air and dust we breathe, and on the money we handle. Can you imagine anything fouler and more thoroughly saturated with disease germs and bacteria than our beloved money? Has it not been passed through thousands of dirty pockets and diseased hands? But that does not deter the most delicate lady and the most rabid bacteria crank from fondling it—but—"be sure and boil the water". To be consistent why not disinfect our greenbacks?

Why not wear filters before nose and mouth when shopping downtown among holiday crowds? Oh, *Sancta Simplicitas*, just think of it—we cannot spend fifteen minutes in such a surging, perspiring mass of humanity without inhaling in the foul air and dust [and] every disease germ in existence; why then do not all the people lie down and die? Because it takes something more in the system than microbes to create disease, namely, lowered vitality and morbid matter; in other words—the disease predisposition. These factors given, the conditions are ripe for the development of germ diseases.

Just as yeast grows in a sugar solution only, so grow and multiply disease germs in disease matter only. Yeast germs will not grow and multiply in clear water because they find no nourishment, nor will disease germs grow and multiply in pure blood and normal tissues in a body possessed of good vitality. They find nothing to subsist upon. The vigorous, vibratory activity of a healthy organism repels and eliminates the invaders without much trouble. These dreaded and maligned little invaders are not nearly so black as painted by medical science; indeed, under certain circumstances, they become our best friends.

They are, in most instances, nothing more or less than nature's scavengers, and to destroy them would be about as sensible as to kill the *white angels* of our street cleaning brigades, who in the performance of their duty are compelled to stir up the dust and dirt.

Fevers and inflammations in the human organisms are closely related to the process of fermentation. Every housewife is familiar with the phenomenon of fermentation. When yeast is added to the saccharine solution, grape juice for instance, a great activity ensues, bubbles arise, the fluid is agitated in violent commotion, the temperature increases, scum forms on the surface, and the sediment at the bottom. If this activity is allowed to continue unhindered, yeast germs, while digesting it, split up the grape sugar into alcohol and carbonic acid. When all the sugar has been thus removed and transformed, the resultant is a fluid of crystalline clearness which we call wine.

The process of fermentation, however, can be arrested at any time by the addition of salicylic acid, formaldehyde, or any other powerful antiseptic. But what happens? If the fermentation is thus suddenly arrested the resulting fluid contains a mass of unfermented sugar, dead yeast germs, and poisonous antiseptics. It has become a nasty, torpid mass, repulsive to sight, smell and taste. In this we have a perfect simile of the *modus operandi* of acute and chronic diseases and their treatment.

When disease germs find in the human body the necessary conditions for growth and propagation—namely, lowered vitality, and their own congenial morbid soil—they multiply very rapidly and develop all the symptoms of that particular germ disease. Similar to the phenomenon of fermentation we observe accelerated circulation, rapid pulse, increased temperature, congestion, and quickened elimination in the form of mucus, pus, perspiration, and other morbid discharges.

The greatly increased vital activity in the system indicates simply that nature, by means of germs, parasites, and fever heat is endeavoring to stir up, consume, and eliminate from the system waste and morbid matter.

If these processes of elimination are allowed to run their course in a natural manner, and when purification and elimination are fully completed, the acute symptoms will subside of their own accord, and after such a *natural cure* the patient is actually rejuvenated, and says that he feels like a *new man.*

As in the case of alcoholic fermentation, it is an easy matter to arrest by antiseptics, antipyretics, and germicides the process of fever and inflammation, but what is the result? Nature is thwarted in her attempt to burn up and eliminate the waste and morbid matter from the system. Drug poisons are added to disease poisons and as a result Nature's acute healing and cleansing efforts are turned into latent chronic diseases.

To quote from our *Naturopath* series:

> When unnatural habits of life, before alluded to, have lowered the vitality and favored the accumulation of waste matter and poisons to such an extent that the sluggish bowels, kidneys, skin and other organs of elimination are unable to keep a clean house, Nature has to resort to other more radical means of purification or **we would choke in our own impurities.** These forcible house cleanings of nature are fevers, catarrh, skin eruptions, diarrheas, boils, abnormal perspirations, and many other so-called *acute diseases.* Sulphur and mercury may drive back the skin eruptions; antipyretics and antiseptics may suppress fever and catarrh. The patient and the doctor may congratulate themselves on the speedy cure, but what is the true state of affairs? Nature has been thwarted in her work of healing and cleansing. She had to give up the fight against disease matter in order to combat the more potent poisons of mercury, quinine, iodine, strychnine, or whatever they may be called.

The disease matter is in the system still—plus the drug poison.

After a time, when vitality has **sufficiently recuperated,** nature may make another attempt at purification; this time perhaps in another direction, but again her well-meant efforts are defeated. This process of suppression is repeated over and over again until the blood and tissues become so loaded with waste material and poisons that the healing forces of the organisms can no longer react against them by means of acute disorders, and then results **the chronic condition,** which, in the vocabulary of the old school, is only another name for *incurable.*

Now we are better prepared to understand the *modus operandi* of vaccination and its relationship to smallpox. If vaccination actually prevents smallpox, it can do so only in one way, and that is **by developing in the system smallpox in the chronic form of the disease.** From the explanation given above we know that *chronic disease* means that the system is so loaded with disease matter and the vitality so low that the vital force is unable to rouse itself to acute eliminative effort. Having disease in the low, cold chronic form means that we are not able to have it in the acute form, but for reasons just given we should much prefer to have a disease in the acute forms and be rid of the morbid encumbrances in a few days or weeks than to be afflicted by the chronic form of the disease for years, or for a lifetime.

Smallpox, like every other infectious disease, is a filth disease. It grows, as we shall see later on, in a scrofulous soil only, and the smallpox eruptions mean "rapid elimination of scrofulous and tuberculous poisons from the system".

Therefore, if we have the choice, we should certainly prefer smallpox to the vaccination. Cheap talk, someone says. Not so, my friend, this is not merely talk—we were put to the test more than once in our own flesh and blood, and therefore we speak from experience and with authority.

In our next number we shall relate the story in detail.

"To vaccinate or not to vaccinate", *that is the question of the day in Chicago*. In order to solve this much discussed problem intelligently and rationally it becomes necessary to understand the true nature of acute and chronic diseases.

Naturopathy claims that germs of themselves alone cannot create disease—if they could, humanity would soon be extinct. Disease germs are present everywhere: on the food we eat, and the water we drink, and air and dust we breathe, and on the money we handle.

When disease germs find in the human body the necessary conditions for growth and propagation—namely, lowered vitality, and their own congenial morbid soil—they multiply very rapidly and develop all the symptoms of that particular germ disease.

*If vaccination actually prevents smallpox, it can do so only in one way, and that is **by developing in the system smallpox in the chronic form of the disease**. From the explanation given above we know that "chronic disease" means that the system is so loaded with disease matter and the vitality so low that the vital force is unable to rouse itself to acute eliminative effort.*

The Anti-Vaccination Crusade II

by Henry Lindlahr, M.D.

Copyright by The Nature Cure Publishing Company
The Naturopath and Herald of Health, XV (5), 257-259 (1910).

In the concluding paragraph of my preceding article on this subject I stated that I myself would prefer smallpox to vaccination, and promised to relate some personal experiences in verification of my assertions.

My oldest boy was unfortunately born at a time when both parents were heavily encumbered with and suffering from hereditary and acquired disease conditions. At birth he weighed only two and a half pounds, and his chance for life seemed very small. The eyes were of a blackish hue, especially in the outer rim, which gradually condensed into a heavy scurf rim, owing to the fact that by talcum powders and home remedies we suppressed Nature's cleansing efforts in the form of skin eruptions.

Henry Lindlahr
(1862-1924)

The first four or five years of his life, he was a sickly, weakly child having regularly every year a few sieges of infantile ailments. We soon learned to treat these, however, in a natural manner and he was not vaccinated.

One day suspicious-looking eruptions appeared and soon spread all over his body. I called in two physicians to verify my diagnosis of smallpox, which they did unqualifiedly.

We applied the natural treatment, which consisted of absolute fasting and cold water applications. The child was kept day and night in the wet packs—in strips of linen dipped in cold water of natural temperature. These were changed when hot and dry. In addition to this he received the indicated high potency homeopathic remedies.

There was hardly a spot on his body unaffected by sores and boils. Constant renewal of the cold packs kept the temperature below the danger point and greatly alleviated the insufferable itching peculiar to the disease.

My wife and I slept in the same room without the least fear of infection, and though not vaccinated since childhood, we remained unaffected.

The wet packs of course greatly furthered the process of elimination and the disease practically ran its course in ten days. From that time on the sores healed rapidly and there remained nothing to indicate the ravages of the disease but a tell-tale mark over his left eyebrow and a few marks on his body.

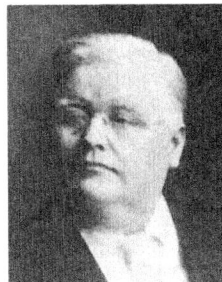

Under this natural treatment of the disease convalescence was rapid and complete, and afterwards the eyes became much clearer and lighter in color.

The very reverse is true after vaccination. We have observed in many children how their beautiful, clear blue eyes after vaccination or antitoxin treatment darkened and developed the signs of chronic catarrhal conditions, especially in the regions of digestive organs and respiratory tract.

Since his recovery from the smallpox the boy has been free from any serious diseases, and his physical development has been the marvel of everyone who knew him before and after the great eliminative crisis. Although he has eaten probably not five pounds of meat in all his life, his physical development is fully equal to that of a child one or two years above his age.

With our younger boy we had a somewhat similar experience. When one year of age he was taken with a severe attack of spinal meningitis. Every half hour his little body was bent backward in the dreadful convulsions peculiar to the disease. Exactly the same treatment was applied as in the smallpox case.

Again, I had two physicians make a diagnosis of the case so that in the future the facts might not be questioned. For nine days it seemed a hopeless fight to everyone who had occasion to witness it. Then both ears broke and began to discharge pus and blood. From that time on all symptoms began to clear up rapidly and on the eleventh day the little patient took his first food. Previous to this he had not received even a drop of milk; nothing but cold water, rendered slightly acid with fruit juices. This was also the only drink administered under the smallpox treatment.

For six weeks the discharge of pus and blood from the ears continued unhindered and unchecked, but rather encouraged and promoted by natural methods of treatment and by the indicated homeopathic remedies.

In this case as in the former the following improvements and physical development was marvelous. While therefore this eliminative crisis the child seemed somewhat dull and dazed in his actions and his looks, he was after recovery much brighter and more active physically and mentally. He is now a little over three years of age, and the very image of health. His picture, a genuine snapshot, appeared on the cover of the first number of *Nature Cure Magazine*. We have 'seldom' seen in men's eyes clearer and freer from defeat than his, and corresponding to this he is a model of physical development.

Compare with this splendid recovery and subsequent improvement in general health, the results after the orthodox serum treatment of spinal meningitis. Statistics say over eighty percent die and the surviving twenty percent are usually in some form or another crippled or invalid for life. Why so?

All acute diseases are natural processes—as we express it—the result of Nature's healing, cleansing efforts, which run a certain well-defined, orderly and natural course. There is a stage of incipiency followed by stages of intense acute activity during which Nature endeavors to burn up, tear down and eliminate by means of fever heat, sores, catarrhal discharges, etc., the morbid matter and poisons from the system. These stages of destruction, cremation and elimination are followed by the stages of reconstruction, or as medical science say, of resolution.

If during any one of these stages Nature's orderly processes are hindered, interrupted or suppressed by ice bags, poisonous drugs, antitoxin, serums, surgical operations, or mental effort, the disease condition is arrested and made a permanent one.

Suppose you are repairing and remodeling your home, and the artisans have demolished the interiors and everything is in a chaotic condition. At this juncture you dismiss the workmen and stop the work of repair, what is the result? Undoubtedly a ruined and desolate home.

Exactly the same is true of a body in which Nature's healing; cleansing and reconstructive efforts are permanently interrupted and suppressed. Deafness, blindness, chronic affections of the kidneys, lungs, heart, brain and other vital organs, epilepsy, paralysis, St. Vitus' dance, and only too often insanity are the inevitable results of such unnatural treatment.

On the other hand, I claim that my boys, through the vigorous eliminations incident to smallpox and meningitis eliminated in a few weeks more scrofulous and psoric taints and poisons from their systems than would have been possible otherwise in many years, or even in a lifetime.

In the following articles on this same subject we shall deal with the chronic after effects of vaccination and with the arguments of its advocates.

We have observed in many children how their beautiful, clear blue eyes after vaccination or antitoxin treatment darkened and developed the signs of chronic catarrhal conditions, especially in the regions of digestive organs and respiratory tract.

All acute diseases are natural processes—as we express it—the result of Nature's healing, cleansing efforts, which run a certain well-defined, orderly and natural course.

If during any one of these stages Nature's orderly processes are hindered, interrupted or suppressed by ice bags, poisonous drugs, antitoxin, serums, surgical operations, or mental effort, the disease condition is arrested and made a permanent one.

THE ANTI-VACCINATION CRUSADE III

by Henry Lindlahr, M.D.

Copyright by The Nature Cure Publishing Co., Chicago

The Naturopath and Herald of Health, XV (7), 385-388. (1910)

Jenner, an English barber and chiropodist, is usually credited with the discovery of Vaccination. The doubtful honor, however, belongs in reality to an old Circassian woman who, according to the historian Le Duc, in the year 1672 startled Constantinople with the announcement that the Virgin Mary had revealed to her an unfailing preventative against the smallpox.

Her specific was inoculation with the genuine smallpox virus. But even with her and the Virgin Mary the idea was not an original one because the principal of isopathy, or curing disease by its own disease products, was explicitly taught a hundred years before by Paracelsus, the great genius of the Renaissance of learning of the Middle Ages. But even he was only voicing the secret teaching of ancient folk lore, sympathy and magic dating back to the Druids and Seers of ancient Britain and Germany.

The Circassian seeress cut a cross in the flesh of people and inoculated this wound with the smallpox virus. Together with this she prescribed prayer, abstinence from meat and fasting for forty days.

As at that time smallpox was a terrible and widespread scourge, the practice spread all over Europe. At first the operation was performed by women and laymen, but when the practice became popular, and people were anxious to pay for it, the doctors began to incorporate it into their regular practice. Popular superstitions run a very similar course to epidemics. They have a period of inception, of virulence and of subsidence. As germs and bacteria become inactive and die a natural death in their own poisonous products, in similar manner popular superstitions die as a natural result of their own falsities and exaggerations.

It soon became evident that inoculation with the virus did not prevent smallpox, but on the contrary frequently caused it, and therefore the practice gradually fell into innocuous desuetude, to be revived by Jenner about 100 years later in a modified form. He substituted cowpox virus for smallpox virus, the *like* for the *same*, in other words the homeopathic principle of *Similia similibus curantur*, for the isopathic principle; "the disease poison cures the disease".

Modern Allopathy applies isopathy in large and poisonous doses of virus, lymph, serums and antitoxins, while Homeopathy, as did ancient mysticism, applies the isopathic remedies in highly diluted and triturated doses only.

From England vaccination gradually spread over all the civilized world and during the 19th century the smallpox disease (variola) constantly diminished in virulence and frequency until today it has become of comparatively rare occurrence. "Therefore vaccination has exterminated smallpox" say the disciples of Jenner.

Is that really so? Is vaccination actually a preventative of smallpox? This seems very doubtful when the advocates of vaccination themselves do not believe it. "What," I hear them say, indignantly, "you mean to insinuate we do not believe in our own theory?" Certainly not, my friends. If you believe that vaccination protects you against smallpox, why are you afraid of *catching it* from those who are not vaccinated? If you are thoroughly protected as you claim to be how can you catch it from those who are not protected? Why do you not allow the other fellow to have his fill of smallpox and then enjoy a good laugh on him? The fact of the matter is you know full well that you are not protected, that you *catch* the disease just as readily as the unprotected.

German statistics are more reliable than those of any other country. In the years 1870-71 smallpox was rampant in the Fatherland and over 1,000,000 people had the disease, and 120,000 died. Ninety-six percent of these had been vaccinated and 4 percent only were not vaccinated.

On account of the great extent and virulence of the epidemic most of the victims had been vaccinated shortly before they took the disease. In 1888 Bismarck sent an address to the Governments of all the German States in which it was admitted that numerous eczematous diseases, even those of an epidemic nature, were directly attributable to vaccination, and that the origin and cure of the disease were still unsolved problems.

In this message to the various legislatures the great statesman says, "The hopes placed in the efficacy of the cowpox virus as a preventative have proved entirely deceptive." Realizing this to be a fact most of the German States have modified and relinquished the compulsory vaccination laws.

"But," our opponents insist, "you cannot deny that smallpox has greatly diminished since the almost universal adoption of vaccination."

Certainly the disorder has diminished but so has also diminished and in fact almost entirely disappeared the plague, the Black Death, cholera, bubonic plague, yellow fever, and numerous other epidemic pests which only recently decimated entire nations. Not one of these epidemics was treated by vaccination or any other form of preventative medicine.

Why then did they diminish and practically disappear?

Not vaccination but the more universal adoption of soap, bath tubs, sanitary measures, plumbing, drainage, ventilation and more hygienic modes of living generally have subdued smallpox and all other plagues. Most of us remember how the yellow fever raged in Havana during the Spanish occupancy. Within two months after the energetic Yankees took possession and gave the filthy city a good scouring, yellow fever had entirely disappeared—without any yellow fever vaccination.

The question is now in order—of all the dreaded plagues of the past why has smallpox alone survived to this day? The true answer is—on account of vaccination. If this scrofulous and syphilitic poison was not artificially kept alive in human blood by vaccination, smallpox would by this time be as rare as cholera and yellow fever.

In a former article of this series we said: "If vaccination protects at all it does so by creating in the body the smallpox disease in the chronic form." We have learned that having a disease in the chronic form means that the healing forces of the system are not strong enough to throw it off by means of an acute form of the same disease. Having smallpox in the chronic form, induced by vaccination, may weaken the system in such a way that it cannot arouse itself to an acute smallpox eruption, necessary to eliminate the scrofulous and syphilitic constitution miasms.

However, if you weaken in this manner the system's reactionary powers against one disease, you weaken its reactionary power against all diseases. In other words, by creating in the body chronic smallpox disease, you favor the development of all kinds of chronic diseases.

Thanks to oft repeated compulsory vaccination of every citizen young and old, we have become a nation universally saturated by the smallpox virus. Is it any wonder that this latent miasm breaks out in acute epidemics once in a while?

Undoubtedly this systematic and almost universal contamination and degeneration of vital fluids and tissues accounts in a large measure for the steady increase of tuberculosis, cancer, syphilis, insanity and for a multitude of other chronic destructive diseases unknown among primitive peoples, free from the blessings (?) of syphilization, mecurialization and vaccination.

Quit sowing the seed, gentlemen, and you will cease reaping the harvest. By the mercurial suppression of syphilis and by means of vaccination, you are perpetuating smallpox.

What has syphilis to do with smallpox? They both are very similar and very closely related in appearance, symptomatology and in their effects upon the organism. Dr. Med. Cruwell, a German physician, who has thoroughly studied the subject says: "Every vaccination with so-called cowpox means syphilitic infection. Cowpox is not a disease peculiar to cattle; it is always due to syphilitic or smallpox infection from the diseased hands of human beings." Cowpox has only been found on the udders of milk cows which came in contact with human hands. Cattle roaming on pasture and prairie, oxen and steers have never been affected by cowpox. If it were a disorder peculiar to cattle, both sexes would be equally affected. Jenner's cowpox was caused by the diseased hands of the syphilitic milkmaid, Sarah Nehnes.

Vaccination of healthy children and adults is often followed by a multitude of symptoms which cannot be distinguished from syphilis, viz.: characteristic ulcers and eczematous eruptions, swellings of the axillary and other lymphatic glands, atrophy of the mammary glands in the breasts of women and of girls above the age of puberty.

This will explain the growing demand for "Bust foods" and "Developers". A perfectly developed bust has become so rare that many hundreds of beauty doctors, and of firms making a specialty of developing the flat-bosomed, realize thousands of dollars annually. One firm in this city, and a small concern at that, has made from $2,500 to $5,000 a year and has over 10,000 names on its constantly increasing list.

When you realize that vaccination dries up the mammary glands, and that almost without exception these 10,000 women had been vaccinated from one to three times before the age of puberty, is it not time to pause and consider?

The statistics of this one small firm is only the report of one out of several hundred doing business all over the country.

Some years ago a disease similar to smallpox or syphilis broke out among sheep in Scotland. As a preventative the sheep were vaccinated but in the course of a few years it was noticed that a great many ewes were unable to nourish their lambs. With the discontinuance of vaccination, this phenomenon disappeared.

Does this help to explain why nowadays over 50 percent of human mothers are incapable of nursing their babies?

For many ages, by means of mercury and iodine, syphilis and gonorrhea have been systematically suppressed so that today the entire civilized portion of the human family is more or less affected by these hereditary miasms.

Evidently constant suppression through many ages has developed these diseases in their present virulent types. This has been systematically accomplished ever since the time that Galen and the Arabian school of medicine substituted the symptomatic treatment of disease by drugs and mineral poisons for the Nature Cure treatment of the old Hippocratic School of medicine.

This explains why luetic diseases, in the civilized form, are unknown among peoples of the earth who do not practice suppression by drugs and operations.

"Why dwell so much upon indelicate subjects of this kind?" some of our lady readers may exclaim. Friends, if these things are good enough to put into your bodies and the bodies of your children, they are good enough to talk about.

Do you know how the wonderful vaccine virus is produced? Previous to Jenner's time, as above described, the product of smallpox sores was directly inoculated from one human being to another, but it was found that this resulted very often in the creation of smallpox in a most virulent form.

Jenner's scheme of using artificially produced cowpox virus had the advantage that the human smallpox and syphilitic poison was somewhat weakened or attenuated in the bodies of healthier animals.

Vaccine is manufactured at present in the following manner: some of the poisonous mass exuding from smallpox or vaccine sore on a human body is rubbed into incisions made in the loins of calves and cows. When the animal becomes covered with vaccine eruptions, the poisonous exudation from these sores is scraped off and prepared as vaccine.

In accordance with our fundamental law of cure which tells us that every inflammatory and feverish condition is a healing and purifying effort of Nature, the organism tries to throw off through the vaccination sores and ulcers, not alone the smallpox virus recently inoculated, but also all other hereditary and acquired miasms and poisons. Regular physicians recognize and apply this law in practice. When they apply *counter irritants* by blisters, Spanish flies, belladonna, cupping, fontanels, etc., they endeavor to remove the internal congestion and inflammation by creating an artificial one on the surface. The Nature Cure physician accomplishes the same thing in a more natural way by wet packs and cold ablutions.

In accordance with this law the ulcerous mass exuding from the vaccine sores contains the miasm, not only of smallpox, but of scrofula, psora, tuberculosis, syphilis, gonorrhea, anthrax, lumpy jaw and whatever else there may be of hereditary and acquired taints and poisons of the system. This nasty mess is then inoculated into millions of innocent victims of a scientific superstition.

When after a while scrofulous, syphilitic or itchy eczemata, swelling of glandular structures, etc., make their appearance in families, which before vaccination were free from these disorders, then people wonder where it all came from, where the poor child *caught it*. We have known fathers and mothers suspected and accused by the family physician of transmitting syphilis to their offspring when as a matter of fact the foul vaccine poison which the doctor himself had inoculated into the child was the real cause of the suspicious sores and eruptions.

It soon became evident that inoculation with the virus did not prevent smallpox, but on the contrary frequently caused it, and therefore the practice gradually fell into innocuous desuetude, to be revived by Jenner about 100 years later in a modified form.

"But," our opponents insist, "you cannot deny that smallpox has greatly diminished since the almost universal adoption of vaccination." Certainly the disorder has diminished but so has also diminished and in fact almost entirely disappeared the plague, the Black Death, cholera, bubonic plague, yellow fever, and numerous other epidemic pests which only recently decimated entire nations. Not one of these epidemics was treated by vaccination or any other form of preventative medicine.

"If vaccination protects at all it does so by creating in the body the smallpox disease in the chronic form." We have learned that having a disease in the chronic form means that the healing forces of the system are not strong enough to throw it off by means of an acute form of the same disease.

In accordance with our fundamental law of cure which tells us that every inflammatory and feverish condition is a healing and purifying effort of Nature, the organism tries to throw off through the vaccination sores and ulcers, not alone the smallpox virus recently inoculated, but also all other hereditary and acquired miasms and poisons.

Vaccination Villainous—It's Compulsion A Crime

by John W. Hodge, M.D.

The Naturopath and Herald of Health, XV (8), 465-467. (1910)

> The sophism of the Jenner-doctrine have, in fact, been so thoroughly exploded that the persistency of its defenders seems to imply a moral, rather than an aberration of a merit; in other words, the collapse of all other supports justifies the suspicion of the hideous fact that the organization of the cowpox syndicate rests upon the deliberate sacrifice of truth to business considerations and corporation interests. —F. L. Oswald, A.M., M.D.

In a recent communication to your columns I called attention to the great number of fatalities from tetanus (lockjaw) following vaccination, which had been reported in the medical and secular press as having occurred during the months of November and December last.

This gruesome death-list, which reached into the hundreds, was for obvious reasons not presented in these columns. In commenting on this wholesale execution of healthy children by doctors who intentionally propagate a filth-disease (cowpox) under the pretense of sanitation, I pointed out the fact that vaccination with the medical faculty is a matter of business, and not one of philanthropy. I stated facts which justify the belief that the money value of vaccination is its only value. I cannot see that the vaccinators have any grounds whatever on which to justify their blood-poisoning operation. I held up to the public view the indisputable fact that all doctors who engage in the coxpoxing business have a pecuniary interest in the procedure which, I have reason to believe, acts as a powerful motive in shaping their opinions and practice in respect to this operation. Perhaps, through stupidity, mulish conservatism, or invincible ignorance, some few physicians may continue to believe in the efficacy of the cowpox procedure, yet, I feel confident that nearly all the doctors who are now engaged in the vaccine enterprise would quickly discard this terrible business of destroying the lives of numbers of healthy children and impairing the health of many others, were not their pecuniary interests so intimately interwoven with it. If it were possible to eliminate the commercial feature from the cowpox enterprise, it is my firm conviction that the consensus of medical opinion would soon declare against it, and the pathetic solicitude on the part of the vaccinists to guard the dear public against the alleged dangers of smallpox epidemics would soon be found drooping. The baby-slashers would go out of the cowpox business, and vaccination, like its congener, various inoculations, would quietly pass into the limbo to which other kindred medical superstitions have been relegated.

Basing my belief on an experience derived from having vaccinated several thousand victims, I am assured that if doctors who are now engaged in the cowpox enterprise were to be held pecuniarily responsible for the ill-effects which result from their vaccine operations, they would very soon abandon the merciless and pernicious practice. But so long as credulous dupes are found who are willing to bare their arms to the vaccine lancet and take the RISK of the operation for the benefit of the doctors, there will be plenty of vaccinators on hand to do this dirty work and take the FEE.

The vaccination practice pushed to the front on all occasions by a certain class of the medical profession, and through political connivance made compulsory by the State, has become not only a great menace to health of the rising generation, but also the most flagrant outrage upon the personal liberty of the American citizen. The inoculation superstition was the chief medical delusion of the eighteenth century.

With few exceptions medical men of that period defended smallpox inoculation and held it up to public attention as the great desideratum for the common welfare. The practice of this horrible medical doctrine spread smallpox broadcast, sent multitudes of victims to untimely graves, and permanently impaired the health of other multitudes.

In the eighteenth century the practice of inoculating healthy people with smallpox pus to *protect* them from smallpox was considered by the medical profession to be a great *blessing* to humanity. In standard medical works of that period the alleged value of various inoculations was always spoken of as one of the best established facts in medical science, just as vaccination is now spoken of by those who practice it.

And yet, alas for human prescience! What was proclaimed as the savior, proved to be the destroyer. In 1840 it was found necessary to make inoculation in England a crime in order to put an end to its use, yet, vicious as that practice proved to be, it was superseded, at the hands of the charlatan Jenner, by a fallacy quite as monstrous. The nineteenth century, notwithstanding its boasted civilization and its much vaunted scientific acquirements, was nearly as much cursed by the vaccinators as was the eighteenth by the doctors who inoculated healthy people with smallpox pus.

The sophism of the Jennerian doctrine has been so thoroughly exploded that the persistence of its upholders seems to imply a moral rather than a mental aberration. In other words, the collapse of all other supports justifies the suspicion of the hideous fact that the organization of the cowpox practice will discard this lucrative enterprise even after they have been made fully aware of its utter uselessness as a prophylactic against smallpox, as well as of its pernicious effects on the lives and health of the rising generation.

Then, too, the connivers at the cowpox swindle dislike to confess that they have so long been duped by the milkmaid's tradition and led to ignore the real cause and neglect the true preventive of smallpox. Once committed to an error, it is amazing with what conservative persistence the medical profession will continue to cling to it. To abandon as worthless or injurious, a measure once adopted as a great *blessing* would seem to be a tacit confession of fallibility and fallibility is a human defect which physicians, as a class, are very slow to admit.

The absurd and senseless dogma which assumes to conserve health by propagating disease is at variance with all established knowledge.

The introduction of the products, diseased animal tissues—miscalled calf lymph—into the circulation of healthy human body is contrary to the teachings of modern surgery and sanitary science, and has no justification in either science or common sense. The cowpox delusion was conceived in ignorance and born of superstition—a dairymaid's whim borrowed by Jenner and palmed off upon the credulity of the medical profession as a never-failing preventive of smallpox.

Since my last communication to the columns, Senator James Henry McCabe of New York City has introduced in our Legislature a compulsory vaccination measure which should be summarily killed by our legislators. Dr. McCabe is a physician, that is, a political doctor whose business combines medicine with politics. Dr. McCabe is also a vaccinist and represents the interests of the cowpox syndicate of New York. At the behest of the cowpox bullies, this politico-doctor would have all citizens subjected by law to the degrading rite of official blood poisoning, which has nothing to recommend it except the fees derived from it by the cowpox syndicate and medical boodlers.

All the compulsory vaccination laws which now disgrace our statue books have been lobbied through the Legislatures by political members of the medical profession. The root and inciting cause of all this vaccination tyranny centres in the inordinate love of money—the mad lust for gold. Money is the universal solvent. It is the symbol of everything which he longs for—power, privilege, office, emoluments, ease, luxury, flattery, respectability, etc. The love of money actuates members of every class, whether in law, theology, politics or trade; but it especially impels the medical vaccinator to plot against the liberty of the citizen, i.e., to reduce the citizen to a condition of dependence where tribute may be exacted of him by legal compulsion.

It is along these lines that members of the medical profession have lobbied Governments and Legislatures, and secured compulsory vaccination laws for which they promised the most and fulfilled the least of any corrupt ring that ever formed a league with the state or cursed a country—and all to *protect* our *dear people* from, an attack on smallpox.

Reader, friend, and fellow citizen, don't you believe that your protection ever occupied the smallest corner in the vaccinator's heart. He sows calf-lymph virus to reap a richer harvest today, and a richer harvest in the future. No question has recently more occupied the attention of sanitarians than that of our means of defense against the arrogations of the cowpox bullies.

Compulsory vaccination ranks with human slavery and religious persecution as one of the most mischievous outrages ever perpetrated on the rights of the human race. It might be seriously questioned if men have ever suffered at the hands of their fellow men a more unqualified evil. It would be difficult to name a redeeming tendency of the delusion that has caused the death of thousands of human beings and polluted the blood of millions of healthy children with the germs of loathsome diseases.

The system of compulsory vaccination is founded upon a hypothesis too preposterous for a moment's serious argument. It arose from the curious dogma that a healthy person is a focus of disease; and that not having been diseased (i. e., vaccinated) he would be the propagator of disease (smallpox) to those who had been diseased (vaccinated) and thus *protected*.

If vaccination protected the vaccinated, they would have no occasion to fear infection. While, if vaccination does not protect the vaccinated from taking smallpox from the unvaccinated, it is a monstrous fraud on human credulity. In either event the vaccinated have no reason to find fault. If they really believe that vaccination protects them, all is well, while if they do not so believe, then they have not the shadow of an excuse for forcing it upon others who do not believe. I venture to think that any logical mind will be able to grasp the force of this argument.

How true it is, that every wrong, in seeking to perpetuate its power, commits *felo de se* [suicide]. The surest way to destroy faith in the vaccination dogma was to resort to compulsion. The attempt to enforce repeated vaccinations upon those who were skeptical as to its value has aroused fierce opposition in every country in which it has been tried. An opposition which, having reason, truth, and history on its side, has conquered in Switzerland and England, and will surely triumph everywhere.

While submitting the above considerations to the readers of *The Naturopath*, I am aware that the policy of presenting medical questions to the general public is vehemently condemned in certain quarters, and attempts to create a priestly craft in medicine are as persistently encouraged. The Legislatures of our various States are annually besieged, in the interests of the cowpox syndicate, by politico-doctors of the McCabe stripe, whose aim is to establish by legislative enactment a medical priesthood, under the plea that the people are too ignorant to judge for themselves. I am not one of those physicians who sympathize with mysticism in medicine. I believe the more rational the public may become on these topics the better for themselves, for medical progress and for the profession.

Vaccination became a question of public policy when the first laws for its enforcement were enacted, and so long as people are taxed to support it, they have the common right of investigation. As a medical tenet they might readily leave it to medical authorities to dispose of, but when the ingenuity of the law is invoked to make it obligatory, and then the public have a right to know what they get for their money. I am, therefore, glad to serve as a medium of instruction. With that object in view I have written this letter.

In commenting on this wholesale execution of healthy children by doctors who intentionally propagate a filth-disease (cowpox) under the pretense of sanitation, I pointed out the fact that vaccination with the medical faculty is a matter of business, and not one of philanthropy.

Basing my belief on an experience derived from having vaccinated several thousand victims, I am assured that if doctors who are now engaged in the cowpox enterprise were to be held pecuniarily responsible for the ill-effects which result from their vaccine operations they would very soon abandon the merciless and pernicious practice.

The introduction of the products, diseased animal tissues— miscalled calf lymph—into the circulation of healthy human body is contrary to the teachings of modern surgery and sanitary science, and has no justification in either science or common sense.

All the compulsory vaccination laws which now disgrace our statue books have been lobbied through the Legislatures by political members of the medical profession.

If vaccination protected the vaccinated, they would have no occasion to fear infection. While, if vaccination does not protect the vaccinated from taking smallpox from the unvaccinated, it is a monstrous fraud on human credulity.

The Anti-Vaccination Crusade IV

by Henry Lindlahr, M.D.

Copyright by The Nature Cure Publishing Co., Chicago

The Naturopath and Herald of Health, XV (8), 489-492. (1910)

A few years ago I happened to attend a public clinic in a Chicago medical college. One of the patients before the clinic was a strong and healthy-looking German girl, about eighteen years of age. Though in general appearance a picture of health, her left hand was a horrible sight; the thumb and parts of the palm and inner hand were disfigured by tuberculous ulceration.

The family health history of this patient was excellent. On either side of the family for generations past there had been no sign of scrofulous or tuberculous diseases. Father and mother and a number of sisters and brothers were living in the best of health. The young woman herself had never in her life suffered with a serious ailment.

All attempts of the assembled students and professors to find a cause for the disease were futile. The sore on the hand had begun to develop about six months before this clinical examination. I approached the young woman, and on looking into her clear blue eyes discovered that the region of the iris corresponding to the upper left arm disclosed a large dark spot, enclosed by whitish lines, in diagnostic parlance, a *closed lesion*. Closed lesions in the iris correspond to scar tissue in the body. As long as a wound, ulcer or catarrhal defect is open and active in the body, it is represented in the iris by dark, blackish shadings. When the lesion in the body is healed and closed, this fact is recorded in the iris by the appearance of whitish lines and clouds in and around the dark shadings. Thus the *closed lesion* in the iris stands for the deposition of new tissues, or scar tissues, in the body.

The region in the iris of the young woman corresponding to the tuberculous hand exhibited whitish clouds of acute inflammatory activity. The scar sign in the region of the upper arm and the peculiar ulceration of the hand suggested to me at once the idea of vaccination. I addressed the patient as follows: "Not long ago, say within a year or two, you have been vaccinated on the left arm, and this was followed by a large ulcerating vaccination sore. The ulcer was cured by medical treatment." Somewhat surprised, she confirmed every part of my diagnosis. She related to us that a year ago, while coming from Germany on an ocean streamer, she had been vaccinated, and that from this developed a large, ugly-looking vaccination sore, which was very stubborn to heal, and which was treated for some time with salves from the drug store.

I then gave it as my opinion to the assembled clinic that the vaccination and the suppression of the resulting ulceration were the direct cause of the tuberculous process on the hand. My diagnosis created considerable hilarity among the allopathic students in attendance on the clinic. It seemed ridiculous to them that anything so thoroughly *orthodox* as vaccination could in any way be held responsible for such serious aftereffects, especially so when the sore of the hand did not appear until six months after the vaccination.

Replying to this objection, I asked why it is that luetic sores on the body and in the throat sometimes do not appear until six months after suppression of the original lesion on the genital organs has taken place, or why cancer does not develop in an organ affected by suppressed itch (as revealed in the iris of the eye) until many years after the suppression of the scabies or common itch disease?

To these questions, of course, orthodox medical science has no answer. The Dean of the college, a very liberal and discerning man, who was conducting this particular clinic, took my part in the controversy saying: "Dr. L. has given at least a very pertinent and plausible theory of this phenomenon, while you yourselves have not given any explanation whatsoever. Therefore gentlemen, please curb your hilarity and do some thinking."

We have met in our practice with many cases of tuberculosis, eczema, pernicious anemia, lockjaw, paralysis, etc., directly traceable to vaccination. The statistics of Anti-Vaccination Societies constantly report thousands of such cases.

In Chicago last year two deaths resulted from smallpox, while hundreds of serious diseases and fatalities could have been traced directly to vaccination. In most cases, however, the detrimental after-effects of vaccination are so insidious and obscure in their development that they are not easily traced back to their true cause—the smallpox or cowpox virus, but it remains for the *diagnosis from the iris of the eye to bring proof positive of these hidden "sequelae".*

Shortly after vaccination the color of the iris darkens, especially so in the regions corresponding to the digestive and respiratory organs. This darkening of the color is noticeable also in cases where according to common parlance vaccination has *not taken*. In fact, the latter persons often show in the eyes more serious *vaccination* defects than those who develop the regular sores. What does this mean? It means simply that in strict accordance with the fundamental laws of cure, those who develop vigorous vaccination ulcers expel through these the vaccine infection. But children who are already encumbered with scrofulous conditions and possessed of weak vitality are frequently not able to develop these purifying ulcerations, they retain the poisonous infection, and in such cases greater deterioration of the organism in general and of the digestive and respiratory tract in particular is the inevitable result.

The saddest part of it is that these unfortunate victims of a scientific superstition are vaccinated over and over again. The more the filthy poison is injected into their circulation, the less *it takes*, to the mystification of the medical fraternity.

A few days ago in the Chicago papers reported the case of a girl who had been vaccinated *ten times* without *results* and then admission to the public schools was refused to the child because she was *not properly vaccinated.*

Ten times the vaccination had *not taken.* How did the doctors know it had *not taken?* It is just possible that internally it had *taken* too much. The diagnosis from the eye probably would have revealed harmful effects. Just think of a little child inoculated ten times with the cowpox virus. Is not that sufficient to completely saturate the little body with the nasty tuberculous poison?

To recapitulate: Those with whom vaccination takes best have taken least of it. They usually succeed in expelling it, but those with whom apparently it has *not taken* may be the ones most seriously affected. The darkening of the digestive and respiratory tracts in the iris of the eye fully explains why vaccination is accountable for all kinds of chronic catarrhal conditions of stomach, bowels, liver, bronchi, throat, and pharynx; why catarrhal affections and decay of the tonsils, chronic bronchitis, pernicious anemia and tuberculosis have increased in every country after the introduction of compulsory vaccination.

Many diagnosticians from the eye claim that diphtheria in its present virulent form and frequency was not known before the introduction of vaccination—that diphtheria as we know it was first described in the year 1820, by Bretonneau, a physician of Tours, France, sometime after the introduction of vaccination—that diphtheria has followed vaccination faithfully from one country to another, and that today it is not known where smallpox virus has not polluted the blood and lowered the vitality of the people. Whether we accept in their entirety these radical charges or not, this much is certain—that diphtheria in its modern virulent form and frequency of occurrence was unknown in any country before the universal practice of vaccination.

This phenomenon is explained by the fact that the vaccination virus, according to the evidence given by the diagnosis of the eye, locates and concentrates principally in the mucous membranes of the bronchi, throat and pharynx. It lowers the vitality of these parts and charges them with the poisonous miasms and taints contained in the cowpox virus. Nature at the first opportunity makes an heroic effort to throw off the scrofulous encumbrance. This may happen when the next cold is *caught*—then the tonsillitis, pharyngitis or laryngitis becomes a genuine diphtheria.

Sometimes we are told that this or that child had diphtheria, but was never vaccinated.

To this we would answer that many times the diagnosis of diphtheria is incorrect. It is always safer for the physician to diagnose the more serious disease. When the case recovers the glory is so much greater. Then, also when vaccinated children produce the diphtheria bacilli in great numbers and pollute with them the air, why should not here and there an unvaccinated child succumb to the infection, especially when hereditarily their blood is contaminated with the vaccine virus back to the third and fourth generation?

It is amusing to note the confusion both of the public and of the scientific mind on the simplest questions of hygiene. The millionaire owner of a dozen palatial quick-lunch rooms in this city is so deeply concerned about the health of his patrons that at stated intervals, under penalty of discharge, he compels every one of his employees to be vaccinated, yet he does not see any wrong in dealing out to his customers wholesale dyspepsia and nervousness in the form of pie, tea and coffee. Where one person in this city dies with smallpox, probably hundreds die from the effects of the deadly Quick-Lunch Counter.

In most cases, however, the detrimental after-effects of vaccination are so insidious and obscure in their development that they are not easily traced back to their true cause—the smallpox or cowpox virus, but it remains for the diagnosis from the iris of the eye to bring proof positive of these hidden "sequelae".

But children who are already encumbered with scrofulous conditions and possessed of weak vitality are frequently not able to develop these purifying ulcerations, they retain the poisonous infection, and in such cases greater deterioration of the organism in general and of the digestive and respiratory tract in particular is the inevitable result.

Those with whom vaccination takes best have taken least of it. They usually succeed in expelling it, but those with whom apparently it has "not taken" may be the ones most seriously affected.

Nature at the first opportunity makes an heroic effort to throw off the scrofulous encumbrance.

Whether we accept in their entirety these radical charges or not, this much is certain—that diphtheria in its modern virulent form and frequency of occurrence was unknown in any country before the universal practice of vaccination.

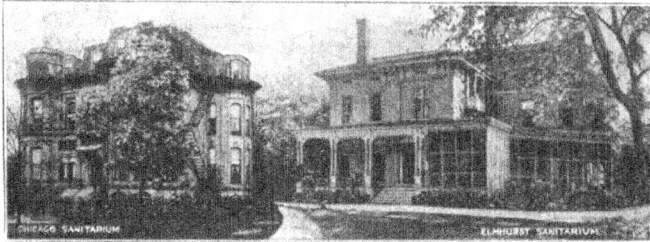

ANTI-VACCINATION LEAGUE OF AMERICA

The Naturopath and Herald of Health, XV (9), 549-550. (1910)

CONSTITUTION

ARTICLE I. NAME

This body shall be known as "THE ANTI-VACCINATION LEAGUE OF AMERICA".

ARTICLE II. OBJECTS

The object of this league shall be:

First—To promote the universal acceptance of this principle that health is Nature's greatest safeguard against disease and that, therefore, no State has the right to demand of anyone the impairment of his or her health.

Second—To take steps to secure the abolition of all oppressive medical laws, and to counteract the growing tendency to enlarge the scope of State medicine at the expense of the freedom of the individual.

Third—To carry on a campaign of education among the people with respect to the evil results of vaccination, including its effects in causing degeneration and in deteriorating the public health.

Forth— To hold an annual conference of members of the League, of delegates and representative of anti-vaccination societies in America, and of such individuals as are interested in the objects of this League.

Fifth—To adopt such means as may seem advisable and practicable to give aid and assistance to societies of individuals engaged in the movement for freedom from compulsory vaccination.

ARTICLE III. MEMBERSHIP

Section 1. All persons who shall have made application to the Secretary, and shall have declared in writing their sympathy with the objects of this League as expressed herein shall be enrolled by the Secretary as associate members of this League, subject to confirmation by the Board of Directors.

Section 2. Any associate member may become an active member of this League on payment of an annual fee of not less than one dollar, and subject to the approval of the Board of Directors.

Section 3. Local, State and Provincial Leagues, on payment of an annual fee of not less than five dollars, subject to the approval of the Board of Directors, may be admitted to this League. Every branch so admitted shall be entitled to three delegates to represent it at the meetings of the Anti-Vaccination League of America.

Section 4. Only active members and duly accredited delegates shall be entitled to hold office and to vote, but all members shall be entitled to attend and have a voice in the meetings of this League.

ARTICLE IV. OFFICERS

Section 1. The officers of this League shall consist of a President, five Vice Presidents, a Treasurer and a Secretary; the same to be elected at the annual meeting of this League and to perform the duties usually assigned to such officers.

ARTICLE V. MEETINGS

Section 1. This League shall meet annually, at a time and place to be determined by the Board of Directors. At least thirty days' notice of such meeting shall be given to all active members and affiliated bodies.

Section 2. The Board of Directors shall have power to call a conference of those interested in the objects of this League at any such time and place as it may see fit.

ARTICLE VI. AMENDMENTS

Section 1. This Constitution may be amended at any annual meeting of this League by a two-thirds vote of the members duly qualified to vote at said meeting, provided that notice of such amendment shall have been submitted in writing, by mail or otherwise, to all active members of this League at least fourteen days prior to said annual meeting.

Section 2. There shall be a Board of Directors, whose duties shall be to carry on the work of this League and to forward its objects *ad interim* between the annual meetings of this League.

BY-LAWS

Section 1. No liabilities shall be incurred by this League or its officers over and above such sums of money as are actually in custody at the time.

Section 2. The Board of Directors shall consist of the President, Vice-President, Treasurer, Secretary and nine other members to be elected at the annual meeting of this League.

Section 3. The Board of Directors may appoint Corresponding Secretaries to forward the objects of this League in their respective localities.

Section 4. The Board of Directors shall make a report of its actions to the annual meeting immediately following such actions.

Section 5. Ten active members and delegates attending any annual meeting shall constitute a quorum for the conduct of the business of this League at such annual meeting.

Section 6. In all matters not otherwise provided for in its Constitution and By-Laws, the proceedings of this League and of its officers and committees shall be governed by parliamentary law as laid down in "Robert's Rules of Order".

Section 7. Any or all of these By-Laws may be altered or amended, or added to by a majority vote at any annual meeting of this League

First—To promote the universal acceptance of this principle that health is Nature's greatest safeguard against disease and that, therefore, no State has the right to demand of anyone the impairment of his or her health.

Second—To take steps to secure the abolition of all oppressive medical laws, and to counteract the growing tendency to enlarge the scope of State medicine at the expense of the freedom of the individual.

Third—To carry on a campaign of education among the people with respect to the evil results of vaccination, including its effects in causing degeneration and in deteriorating the public health.

Vaccination and Cancer

by F. M. Padelford, M.D.

The Naturopath and Herald of Health, XV (11), 659-660. (1910)

That cowpox vaccination furnishes any immunity from smallpox is disputed, and this, too, by authorities whose scientific standing is second to none. Among those who do deny the value of the practice are: Prof. Alfred Russel Wallace, Dr. Adolph Vogt, professor of Hygiene and Sanitary Statistics in the University of Berne; Dr. Charles Creighton, author of exhaustive works on the subject; Dr. E. M. Crookshank, professor of Comparative Pathology and Bacteriology in King's College, London; Dr. Charles Ruata, professor of Materia Medica in the University of Perugia, and others whose names it is here unnecessary to state.

Regardless of verbal assertions to the contrary, practically every present day disciple of Edward Jenner believes that the immunity from smallpox which results from what is commonly known as vaccination is of comparatively short durations, probably two years or less.

For the sake of argument let us admit that for a period of not more than two years vaccination with the proper lymph—whatever this brand may be—will establish a relatively high degree of immunity from natural smallpox. But because this may be so, is it reasonable or just to demand that all children shall be subjected to the dangers which must exist if living germs of disease are introduced into their bodies?

By the prompt and rigid quarantine of such cases of smallpox as do occur, the vast majority of these little ones should be protected from exposure to the disease. Then when we vaccinate universally we are poisoning a race to protect a few from a malady whose ravages were never so great as to excite the alarm that now exists because of cancer.

It has long been suspected that vaccination might be an etiological factor in the causation of this fearsome complaint. While, as yet, direct proof that such is the case is lacking, much evidence has accumulated which seemingly shows that this fear is far from being unwarranted.

The published reports of the New York State Cancer Laboratory contain much that should be taken into account while this phase of the subject is under consideration.

In the *Sixth Annual Report*, on page 52, under the heading, "Cancer and the Acute Exanthemata",* the following may be found. (It should be noted that of all the diseases of this class only vaccinia and smallpox are mentioned as possessing any pathological similarity to the cancerous condition.)

"Although at first sight there would scarcely appear to be any relation between the cancerous process and the acute exanthemata, yet this

---

*Exanthemata is a skin rash that accompanies a disease or fever. *Ed.*

analogy between the two groups of diseases has been strongly advocated, principally by Bosc, Gaylord, Borrel, and von Wasielewski; the first two observers basing their advocacy on the ground of the similarity of some of the inclusions in the two processes, and Borrell and von Wasielewski on more general grounds."

"It will perhaps be of interest to follow more closely the relation which exists between the two processes. Those who discovered a resemblance between the inclusions found in cancer and those observed in smallpox and vaccinia were the first to call attention to the analogy between the two processes. It was Gorini, namely, who first detected points of similarity between certain larger forms of the vaccine body which had been previously described by L. Pfeffer, Guarnier, and Clarke, but Gorini was able to trace a gradual transformation between the larger typical vaccine bodies and these larger inclusions, which resemble the inclusions in cancer.

Sheep-pox is characterized by the development of both epithelial and connective tissue nodules in the subcutaneous tissue."

On page 62 of the report for 1900, it stated: "We found that the organism of vaccinia, while undergoing development, shows essentially the same phases we had already noted in the organism observed in fresh scrapings of cancer and in the peritoneal fluid and blood of cancer cases."

In the fourth report Dr. Gaylord states that "in one case of general carcinosis small amoeboid bodies were found in the blood immediately after it was withdrawn from the patient. These conformed very closely in appearance to similar bodies described by Pfeiffer and Reed in the blood of vaccinated children and monkeys".

J. Jackson, M.D., an English pathologist, is quoted as having written ten years earlier that, according to his experience, "Every parasitic form which occurs in vaccinia occurs also in cancer".

These facts will be regarded as significant or not according to the bias of the individuals who reads them. They certainly justify a suspicion that while there may not be any direct relationship between vaccination and cancer, yet the practice of inoculating generation after generation with the complex product known as vaccine lymph may ultimately so modify the metabolic processes that cancer is likely to develop.

To prove that this is so should not be required of those who oppose the operation. But to prove that it is not so should certainly be demanded of those who would and do compel it.

Vaccination is an experiment. The practice originated in a superstition of ignorant people, and during the century and twelve years that it has endured it has caused an endless amount of sickness, of suffering, and of death.

From the beginning its advocates have exaggerated its value, denied its dangers, and concealed it disastrous results. When its value has been questioned, they have offered generalities in place of facts, and have resorted to both ridicule and abuse. Why?

The Homoeopathic Recorder
Fall River, Massachusetts

Then when we vaccinate universally we are poisoning a race to protect a few from a malady whose ravages were never so great as to excite the alarm that now exists because of cancer.

"It will perhaps be of interest to follow more closely the relation which exists between the two processes. Those who discovered a resemblance between the inclusions found in cancer and those observed in smallpox and vaccinia were the first to call attention to the analogy between the two processes.

They certainly justify a suspicion that while there may not be any direct relationship between vaccination and cancer, yet the practice of inoculating generation after generation with the complex product known as vaccine lymph may ultimately so modify the metabolic processes that cancer is likely to develop.

Vaccination is an experiment. The practice originated in a superstition of ignorant people, and during the century and twelve years that it has endured it has caused an endless amount of sickness, of suffering, and of death.

PUBLIC HEALTH TRACTS

by Benedict Lust, N.D.

The Naturopath and Herald of Health, XV (11), 661-662. (1910)

Vaccination or Sanitation? The question of the hour!

Dr. Edward Jenner discovered (as is said) that vaccination, once performed with one mark, prevented smallpox for life.

—*The people found that it did not.*

The doctors then discovered that vaccination, with four good marks, prevented smallpox for life.

—*The people find that it does not.*

The doctors next discovered that vaccination, if properly done, mitigated smallpox.

—*The people find that it does not.*

The doctors afterwards discovered that re-vaccination would prevent smallpox, if efficiently or successfully performed.

—*The people find that it does not.*

The doctors then discovered that efficient vaccination in infancy, and successful re-vaccination at the age of fourteen, prevented deaths from smallpox.

—*The people find it otherwise.*

The doctors found that vaccination was the means of communicating serious and loathsome disorders such as skin disease, scrofula, syphilis and leprosy.

—*The people had already made the same discovery.*

The doctors have discovered that arm-to-arm vaccination has lost its protective virtue and are recommending vaccination from the calf, and in India from the buffalo and donkey.

—*The people say that vaccination cannot lose a protective virtue it never possessed.*

The doctors, in a desperate effort to reinstate a mischievous and discredited system, are, as a last resort, recommending "glycerinated" vaccine virus.

—*The people declare that this is only a new imposture.*

The doctors discovered that a smallpox panic is a golden shower to them in the shape of vaccination fees and medical attendance on the re-vaccinated sufferers.

—*Which the people cannot deny.*

The doctors have discovered that in order to keep up vaccination, the articles of the vaccine creed must be continually changed.

—*The people find the same.*

The doctors are threatening to inoculate us against cholera, hydrophobia, consumption and diphtheria, by means of foreign lymph, antitoxins and viruses, all of which are disease products.

—*The people ask, is it all for money?*

The doctors found that the people would not submit to vaccination without coercion by fines, seizure of goods, or imprisonment.

—*From which oppression the people demand deliverance.*

The people find that smallpox is not to be got rid of by mixing cowpox with the blood, but by making homes healthy.

—The doctors aver that they have found to the contrary.

The people are discovering that defective drainage, overcrowding, badly constructed dwellings, ill-ventilation, un-wholesome food and deficient water supply are the exciting causes of smallpox epidemics.

—The doctors must be compelled to make the same discovery.

Any medical theory which sets aside the laws of health and teaches that the spreading of natural or artificial disease can be advantageous to the community is misleading, mischievous, and opposed to common sense. Any teacher, whatever his assumption of authority, title or degree, who inculcates such doctrine, is a perverter of common sense and an enemy of the human race. The first duty of a parent is to protect his offspring and to resist every attack upon their health at any and every cost, no matter from what quarter it may come. How long will our feelings of justice and right permit us to submit to have our children's blood poisoned, in order that the claim of medical infallibility may be saved, and medical domination may be upheld?

Any medical theory which sets aside the laws of health and teaches that the spreading of natural or artificial disease can be advantageous to the community is misleading, mischievous, and opposed to common sense. Any teacher, whatever his assumption of authority, title or degree, who inculcates such doctrine, is a perverter of common sense and an enemy of the human race.

How long will our feelings of justice and right permit us to submit to have our children's blood poisoned, in order that the claim of medical infallibility may be saved, and medical domination may be upheld?

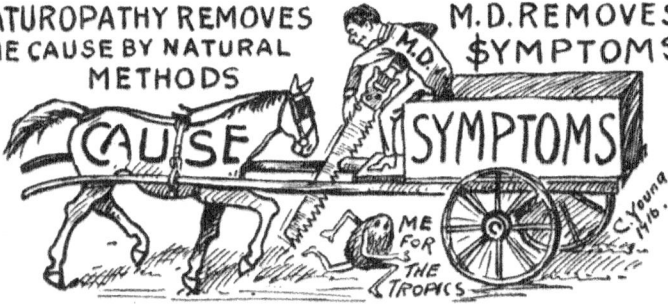

1911

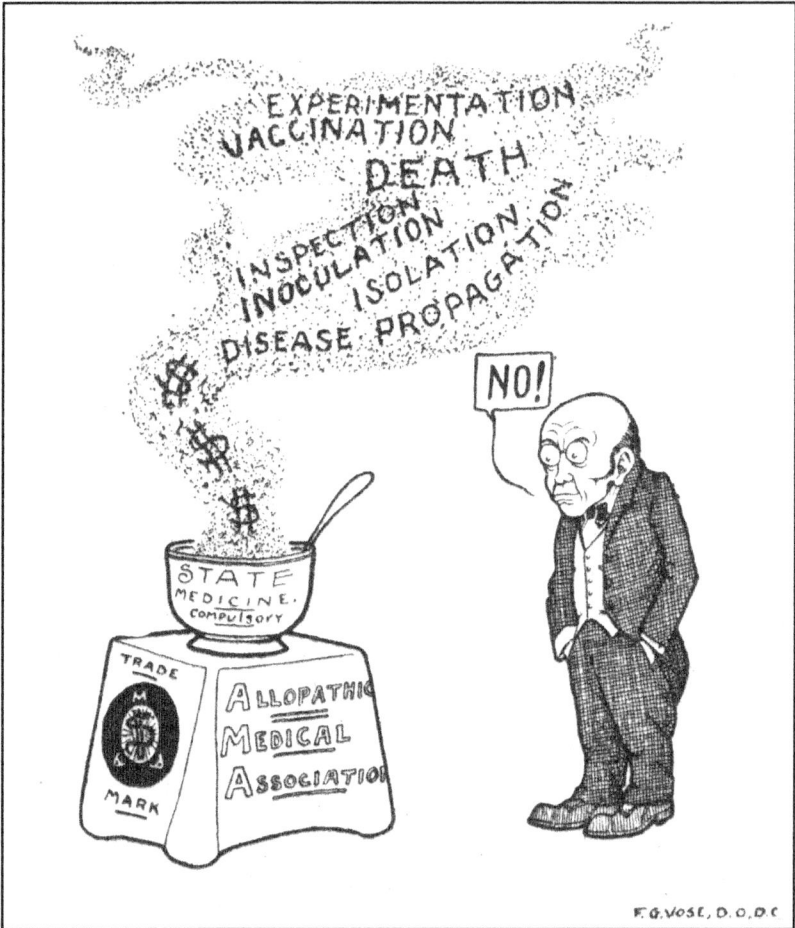

How Smallpox Was Banished From Leicester

by John W. Hodge, M.D.

The Naturopath and Herald of Health, XVI (1), 26-33. (1911)

A stereotype assertion which is a frequent requisition with doctors addicted to the vaccine practice and emoluments is that "vaccination prevents smallpox; that nothing else does". In the following pages I propose to prove that both these assertions falsify the facts.

The assertion that vaccination prevents smallpox is an assumption; that smallpox has been prevented without resort to vaccination is a fact. That smallpox can be readily and effectively controlled and spread in a populous municipality prevented without recourse to *preventive* vaccination has been clearly and repeatedly demonstrated on a large scale for a long period of time in the town of Leicester, England.

Thirty Years Of Rapidly Decreasing Vaccination In Leicester And The Lesson It Teaches

The big manufacturing town of Leicester with her resident population of 250,000 denizens affords most conclusive proof of the utter uselessness and the actual perniciousness of so-called protective vaccination.

The experience of Leicester has furnished evidence so convincing and conclusive against vaccination that vaccinating doctors, Health Board officials and vaccine manufacturers carefully avoid dealing with it except to prophesize evils for Leicester which have never come to pass.

Before me are the official government records of this big manufacturing town which show that from 1853 down to the year 1872 Leicester was one of the most completely vaccinated towns in the British Kingdom, the number of vaccinations owing to the alarm after severe epidemics of smallpox, having several times exceeded the number of recorded births. During the years which immediately proceeded the year 1871, 95 percent of the births of Leicester were officially recorded as having been satisfactorily vaccinated. Yet, in 1871, when at the very height of her good vaccination record, Leicester was rudely attacked by an epidemic of smallpox with extreme severity, its deaths from this disease during that year numbering more than 3,500 per million of population, or about a thousand per million more than the smallpox mortality of unsanitary London during the same epidemic. If ever a crucial test-experiment existed, it was that of Leicester, in which an almost completely vaccinated community suffered far more from smallpox than did poorly vaccinated and terribly unsanitary London with her crowded slum-population on the average of the last forty years of the eighteenth century.

LEICESTER LEARNS A WHOLESOME LESSON AND STRAIGHTWAY THROWS OFF THE GALLING COWPOX YOKE

The fearful mortality from smallpox in completely vaccinated and presumably well protected Leicester during the years 1871-1872 had the effect of destroying the people's faith in protective vaccination. The result was that poor and rich alike, the toilers, the aristocrats and the municipal authorities began to refuse vaccination for their children and themselves. This refusal continued until 1899 when, instead of 95 percent, the vaccinations reached only about 5 percent of the total births. As evidence of the rapidity with which vaccination fell off, it may be stated that of the children born in Leicester during the eight years ending in 1895, only three percent were vaccinated, as is shown by the official records. As this ominous decrease of vaccination went steadily on despite the compulsory vaccination acts, the pro-vaccinists gravely prophesied again and again that, once smallpox contagion gained entrance to this unvaccinated municipality with its great mass of *highly inflammable material,* the *dread disease* would spread through the town like wild fire on a prairie and would surely *decimate* (that's the word) the population. But alas for medical prescience and professional wisdom dire predictions of the boomers of Dr. Jenner's quack-nostrum proved to be but silly croakings.

Smallpox has been introduced into unvaccinated Leicester again and again, but it has never spread beyond a few mild cases, and from the day she abandoned vaccination to this no other town in the British Kingdom of approximately equal population has had so low a mortality from smallpox as has this almost completely unvaccinated and, as the pollutionists contend, *unprotected* population. From the time at which vaccination was first abandoned to the present, the annual death-rate from all causes in Leicester has fallen from about 25 per thousand in the five years ending in 1875, to about 14 per thousand in the five years ending in 1906. The official report on the health of Leicester for 1909 gives the general death-rate for that year as 12.9.

The very high standard of public health attained by unvaccinated Leicester since her declaration of independence and the failure of smallpox, when introduced into the borough by vaccinated tramps, to make any serious headway among the unvaccinated denizens, together with the extreme mildness of the few cases of smallpox which did occur among the unvaccinated, proved to demonstrate the utter uselessness of vaccination as a preventative of smallpox.

Although, as heretofore stated, it has been for many years predicted by the vaccine hypothesists that the introduction of a case or two of smallpox into unvaccinated Leicester would operate like a spark in a powder-magazine, and an overwhelming calamity would be the inevitable result. Experience has completely falsified all these ominous predictions and entirely upset the Jennerian theory that smallpox is especially dangerous to the unvaccinated. Surely the experience of unvaccinated Leicester has clearly demonstrated that vaccination, if it does anything at all, increases liability to smallpox, and renders it more fatal, and that the only effective plan by which to abolish the *dread disease* (smallpox) from a municipality is to do as Leicester did. This is: abandon vaccination and devote attention and energy to sanitation and to the isolation of such few cases of smallpox as are wont to occur in the absence of *preventative* vaccination. The happy experience of this great and populous borough in its dealings with smallpox during the past 38 years should be all sufficient to carry the conviction to any logical and unbiased mind that *preventative* vaccination is an absurd, senseless, futile and pernicious process. Yet, strange to tell, this wonderfully clear and conclusive test-experiment which proved beyond peradventure [perhaps] the utter uselessness and worse than uselessness of vaccine inoculation as a prophylactic measure against smallpox infection goes unheeded and ignored by the self-serving partisans of the Jennerian doctrine, who as a class seems to be either phenomenally stupid and grossly ignorant, or else willfully blind to the true history of the effects of vaccination. Any doctor addicted to the vaccine practice who has not studied these decisive statistics on this subject of vital importance to the whole human race, is guilty of culpable negligence and is not entitled to hold an opinion on the subject of vaccination. Any candidate for election to a State Legislature who has not devoted the necessary time required for the careful study of the cases of Leicester and Japan, but is ready to vote for coercive legislation for the enforcement of this disease transmitting practice upon those who know infinitely more of the question than he does, is an incompetent, utterly unworthy the support of any intelligent self-respecting constituency. Regrettable as it is to have to say it, there have been many such candidates elected to our State Legislatures.

C. K. Millard, M.D., medical officer of health of Leicester, who is an avowed adherent of the Jennerian doctrine, read a paper on "The Leicester Method of Dealing with Smallpox" before the Incorporated Society of Medical Officers of Health on March 10, 1904. From Dr. Millard's paper, which was published in July, 1904 issue of *Public Health*, I quote the following extract: "The people of Leicester, by abandoning compulsory vaccination, have taken the law into their own hands, and have set expert medical opinion at defiance; but that is no reason why we should refuse to study their experiment and learn from it all we can." (Vide, *Public Health*, July 1904, p. 627)

In this *Report on the Smallpox Epidemic in Leicester in 1903*, at page 10, Dr. Millard says: "The name of Leicester has come to be inseparably connected with the agitation against compulsory vaccination, and in no other large town have the vaccination laws been so completely set at defiance. For the last 20 years, in fact, they have been practically a 'dead issue', all attempts at compulsion having been openly abandoned. Prior to that period, however, Leicester ranked as a well-vaccinated town."

During the quinquennium (1872-1876) when Leicester was a well-vaccinated town, the general average death-rate from all causes was 25.18. The population of the borough at that time was less than 100,000. During the last 35 years the general death-rate in Leicester has steadily decreased, *pari passu*, with the decrease in vaccination, until at the time of the annual report for 1908 it had reached the phenomenally low figure of 12.98, while in 1909 it had fallen to 12.90. Leicester's population in 1909 numbered nearly 250,000.

It is therefore seen that well-vaccinated Leicester of 1872-1876 had a general death-rate almost double that of unvaccinated Leicester of 1909, although the population had nearly trebled since 1876.

Since vaccination was abandoned in Leicester the infant mortality in the borough has been steadily decreasing until it reached in 1908 the unprecedentedly low figure of 129.7 per 1,000 births.

This control-experiment by vaccinated Leicester, a town which has for a quarter of a century been declared by the partisans of the vaccine nostrum to be "a nidus for smallpox to settle in and propagate itself", had demonstrated beyond cavil that vaccination is not only wholly unnecessary and utterly useless as an anti-variolous measure, but also that it is actually pernicious and disastrous in its effects upon the public health. Dr. Millard tells us that "Vaccination reached its lowest point in Leicester in 1895, when only 75 vaccinations were registered out of 5,000 births." This means that only 15 children out of every 1,000 born in Leicester were vaccinated. Dr. Millard says: "The last census taken showed that there were over 80,000 unvaccinated people in Leicester, consisting principally of children and young adults. In accordance with the Jennerian doctrine that the vaccinal condition of a community is the predominant factor in determining the incidence of smallpox and the severity of the disease, prophesies have been freely and confidently made as to the disastrous consequences which would surely and speedily follow on what the late Dr. Ernest Hart called Leicester's *gigantic experiment*.

Retribution in the shape of a dire epidemic and a terrible *massacre*, especially of the children, has been repeatedly and blatantly prognosticated by the wise wigs of old school physic; but up to the present time these grave prognostications have not only all been unfulfilled, but, on the contrary, Leicester, since having thrown off the cowpox yoke, has enjoyed a phenomenal immunity from smallpox unequalled and unapproached by any well-vaccinated municipality of its approximate size in the world.

On page 8 of his official "*Report on the Smallpox Epidemic of Leicester in 1904*", Dr. Millard says: "Probably the most noteworthy feature of the epidemic was the very mild cases of the disease as evidenced by its remarkably low fatality, only four cases proving fatal, which is equivalent to a fatality on 321 cases of only 1.24 percent. Such a record is, I believe, almost unique. However, one of the four fatal cases was an imported one—the child of a tramp—which was not infected in Leicester, merely happening to sicken with the disease whilst passing through the town. "Such a small loss of life," observed Dr. Millard, "is of course very satisfactory and is all the more remarkable as occurring in Leicester where such a large proportion of the population is unvaccinated."

Think of a case-fatality from epidemic smallpox of less than one percent in a populous town which has repudiated Jenner's quack-nostrum more than a quarter of a century previously and has persistently rejected it ever since!

When the smallpox epidemic of 1904 struck Leicester, had it been a well-vaccinated borough as it was in 1871, when 95 percent of the births were cowpoxed, what high-sounding encomiums would have been lavished upon the memory of the "immortal" Jenner and his great *life-saving discovery.*

The Unvaccinated Not A Source Of Danger

On page 12 of this same official report, under the sub-caption, "School Infection", Dr. Millard says:

> In view of the fact that over 80 percent (probably nearly 90 percent) of the children attending the public elementary schools in Leicester have never been vaccinated, and that school attendance, as is well known, provides, very favorable conditions for the spread of infection, it was certainly to have been expected that considerable spread of the disease would have occurred amongst children infected at school. Fortunately, however, such was not the case.

"It will be recollected," adds Dr. Millard, "this in the 1903 epidemic there was also surprisingly little infection through the medium of schools. On the other hand, *great spread took place through the medium of slight cases which had escaped detection,* and such cases occurred in *vaccinated subjects.*" (The italics are mine.)

From the above official statement of a defender of vaccination it is obvious that the *vaccinated, not the unvaccinated,* constituted the real element of danger in the spread of smallpox. Here we have the recorded admission of an unflinching defender of Jennerism that vaccination utterly defeated the principal objects it had intended to accomplish, namely, the prevention of smallpox infection. In view of such testimony as this from the pen of a partisan of vaccination, what respect can intelligent people have for the ignorant and absurd dictum of the Jenner-bigots that "an unvaccinated school-pupil is a focus of infection and a menace to the public health"?

These experiences which were about the same in both the Leicester epidemics, which occurred long after vaccination had been abandoned, conclusively prove the absurdity of the pretense that "an unvaccinated child is a focus of infection", or "a menace to the community in which he resides". That vaccinated subjects constituted the principal element of danger and were the real foci of infection in both the above-mentioned epidemics of smallpox are thus frankly attested by a staunch advocate of the Jennerian rite in his official reports, as medical officer of health for Leicester.

As a characteristic specimen of the wild and haphazard assertions of the medical promoters of Jenner's quack-nostrum, I present the following extract from a classical work, entitled, *Vital Statistics*, by Charles Pearce, M.D., M.C.R.S.: "Sir Duminie Corrigan, M.D., when acting as one of the committee in 1871, on the Vaccination Act, said: 'An unvaccinated child is like a bag of gunpowder which might blow up the whole school, and ought not, therefore, be admitted to a school unless he is vaccinated.'" In my opinion this Dr. Corrigan is like a bag of wind which might blow up and blow out what little gray matter he has in his brain-pan. Bearing in mind the recorded experience of the 80,000 unvaccinated school-pupils in Leicester during the smallpox epidemics of 1903-4, what could appear more monstrously absurd than the above-quoted quixotic deliverance of an otherwise presumable sane physician? Dr. Corrigan's case furnishes an apt illustration of the peculiar state of mind under which the victims of the Jennerian delusion are laboring in their efforts to bolster up a discredited and waning cause. Is it not passing strange that a presumably intelligent physician, apparently sane on other subjects, should cherish the obvious delusion that a healthy child is dangerous to anybody by reason of its not having been vaccinated (diseased)?

As additional proof of the absurdity of the claims of the vaccine theorists, I again quote from Dr. Millard's report (page 6), the following extract: "It is a curious coincidence that in the two years, 1903 and 1904, in which the epidemics occurred, the general death-rate of Leicester was the lowest on record." Had the vaccine bigots been permitted in 1903 and 1904 to foist their disease-transmitting imposture upon the people of Leicester, who can believe that such happy results as were achieved without vaccination could have been possible with it?

SMALL MORTALITY AMONG THE UNVACCINATED

On page 19 of his official report of the 1904 epidemic in Leicester Dr. Millard tells us: "The loss of life caused by the epidemic was astonishingly small. There were only four deaths, one a man of broken-down habits, and three children; one of the latter was a baby five weeks old, and one was the child of a tramp. The last case did not belong to Leicester, and was not infected in Leicester, so that this death might fairly be deducted. There was also, I am pleased to say, very little disfigurement or injury produced by the disease in those who recovered, the great majority showing no scarring whatever. On the whole, therefore, Leicester is certainly to be congratulated on having once again escaped so lightly."

In view of these official data recorded and vouched for by an ardent defender of vaccination, what becomes of the time-worn assertion that vaccination, when it fails to protect from smallpox, renders that disease milder and less fatal? Where is the well-vaccinated and revaccinated population in the world that can boast of a case-fatality in a variolous epidemic of less than one percent, which was the rate in unvaccinated Leicester in 1904, a municipality having a population of about a quarter of a million? Will some obliging apologist for vaccination kindly tell us what it was that made smallpox so *mild* and *manageable* in unvaccinated Leicester? Will some promoter of the Jennerian delusion please refer us to some *well-vaccinated* population which can boast of a smallpox fatality-rate so "astonishingly small" as that of *unvaccinated* Leicester? In view of Leicester's experience, what becomes of the stock-argument of the provaccinists that vaccination mitigates smallpox? Leicester's experiment flatly belies every claim that has ever been trumped up for vaccination as a preventative or a mitigant of smallpox and proves beyond peradventure [perhaps] that the vaccine practice is worse than useless except for the purpose of supplying doctor fees and furnishing business for undertakers.

In view of Dr. Millard's official statement that there was in Leicester "very little permanent disfigurement or injury produced by the disease in those who recovered", what becomes of the stock argument of the apostles of Jennerism that the disappearance of "pocked-marked faces" at certain periods of time was the result of protective vaccination? If pock-marked faces after epidemics of smallpox in an unvaccinated population are so rare, as Dr. Millard tells us they have been in Leicester, how do the vaccine theorists account for the rarity of cases of facial blemish in the absence of vaccination? Had vaccination been in vogue in Leicester at the time referred to, it would have been credited by its shifty advocates with the mighty achievement of having averted the dreaded facial disfigurement incident to modified smallpox.

In his official report Dr. Millard further says: "Leicester, as we have seen, is a notoriously badly vaccinated community, and probably contains a larger proportion of unvaccinated persons than any other large town." (*Public Health,* July 1904, p. 614)

In reference to the Leicester epidemic of 1904, Dr. Millard says: "The money-cost of the epidemic to the rates was probably not much more than would have to be spent *every year*, if vaccination and re-vaccination were systematically carried out on the whole healthy population." (Loc. Cit., p. 626)

Such a damaging admission, coming from the mouth of a medical man pledged to vaccination and presiding over the health department of a populous municipality which more than a quarter of a century ago discarded vaccination and has persistently refused it ever since, is pretty conclusive testimony against the contention of his fellow-vaccinists who assume that the prevalence which smallpox would attain in the absence of vaccination would bring to them far greater pecuniary profit than vaccination does. The experience of unvaccinated Leicester flatly confutes the preposterous claim of the disease-inoculators that health can be conserved by the propagation of disease.

Dr. Millard tells us further that "in Leicester during the twenty-four years that notification has been in force, the average annual number of smallpox cases has been only thirty-seven. The average number of children born annually has been 5,000, so that (allowing for probable deaths) at least 8,000 vaccinations (including re-vaccinations) to prevent thirty-seven cases of smallpox." (Loc. Cit.) Even if vaccination were a certain preventive of smallpox, think of the glaring absurdity of imposing more than 216 disease-imparting operations upon healthy people to prevent one case of smallpox! What an act of insanity it would be to implant the infective products of undefined disease into the bodies of 8,000 healthy children in order to prevent the possible development of a very few mild cases of smallpox! Could absurdity go further than this?

Last year I received from Dr. Millard, medical officer of health for Leicester, a copy of his then last (1908) official report. In prefacing this report, Dr. Millard says: "The retrospect is on the whole a satisfactory one, the death-rate being only 12.98 per 1,000. A comparison with other great centres of population continues to be very favorable to Leicester. During the ten years (1898-1907) only one town in the kingdom had a lower average death-rate than Leicester."

On page 26 of the same official report, Dr. Millard tells us that in Leicester "compulsory vaccination had practically been all but abolished", and that "there has in 1908 been a decrease in the number of vaccinations as compared with previous years". He remarks that "during the year (1908) no cases of smallpox have occurred in Leicester".

From Dr. Killick, who still holds the position of medical officer of health for Leicester, I have just received his last report upon the health of Leicester for the year 1909. From page 27 of this report I quote the following extract: "The disease (smallpox) did not appear in Leicester during 1909 and it is now three years since the last case was reported and five years since a death from smallpox occurred in Leicester." As the experience of Leicester during the epidemics of 1903 and 1904 was very different from what had been expected by many people, and as it has an important bearing upon the vexed question of the necessity of compulsory vaccination, it may be well to quote the figures of the epidemics. In the 1903 epidemic there were 394 cases of smallpox with 21 deaths, yielding a case-mortality of 5.3 percent.

In the 1904 epidemic there were 321 cases, with 4 deaths, yielding a case mortality of only 1.2 percent. Several of our large cities suffered from more or less extensive epidemics about this period, but in none other was there such a low case-mortality as 1.2 percent recorded. In view of the large proportion of unvaccinated persons in Leicester such a result is especially remarkable." Thus does unvaccinated Leicester continue to maintain her enviable position in the fore-front rank as one of the two healthiest great manufacturing towns of the British possessions? Since having abandoned the Jennerian rite, Leicester has uninterruptedly enjoyed greater immunity from smallpox and has a lower death-rate therefrom than any well-vaccinated great centre of population in the world into which smallpox has gained admission. The experience of unvaccinated Leicester is an eye-opener to the people and an eye-sore to the pro-vaccinists all over the world. Here is a great manufacturing town, having a population of nearly a quarter of a million, which has demonstrated by a crucial test of an experience extending over a period of more than a quarter of a century that an unvaccinated population has been far less susceptible to smallpox and far less afflicted by that disease since it abandoned vaccination than it was at a time when 95 percent of its births were vaccinated and its adult population well re-vaccinated. More than this, Leicester's death-rate from all causes has been greatly reduced since vaccination was abandoned. If for the sake of argument it be conceded that vaccination is capable of protecting its subjects from smallpox infection for a period of a few years, I submit to any intelligent, fair-minded physician that "the Leicester method of dealing with smallpox", a method in which notification, isolation, quarantine, disinfection and sanitation are key-notes, having proved itself quite sufficient for the control of epidemic smallpox without resort to general vaccination, is a far more ideal method of prophylaxis and one infinitely more in accord with the recognized principles of preventative medicine, hygiene and sanitary science than the generally practiced system of "stamping out" a little smallpox by "stamping in" a great deal of vaccinia.

Epitomized Statement Of Leicester's Experience With Smallpox And Vaccination

The case of Leicester, which is of world-wide interest, may be summarized as follows:

1. In 1872 with a population of less than 100,000, Leicester had several thousand cases of smallpox, 346 of which cases resulted fatally, notwithstanding a high vaccinal average of about 95 percent of the total births for the immediately preceding quinquennial period, as shown by the official record.

2. The annual average death-rate at that period for all ages from all causes was 27 per thousand, and from the seven principle infectious diseases (including smallpox) was over 8,000 per mil-

lion. With such overwhelming proof of the absolute uselessness of vaccine inoculation as a prophylactic measure against small-pox, vaccination began to fall into disfavor and disuse with the people of Leicester.

3. Concurrently with increasing vaccinal default and the carry-ing out of sanitary measures the general death-rate in Leices-ter steadily declined and the number of smallpox cases soon became infinitesimally small. During the last few years the gen-eral death-rate has averaged about 14 per thousand per annum, and in 1905, 13.4 per thousand while in 1908 it was only 12.98 and in 1909 only 12.90 per thousand, so that most unhealthy, now ranks among the healthiest and cleanest of the great manu-facturing towns of the British Kingdom.

4. This astonishing hygienic progress and remarkably low fatality-rate in Leicester are largely attributable to a declining infantile mortality, which has during the last thirty-three years fallen from an average of over 240 deaths per 1,000 births, with a higher percentage of infantile vaccination (1868-1872), to less than 150 deaths per 1,000 births in 1905 and 126.6 in 1909. During last year but 660 of the 250,000 citizens of Leicester were vaccinated. This means that only one out of every 378 persons was vaccinated.

5. None of the credit for this improved state of affairs can be fairly ascribed to vaccination, seeing that during the fourteen years, 1891 to 1904, primary vaccination amounted to only about 5 percent of the recorded births, and scarcely any re-vaccinations were performed. In the year 1909 the vaccinations in Leicester amounted to but 12.1 of the births registered.

6. An unvaccinated child-population of vaccination-age of between 80,000 and 100,000 remains in the town, declares Dr. Millard in his official report.

7. Although smallpox has been frequently imported into Leicester, it has failed to *decimate* this alleged *inflammable material*, and the people have the utmost confidence in *the Leicester system* of sanitation, notification, isolation and disinfection, which—without recourse to vaccination—has served them so well for so long a period of time.

8. As proof of their great abhorrence of vaccination, I may state that thousands of otherwise law-abiding and blameless citizens of Leicester have submitted to insult, fine and imprisonment rather than submit their children to the Jennerian imposture. The homes of defaulters, who were unable to pay repeated fines for their very natural and proper resistance to their cruel and despotic law, have been seized and sold. Millions of pounds

of the public funds have been squandered on this useless and mischievous medical fallacy.

9.   At the present writing the official records show the names of more than 15,000 parents in Leicester who are legally liable to be summoned to court. The feeling of repugnance against vaccination is stronger in Leicester to-day than ever before.

10.   Leicester stands out conspicuously at the present day, a shining example to the whole world of the fact that prophylaxis against smallpox is to be realized through the attainment of health by means of personal hygiene, isolation and municipal sanitation and not by the inoculation of diseased products of man and beast into the healthy human body. Whereas, the legitimate aim of therapeutics is to restore the sick to a state of health, and that of hygiene to maintain our bodies in a state of health by right living and salubrious environment, vaccination undertakes the absurd and dangerous experiment of modifying our robust, healthy bodies in order to adapt them to an insalubrious environment.

Niagara Falls, N.Y.

The people of Leicester, by abandoning compulsory vaccination, have taken the law into their own hands, and have set expert medical opinion at defiance; but that is no reason why we should refuse to study their experiment and learn from it all we can.

Although smallpox has been frequently imported into Leicester, it has failed to decimate this alleged inflammable material, and the people have the utmost confidence in the Leicester system of sanitation, notification, isolation and disinfection, which—without recourse to vaccination—has served them so well for so long a period of time.

Sir Duminie Corrigan, M.D., when acting as one of the committee in 1871, on the Vaccination Act, said: 'An unvaccinated child is like a bag of gunpowder which might blow up the whole school, and ought not, therefore, be admitted to a school unless he is vaccinated.'

What an act of insanity it would be to implant the infective products of undefined disease into the bodies of 8,000 healthy children in order to prevent the possible development of a very few mild cases of smallpox!

VACCINATION, A DANGEROUS OPERATION

by Samuel Saloman

The Naturopath and Herald of Health, XVI (3), 170-173. (1911)

Vaccination is becoming more and more a vital public question. Many of those who have in the past submitted without protest to the operation have in the last few years made inquiries into the matter, with the inevitable result that in those sections where the practice is not compelled by the law, vaccination is becoming more and more neglected. In those communities cursed by compulsory vaccination laws, protests from individuals and organizations are being heard against the practice, growing louder and louder as the repeated failures of vaccination and the dangers inherent in the operation are coming to view, and public-spirited, liberty-loving citizens are everywhere bending their every effort to have such pernicious legislation repealed. Where such is for the moment impossible, individuals are resorting to every possible expedient to evade the law.

To reassure the public, circulars are issued by the Boards of Health, national as well as local, setting forth the seriousness of smallpox as an epidemic disease, the certain prevention of such disease through vaccination and revaccination, and the harmlessness of such operation.*

A considerable amount of literature has also been issued by those on the other side of the question, discussion of the question in the press and on the platform is had wherever possible, and the public no longer lacks, or should lack, full information concerning vaccination.

Without wishing in any way to disparage the efforts of antivaccinists, many of whom have suffered severely by reason of their outspoken convictions; it seems that full opportunity has not been taken of most damaging admissions as to vaccination by leading medical men in their published works, in the columns of medical periodicals, and in government documents and reports. What should make such statements of particular value to anti-vaccinists is the fact that the authors thereof place implicit confidence in the practice.

Particularly valuable in this respect is Osler's *Practice of Medicine*, employed as a textbook in leading medical colleges. Dr. William Osler, for years honorary professor of medicine at Johns Hopkins University, now *regius* professor of medicine at Oxford University, looked up to everywhere as one of the fixed stars in the medical firmament, warmly defends vaccination at every opportunity, yet his book, above mentioned, only bristles with antivaccinist arguments. Dr. Osler, it will be remembered, is he who issued this alleged humorous challenge to the "Priests of Baal,"

---

*There is a current internet campaign to sanitize vaccination with popups alluding to the harmlessness of vaccines. —Ed.

the British antivaccinists, at Edinburgh on July 3d of last year, I will go into the next severe epidemic with ten selected vaccinated persons and ten selected unvaccinated persons. I should prefer the latter—three members of Parliament, three anti-vaccination doctors, if they could be found, and four anti-vaccination propagandists. And I will make this promise—neither to jeer nor to jibe when they catch the disease, but to look after them as brothers, and for the four or five who are certain die, I will try to arrange the funerals with all the pomp and ceremony of an anti-vaccination demonstration."

As to the above, according to the *Vaccination Inquirer* (British) of August 1, 1910: "A somewhat similar challenge was made by the Leith medical officer of health a year or two ago. It was immediately accepted, and that was the end of the matter."

As to the value of vaccination as a preventive of smallpox, Osler says:

Sanitation cannot account for the diminution in smallpox and for the low rate of mortality. Isolation, of course, is a useful auxiliary, but it is no substitute. Vaccination is not claimed to be an invariable and permanent preventative of smallpox, but in the immense majority of cases successful inoculation renders a person for many years insusceptible.

This is, of course, contrary to the teachings of history, wherein is shown that vaccinated communities, all other conditions being equal, suffered as severely from smallpox as communities where vaccination was entirely neglected. Again, though he repeatedly employs the words "successful inoculation", he neglects to point out the way such success can be secured.

Under the [subheading] of Technique he states that "a person exposed to the contagion of smallpox should always be revaccinated", practically an admission that vaccination protects when there is no need of protection and fails to protect when the protective power of vaccination should be manifested. "This," he continues, "if successful, will usually protect but not always. The cases in which smallpox is taken within a few years of vaccination are probably instances of spurious vaccination." Revaccination, according to this artful medical dodger, will protect when it will protect and will not, when it will not; an explanation not especially illuminating. He, in common with provaccinists everywhere, takes advantage of the loophole of escape offered by claimed *spurious vaccination*. In other words, if a vaccinated person is brought in contact with smallpox and escapes infection, set his escape down to *successful* vaccination; if he takes the disease, put it down either to *unsuccessful* vaccination or to *spurious* vaccination.

As to whether vaccination is a harmless operation or not, Osler is a trifle more explicit. He is honest enough to admit that vaccination is not, as claimed, a harmless operation, accompanied by no more danger or discomfort than follows the scratch of a pin, but that "constitutional symptoms of a more or less marked degree follow the vaccination." The symptoms referred to are as follows:

> Usually on the third or fourth day the temperature rises, and may persist, increasing until the eighth or ninth day. There is a marked leukocytosis. In children it is common to have with the fever restlessness, particularly at night, and irritability, but as a rule these symptoms are trivial. If the inoculation is made on the arm, the axillary glands become large and sore; if on the leg, the inguinal glands.

This, as well as what follows, has reference to the operation of vaccination properly performed and with vaccine of unquestioned purity, if such can possibly be obtained. If you will take the trouble to look into the question of vaccine production, you cannot possibly escape the conclusion that it is not as easy to secure *pure* vaccine as it is to get undefiled filth.

Sometimes, according to the esteemed authority above referred to, far more serious results follow vaccination, in quite a few cases resulting in death or lifelong disease. Quoting further:

> It is not uncommon to see vesicles in the vicinity of the primary sore. Less common is a true generalized pustular rash, developing in different parts of the body, often beginning about the wrists and on the back. The secondary pocks may continue to make their appearance for five or six weeks after vaccination. In children the disease may prove fatal. They may be most abundant on the vaccinated limb, and usually occur about the eight or tenth day.

> Complications: In unhealthy subjects or as a result of uncleanliness, or sometimes injury, the vesicles inflame and deep excavated ulcers result. Sloughing and deep cellulitis may follow. In debilitated children there may be with this a purpuric rash. Acland thus arranges the dates at which the possible eruptions and complications may be looked for:
> 1. During the first three days: erythema, urticaria, vesicular and bullous eruptions, unvaccinated erysipelas.
> 2. After the third day and until the pock reaches maturity: urticaria, lichen urticatus, erythema multiforme, accidental erysipelas.
> 3. About the end of the first week: generalized vaccinia, impetigo, vaccinal ulceration, glandular abscess, septic infections, gangrene.
> 4. After the involution of the pocks: invaccinated diseases— for example, syphilis.

Quite a few complications, it must be admitted, to follow a supposed harmless operation. If the risk attending the operation were generally known, vaccination would not have the vogue it has to-day, even among those who implicitly believe in the cowpox delusion.

Referring to the possible transmission of some of the serious diseases through the agency of vaccination, Osler states that "syphilis has undoubtedly been transmitted by vaccination, but such instances are very rare". In this particular he differs from some of the greatest authorities on syphilis, who are of the opinion that vaccination has been responsible for more cases of syphilis than many imagined.

So, with tuberculosis, he states that "the risk of transmitting tuberculosis from the calf is so slight that it need not be considered". Yet in another paragraph, referring to the influence of vaccination on other diseases, he says "A quiescent malady may be lighted into activity by vaccination. This has happened with congenital syphilis, occasionally with tuberculosis."

Here is an admission that is most valuable to the cause of the anti-vaccinists for it is easy to prove that the diseases mentioned are most widespread, particularly tuberculosis. According to Von Bering, generally accepted as one of the leading tuberculosis authorities, tuberculosis is the most widespread of all diseases. That being the case, vaccination is the influence that light quiescent maladies like syphilis and tuberculosis into activity, the sooner we dim the light of vaccination the better it will be for humanity.

In the light of the facts above mentioned, it would seem that conscientious physicians would inquire fully into the history of the child and antecedents before vaccinating. It should not be necessary to state that such is very rarely the case. I happen to know of quite a few cases where the parent of the child informed the physician that vaccination might be prejudicial to the health of the child, that the child has been in poor health since birth, and has been laughed at for the information. The physician in such a case has nothing to lose. Looking at the matter from a material viewpoint, he has everything to gain. If serious complications follow the vaccination, due to any of the many causes before enumerated, it means a substantial sum in the physician's pocket as a result. Though Osler denies that syphilis and tuberculosis may be invaccinated—that is, generally—he concedes that tetanus (lockjaw) may be and undoubtedly is introduced into the system with the vaccine. He makes the positive statement that the vaccine pus may be impregnated with the germs of tetanus. As to that he says:

"McFarland has collected 95 cases, practically all American. Sixty-three occurred in 1901, a majority of which could be traced to one source of supply, in which R. W. Wilson demonstrated the tetanus bacillus. Most of the cases occurred about Philadelphia. Since that date McFarland tells me that very few cases have been reported. The occurrence of this terrible complication emphasizes the necessity of the most scrupulous care in the preparation of the animal virus, *as the tetanus bacillus is almost constantly present in the intestines of cattle.*" (Italics mine.)

If full confirmation is needed as to the above, it can be found in a government report issued within the last few years (*Bulletin 12, Hygiene Laboratory, 1903*), which contains this paragraph:

> Tetanus may become a contaminating element of vaccine before it leaves the heifer. During the period of three to five days which elapses between the vaccination of the heifer and the removal of the virus there is opportunity for tetanus to find a lodgment in the eruption of the heifer's body surface, provided tetanus is present in the stall or stable surroundings of the animal.

Judging by the number of cases of tetanus that have come to light in the last couple of years following vaccination, attention should be directed to vaccination as the direct cause. Instead of holding vaccination responsible for the lives blotted out by tetanus, the profession prefers to delude the public, possibly themselves, into the belief that tetanus has in the cases reported been due rather to infection from without. If so terrible a complication can possibly follow vaccination, all reported cases of tetanus following vaccination should be thoroughly investigated, and if the physician performing the operation or the manufacturers of the vaccine are found to be responsible they should be severely punished. If vaccination is to be forced upon the public despite its wishes in the matter, someone should be held accountable for any untoward results.

Revaccination, according to this artful medical dodger, will protect when it will protect and will not, when it will not; an explanation not especially illuminating. He, in common with provaccinists everywhere, takes advantage of the loophole of escape offered by claimed "spurious vaccination". In other words, if a vaccinated person is brought in contact with smallpox and escapes infection, set his escape down to successful *vaccination; if he takes the disease, put it down either to* unsuccessful *vaccination or to* spurious *vaccination.*

"A quiescent malady may be lighted into activity by vaccination. This has happened with congenital syphilis, occasionally with tuberculosis." —William Osler, M.D.

Does Vaccination Grant Immunity From Or Lessen the Severity Of Smallpox?

by Joseph P. Rinn

The Naturopath and Herald of Health, XVI (4), 205-211. (1911)

M r. Chairman, Ladies And Gentlemen*

Before addressing you on the subject of vaccination, I wish it clearly understood that I am a believer in scientific medicine, and not in any way in sympathy with those soft-hearted persons that attempt to restrict or hamper investigations tending to find means to alleviate human suffering, even though the liberty permitted in such investigations is occasionally abused.

It is because I am a believer in scientific medicine that I am to-day opposing vaccination, as I believe that the accumulated evidence of a century shows conclusively that it is unscientific, unsanitary, a propagator of disease, and with no power to either grant immunity from or lessen the severity of smallpox.

The time has passed when the medical profession can assume a dogmatic attitude of infallibility toward the public, as the intelligent laity has opinions on medical subjects that are well grounded upon facts, and they are just as capable of weighing evidence as the medical profession. The mere fact that a profession has a financial interest and bias generated through such a cause should forever bar it from being the sole judge of evidence that would be likely to affect its interests. The history shows that the medical profession is one of great mistakes and wrong diagnosis, and if they are not intelligent enough to reform themselves on the question of vaccination in the face of unmistakable evidence, it will be eventually done by the laity, not only in vaccination, but in many other lines, and in so radical a manner as may hamper the legitimate progress of scientific medicine.

In the *American Journal of Obstetrics* of July, 1908, you will find an address by Dr. J. M. Baldy, president of the American Gynecological Society of Philadelphia, in which he says: "The general administration of anesthetics as performed to-day is the shame of modern surgery, is a disgrace to a learned profession, and if the full, unvarnished truth concerning it were known to the laity at large, it would be but a short while before it were interfered with by legislative means, and properly so."

This testimony is from a prominent medical man and speaks for itself.

In the *Bulletin of the Academy of Medicine* in Pittsburg, for Febru-

---

*Lecture held February 5, 1911, before the Brooklyn Philosophical Association.

ary, 1908, Dr. Henry Bates, Jr., of Philadelphia tells of his investigation into what is taught in medical colleges in the United States, and it seems astounding to the intelligent laity that such conditions could prevail as that of no standardization of studies in our colleges of medicine, and yet that men with hardly any knowledge to speak of in medical science can be let loose in the community to gain experience on humanity. Dr. Bates showed that in some colleges they required 2,221 hours of study on general surgery, and in others only 78 hours; that in some colleges they required 1,900 hours of study on general medicine, and in others only 78 hours; that 646 hours of pathology study was required in some, and only 48 hours in others; that some have 756 hours on chemistry, and others only 78 hours; that some colleges required 1,248 hours of anatomy study and others only 125 hours; that some colleges required 750 hours of study of physiology and others only 56 hours.*

In spite of this laxity on the part of the medical profession, these half-trained students who gain a smattering of knowledge out of books, taught to them in many instances by others that had gained their knowledge out of books, are given certificates as doctors by these colleges, and immediately assume an attitude of dogmatism to the public on subjects such as vaccination, of which they have but little knowledge.

A book, recently published in New York by Dr. Norman Barnesby, called *Medical Chaos and Crime*, shows such a startling condition of affairs in the medical profession in this country as would seem impossible if it were not substantiated by evidence that cannot be questioned.

In view of these facts what daring assurance it is on the part of medical men to insist that the laity shall not be permitted to pass judgment upon the evidence offered by facts as to the value or lack of value of medical remedies.

In all ages the medical profession has endorsed what was afterward proven of no value. In 1750 the Royal College of Physicians of Great Britain endorsed inoculation as the best-proved thing in medicine, that is, the inoculation of a person with matter from a smallpox patient as a preventative of smallpox, and even when this created epidemics of smallpox they wrote books upholding its value, as they do now for vaccination until the British government had to make it a penal offense to perform it. In 1802 the medical profession, with but little scientific investigation, accepted the theory of vaccination of Dr. Edward Jenner, and went before the House of Commons in England and stated that vaccination by Jenner's principles of cowpox granted immunity for life from smallpox. Again they endorsed the principle of arm-to-arm vaccination, until the spread of

---

*The 1910 *Flexner Report*, by Abraham Flexner, reported on the practices and standards of medical education for all of the medical schools resulting in the closure of 161 schools and demise of the Eclectic, Homeopathic and Naturopathic medical schools. —*Ed.*

syphilis and tuberculosis from it became so pronounced that, as shown by Prof. Charles Creighton in the ninth edition of the *Encyclopedia Britannica*, they had nearly twenty epidemics of syphilis in different countries.

Now the medical profession insists that vaccination is efficacious in smallpox, although it is a well-known fact that sanitation and isolation are always insisted upon by them in smallpox, and at no time or place can they show that vaccination alone, without sanitation, has had the slightest effect on smallpox. In Jenner's day they upheld the belief that vaccination granted immunity for life, and even though this was positively disproved by 1805, they went before Parliament in England and induced them to grant money for vaccine establishments and an additional reward of twenty thousand pounds to Dr. Jenner in 1807.

Dr. William Rowley, physician to St. Marylebone Infirmary, in a work published in 1805 called *Cowpox Inoculation*, and which reached a third edition in 1806, gave particulars of 504 cases of smallpox and injury after vaccination with 75 deaths. He said to his medical brethren in his book, "Come and see. I have lately had some of the worst species of malignant smallpox in Marylebone Infirmary, which many of the faculty have examined and known to have been vaccinated."

For two days Dr. Rowley had an exhibition in his lecture room of a number of children suffering from terrible eruptions and other diseases after vaccination.

In 1806 Dr. D. Moseley, physician to Chelsea Hospital, published a book giving many cases of persons who had been properly vaccinated and had afterward had smallpox, and also several cases of severe illness, injury and even death from vaccination, and these failures were admitted by the Royal Jennerian Society in their report in 1806.

Dr. Maclean, in the *Medical Observer* of 1810, gave a history of 535 cases of smallpox after vaccination, of which 97 proved fatal. He also gave 150 cases of disease after vaccination with the names of ten medical men and two professors of anatomy who had suffered in their own families from vaccination.

Here we have records of persons vaccinated in Jenner's day who caught the smallpox and died from it, as well as dying from vaccination itself, and in that age when they weakened a person who was ill by persistently bleeding him as a cure, we can understand how they had not the ability to find out the scientific fallacy of vaccination, because about that period the general decline of all diseases set in through improvement in sanitation and better knowledge of hygiene. They naturally credited vaccination with being of great value and insisted that the failures were experienced because the vaccine did not take, or because vaccination only granted immunity for twenty years. The ridiculous principle of revaccination has been insisted upon by medical men ever since, but the evidence that vaccination did not protect nor lessen the severity of smallpox has been forced upon the profession time and again by the facts, but each time they cried, "Vaccinate oftener" and it will be all right. From twenty years immunity it went to fifteen, then to ten years, seven years, five years, and in some places they now stand for every two years, others every year, and in others as often as vaccination will take.

Of later years the medical claim has been that vaccination grants immunity from or lessens the severity of smallpox, but if it grants immunity in any degree, we should scientifically know in what degree or simply state that it lessens the severity of the disease. The Chicago Health Department issues a Bulletin, in which it says: "After many years of experience with smallpox and vaccination, the Chicago Health Department hereby declares: "True vaccination—that is, repeated until it no longer takes— always prevents smallpox. Nothing else does."

Now, experiments in the Italian army in epidemics tend to show that smallpox attacked those in whom vaccination took twice as often as in soldiers in whom it did not take, and that the deaths were much greater among those in whom vaccination took than in those in whom it did not take.

Dr. Adolf Vogt, professor of hygiene and sanitary statistics in the University of Berne, one of the greatest statisticians on medical science in Europe, proved in his arguments presented to the Royal Commission of Great Britain in its investigation in vaccination that resulted in the abolition there of compulsory vaccination, that a previous attack of smallpox and vaccination that took made a person more susceptible to another attack than if they had never had smallpox or been vaccinated.

In order to test the belief of the medical profession that is so strongly asserted by the Chicago Board of Health, as to the immunity given by vaccination that takes, I recently offered a reward of one thousand dollars to any hospital that would furnish five doctors who would submit to being vaccinated by vaccine virus supplied by the New York City Board of Health, and who would, after having said vaccination passed upon as having taken perfectly, permit the inoculation in their bodies of smallpox matter by physicians selected by me, and if at least 60 percent or three out of the five physicians did not contract smallpox, I would forfeit to the hospital or any charity the sum of one thousand dollars. Although this offer has been [broadcast] over the entire country for a month, no hospital or physician has accepted it, and yet they will not stop claiming that vaccination, when it takes, will grant immunity, although I am still willing to test its efficacy for even thirty days.

The fact is, the medical profession knows little or nothing about the vaccine virus that they use, and hardly a man among them could conscientiously assert that he knows what kind of virus he is using on his patients. They call Jenner the founder of vaccination, and in all their medical works praise him; yet I challenge the medical profession to show that any vaccine factory in this country, or any Board of Health, is manufacturing virus according to the principle laid down by Jenner in his book published in 1801, entitled, *An Inquiry into the Causes and Effects of Variola Vaccinae.*

What are they using for vaccine virus? Horse grease cowpox, as first advocated by Jenner, or pure horse grease, as he later in life adopted. Jenner distinctly proved that *spontaneous cowpox* was useless, and warned the profession against its use, and yet the advertisements of the prominent vaccine firms state that their seed virus is from cows having spontaneous cowpox. Other firms are and have been using virus from cows that were inoculated by pure smallpox from human beings. Now if Jenner is father of the vaccination theory, and the medical profession has never disavowed its belief in it, by what right or by what discovery since made do they depart from the Jennerian principle of vaccine virus and then enforce it upon us by law?

Pure Virus

The medical profession is constantly quoting "pure calf lymph from healthy calves". How can calves be healthy when they have to be diseased with cowpox in order to get the virus? The scab from a running sore is scraped away and the pus or running matter is collected and this is what vaccine virus is that is put into your healthy bodies.

This is a direct violation of the principle of asepsis in surgery, which is advocated by scientific medicine and which stands for this: that no foreign organisms shall be permitted to go into any cut part on the human body, and aseptic medicines are used in all operations to prevent what is done in vaccination. Any surgeon that would put pus or matter from a running sore into a freshly cut body in an operation, would now be considered a fit subject for a lunatic asylum, and yet they do this very thing in vaccination and never seem to realize its dangers. When accidents and deaths occur from vaccinations, they always claim that the vaccination was improperly done or that the person was not clean, but always deny that the vaccine itself could be diseased and could cause the fatal result. I challenge them to produce vaccine virus free from bacterial taint, and I shall now give medical evidence that shows that all or nearly all the vaccine virus is tainted with germs of disease, and I hereby publically offer to wager one thousand dollars that I can go on the market and buy vaccine virus of different makes and that 95 percent will be found contaminated with germs of disease.

In the *British Medical Journal* of July 5, 1902, in an editorial on "The Bacteriology of Vaccine and Variola" it is stated as follows: "Dr. Pfuhl, writing in 1898 of his experience in the official station at Hanover, says: 'Strictly germ-free vaccine lymph will, in my opinion, always belong to the region of Utopia. As a result of my own experience I always found that every sample of lymph contained bacteria in greater or smaller numbers.'"

A few years ago the Columbus Medical Laboratory of Chicago made a thorough analytical test of the vaccines from all known propagators of the United States, bought on the open market, and they only found one that was free from pus bacteria and other pathogenic micro-organisms.

Bulletin No. 12, United States Hygienic Laboratory, Washington, D.C., Dr. Rosenau on "Bacteriological Impurities in Vaccine Virus" states as follows:

> It is impossible to use germicidal agents in the treatment of vaccinal eruptions of calves; as such substances would kill the potency of the virus. Therefore, it is evident that even the greatest care will not ensure virus against *foreign organisms*. We found pus cocci (germs of sepsis) and other bacteria in both the dry points and the glycerinated virus. It will be seen that there is practically no vaccine on the market free from bacterial contamination. Tetanus spores may live a long time in vaccine virus. We found them alive and virulent on dry points after 295 days, and in the glycerinated virus sealed in capillary tubes 355 days. Tetanus may become a contaminating element of vaccine virus before it leaves the heifer.

Is it necessary to produce any more evidence of the falsity of the statement of the medical profession, when they claim the vaccine virus is not responsible for the many deaths we have had from lockjaw, or as it is medically called tetanus?

I can give the names and addresses of over one hundred persons who died from lockjaw in 1909 and 1910, shortly after vaccination, who were in apparently good health when vaccinated.

The *Scottish Medical and Surgical Journal* of April, 1900, on page 330 says, "A party of Esquimaux [Eskimo] who visited Berlin and were vaccinated there, developed a general disease resembling or identical with smallpox, and perished of it."

Does this show whether vaccination is dangerous or not? I shall now proceed to prove from facts and figures in the United States, Italy, Great Britain and Japan that the arguments for vaccination are false and that the more we vaccinate, the more danger from smallpox.

In the *New York Medical Record* of July 22, 1899, page 133, we have a detailed account of vaccination in Italy that in all these years has not been disputed by medical men. It is written by Dr. Charles Ruata, professor of hygiene and materia medica in the University of Perugia. Prof. Ruata says: "Italy is one of the best vaccinated countries in the world, if not the best of all. Our young men, with few exceptions, at the age of twenty must enter the army, where a regulation prescribes compulsory vaccination. For twenty years before 1885, our nation was vaccinated in proportion of 98.5 percent, but notwithstanding the epidemics that we have had been so frightful that nothing before the invention of vaccination could equal them.

During 1885 we had 12,000 deaths from smallpox; in 1886, 19,000; 1887, 16,249; 1888, 18,110; and in 1889, 13,413."

Referring to the Italian army Prof. Ruata says: "Vaccination had been performed twice a year in the most satisfactory manner for many years past. The soldiers not protected, because the vaccination did not take, were less attacked by smallpox than those duly protected by the good results of their vaccination, and the death-rate in those with good results was greater than among those in whom vaccination did not take, and there was double the number of cases of smallpox among those in whom vaccination took than among those in whom it did not take." Does this show that vaccination granted immunity from smallpox or lessened the severity of the attack? It shows if evidence counts for anything, that vaccination is a menace and a danger rather than a protector from smallpox.

GREAT BRITAIN

Now what do the records of Great Britain show? Compulsory vaccination began in 1853; the laws were made more stringent in 1867 and again more stringent in 1871.

Dr. C. T. Pearce in his book on *Vital Statistics*, published in 1877, says: "Since 1853 we have had three epidemics of smallpox, each more severe than the preceding one."

First epidemic (1857-1859), the number of deaths was 14,244; second epidemic (1863-1865), 20,059; and third epidemic (1870-1872), 44,840.

Increase of population from first to second epidemic was 7 percent, and increase in smallpox was 50 percent. The increase of population from second to third epidemic was 10 percent and the increase in smallpox was 120 percent. Vaccination increased, so did smallpox and deaths.

Prof. Alfred Russel Wallace in his book *The Wonderful Century* has riddled the arguments for vaccination. He selects the army and navy of England, which have been pointed to with pride by the vaccinationists as showing the best results for vaccination. He compares the results of vaccination among 220,000 men of the army and navy, all thoroughly vaccinated and revaccinated regularly, as against the town of Leicester, with 200,000 that discarded vaccination after the smallpox epidemic of 1871, and depended solely on sanitation and isolation, and showed that in nineteen years, from 1878 to 1896, unvaccinated Leicester had so few deaths from smallpox that the registrar-general of Great Britain recorded it as equivalent to 10 per million of inhabitants, whereas the results in the army and navy were nearly three times that of Leicester. This is surely a test of the vaccination theory, and it is a striking proof that sanitation and isolation is far superior to vaccination. For twelve years in Leicester, from

1878 to 1889, there was less than one death per annum from smallpox in a population of 200,000. Yet in the epidemic of 1871-1872, when Leicester was well vaccinated, it had 327 cases of smallpox per 10,000 population and 35 deaths, and in the same epidemic Birmingham, its neighbor, had 213 cases of smallpox per 10,000 population, and 35 deaths. Then Leicester discarded vaccination and Birmingham kept it up, so that when the next smallpox epidemic came in 1891-1894, Birmingham was thirty times as well vaccinated as Leicester, with the following results: Birmingham had 63 cases per 10,000 population and 5 percent death, while Leicester had only 19 cases per 10,000 population and one and one-tenth percent death. In the same epidemic Warrington, another well vaccinated town, had 123 cases per 10,000 population and 11.4 percent deaths. Here we see that in the unvaccinated town of Leicester the cases were six times less in number and eight times less in the death-rate than in the well vaccinated towns of Birmingham and Warrington.

From 1872-1876, when Leicester was a well-vaccinated city, the average death rate from all causes was 25.18, but with the decrease in vaccination it has fallen to 12.90 in 1909, although the population has doubled. Since vaccination was abandoned, infant mortality has steadily decreased until in 1908 it reached the low figure of 129.7 per 1,000 births, a record that cannot be approached in thoroughly vaccinated places. In the smallpox epidemic of 1903 they had 394 cases with 21 deaths, or 5.3 percent mortality, and in 1904 they had 321 cases and only four deaths, or a fatality of 1.24 percent. No such record has ever been made in thoroughly vaccinated cities of the same size in the world, and yet this occurred in unvaccinated Leicester, where, if the theory of vaccination were true, the epidemic should have spread like wildfire and with great loss of life. They have not had a case of smallpox since then in three years, and yet medical men persist in advocating the necessity of vaccination in spite of the risk to life and health through contamination from diseased vaccine virus.

UNITED STATES

Now, what are the records in the United States Army? The only accurate statistics we have in the United States are reports of the United States marine hospital service from December 28, 1899 to 1990 show that there were 11,448 cases of smallpox among a body of picked men in the army and navy, where it was obligatory that they should all be vaccinated and revaccinated regularly.

The records of the army in the Philippines are, according to Lieutenant Colonel Henry Lippincott, Chief Surgeon, Department of the Pacific and Eighth Corps, as given in the *Medical Record of Philadelphia*, April 14, 1900, volume 5, page 829, another striking example of the lack of value of vaccination. Lieutenant Colonel Lippincott's paper says:

Smallpox is endemic among the Filipinos, and although often malignant and fatal, never caused them to avoid or take steps to prevent disease. With them, the smallpox is like the measles with the Mexicans—persons with mild cases wandering about the cities and towns when we entered Manila. Of course, all this was stopped when our army took control, and the most energetic means adopted to prevent the spread of the disease. This was done also for our army—vaccination and revaccination many times repeated, went on as systematically as drills at a well-regulated post ... I believe I can say that no army was ever so well looked after in the matter of vaccination as ours.

You have here a definite statement of how carefully the soldiers were vaccinated, and yet from the annual reports of the Surgeon General to the United States government, we find that in the period of five years from 1897 to 1902 there were 737 cases of smallpox among the army in the Philippines, with 261 deaths, a mortality of over 35 percent, nearly double the mortality that took place before the days of vaccination, when the sanitary conditions were vile and the people ignorant of hygiene. The facts of these figures of cases of smallpox and deaths in the Philippines were substantiated on January 4, 1911, by a letter from the War Department written by Albert G. Love, Captain of the Medical Corps of the United States Army.

Since we took control of the Philippines, disease of all kinds have been reduced by sanitation and isolation, which had never been followed in the treatment of disease before we took control, yet vaccination is credited with being the factor that produced the results in smallpox. If that is so, what did it [do] in the other diseases? If sanitation alone was not the cause of the abolition or reduction of smallpox there, why did our thoroughly vaccinated soldiers suffer a mortality of 35 percent in smallpox in the five years from 1898 to 1902, while the sanitary efforts put into practice had not yet produced its effects? If vaccination should get the credit for results in smallpox in the Philippines, why does Leicester with no vaccination stand as the leader in having the lowest record for smallpox cases and smallpox mortality, as well as about the lowest average death rate and the lowest infant mortality of any large city in the world?

Japan

Considerable lying has been done in the medical papers about Japan, and that country is constantly quoted as giving evidence of the value of vaccination. In the July 25, 1908 [issue} of the English publication called *Health*, it is stated as follows: "Any attempt to evade revaccination at stated periods in Japan, is made a serious offense. The result is that smallpox, once the curse of the islands, is now all but unknown and similar

results are reported from every country in which vaccination is made compulsory and rigidly enforced."

Now, this is the class of statements that are constantly appearing in
the medical papers, and which are undoubtedly read by many medical
men and believed to be true; yet I have given you the figures on Italy,
Great Britain and the United States, which absolutely disprove the statements by this medical paper. In order to obtain the exact facts as to the
real situation in Japan, Dr. J. W. Hodge of Niagara Falls, N.Y., one of the
greatest students of vaccination in this country, wrote to Mr. S. Kubota,
director of the Sanitary Bureau of Japan, and he learned from him that in
the very year that this medical publication said that smallpox was all but
unknown in Japan, they had 18,067 officially recorded cases of smallpox
and 5,837 deaths, a mortality of 35 percent, or more than double the mortality resulting from smallpox before vaccination was heard of.

The following facts were also learned by Dr. Hodge: Compulsory vaccination began in Japan in 1872, but notwithstanding rigid enforcement
of the law, Japan suffered many thousand deaths annually from smallpox,
following successful vaccination. The medical men insisted that if the
people had been revaccinated, the deaths might have been avoided, so
in 1885 they passed more astringent laws, whereby revaccination every
five to seven years was made compulsory, and in pursuance of this law,
25,474,370 vaccinations, revaccinations, and revaccinations were officially recorded as being performed in Japan between 1885 and 1892; about
two-thirds of the entire population were revaccinated within the period
stated.

Now, even the most ardent vaccinationists could hardly desire any
more than this as a test of the value of vaccination, yet the official records
show that during the seven years mentioned from 1886 to 1892, they had
156,175 cases of smallpox and 39,979 deaths. By a compulsory law every
infant born in Japan must be vaccinated within the first year of its birth,
and in case it does not take the first time, it must be followed by three
additional operations within the year, and every five to seven years thereafter. In the event of an outbreak of smallpox, the Japanese authorities
rigidly enforced general revaccination, irrespective of previous vaccinations. Now, in spite of these precautions, what has been the result? The
official records show that from 1892 to 1897 Japan had 142,032 cases
of smallpox and 39,536 deaths. Another Act of Parliament passed in
1896, made revaccination repeated every five years compulsory on every
Japanese subject regardless of station. This Act, like its predecessors, was
rigidly enforced under severe penalty; yet, in the very next year, 1897, they
had 41,946 cases of smallpox and 12,276 deaths. This was a mortality of
32 percent, nearly double the mortality from smallpox before vaccination
had been heard of. The official records show that from 1889 to 1908 they
had 171,511 cases and 47,919 deaths. I submit without further argument
that the evidence I have produced shows that vaccination neither grants
immunity from smallpox nor lessens the severity of the disease.

It is because I am a believer in scientific medicine that I am to-day opposing vaccination, as I believe that the accumulated evidence of a century shows conclusively that it is unscientific, unsanitary, a propagator of disease, and with no power to either grant immunity from or lessen the severity of smallpox.

The history shows that the medical profession is one of great mistakes and wrong diagnosis, and if they are not intelligent enough to reform themselves on the question of vaccination in the face of unmistakable evidence, it will be eventually done by the laity, not only in vaccination, but in many other lines, and in so radical a manner as may hamper the legitimate progress of scientific medicine.

Now the medical profession insists that vaccination is efficacious in smallpox, although it is a well-known fact that sanitation and isolation are always insisted upon by them in smallpox, and at no time or place can they show that vaccination alone, without sanitation, has had the slightest effect on smallpox.

The ridiculous principle of revaccination has been insisted upon by medical men ever since, but the evidence that vaccination did not protect nor lessen the severity of smallpox has been forced upon the profession time and again by the facts, but each time they cried, "Vaccinate oftener" and it will be all right. From twenty years immunity it went to fifteen, then to ten years, seven years, five years, and in some places they now stand for every two years, others every year, and in others as often as vaccination will take.

The medical profession is constantly quoting "pure calf lymph from healthy calves". How can calves be healthy when they have to be diseased with cowpox in order to get the virus? The scab from a running sore is scraped away and the pus or running matter is collected and this is what vaccine virus is that is put into your healthy bodies.

This is a direct violation of the principle of asepsis in surgery, which is advocated by scientific medicine and which stands for this: that no foreign organisms shall be permitted to go into any cut part on the human body, and aseptic medicines are used in all operations to prevent what is done in vaccination.

(cont'd)

The only accurate statistics we have in the United States are reports of the United States marine hospital service from December 28, 1899 to 1990 show that there were 11,448 cases of smallpox among a body of picked men in the army and navy, where it was obligatory that they should all be vaccinated and revaccinated regularly.

AN OPEN LETTER

by Major Thomas Bourden

The Naturopath and Herald of Health, XVI (5), 303-305. (1911)

TO THE GOVERNOR AND MEMBERS OF THE LEGISLATURE OF THE STATE
OF CONNECTICUT

Gentlemen: The year 1911 affords an opportunity for the opponents
of the compulsory enforcement of vaccination, by law or otherwise,
to renew their efforts to secure their just rights at the hands of a new
General Assembly.

That their efforts may meet with complete success this year is to be
wished for, but, should victory in their fight for pure blood and sanctity
of the body, be further postponed, it is certain that the right to accept or
reject vaccination without fear or favor of any man or set of men will, in
the end be gained.

The violation of the body of a healthy person and the defilement of
the pure blood of a child or adult by pus inoculation as in vaccination,
and without their consent, is an assault and a crime in the nature of rape.
A law compelling such a procedure is unjust and opposed to the dictates
of common sense.

In the very nature of things the practice of vaccination under compulsion must cease; and from the widespread and rapidly growing opposition
to the practice, both at home and abroad, among physicians as well as laymen, it is safe to say that the time is not far distant when it will be deemed
a crime for a person to vaccinate another. Hardly a day passes [that one]
sees the announcement of some new vaccine virus for employment against
diseases other than smallpox; and could the doctor have his way, there
would soon be laws enacted to compel vaccination with all sorts of vaccine for every sort of ailment.*

The introduction of a virus, which has power of reproduction indefinitely—a poison—whether of human or animal extraction, directly into
the blood is not natural, not in harmony with nature's methods, and cannot be productive of anything but evil, and, in spite of the fact that it is
the fashion now, time will come, and soon, when the evil wrought and the
futility of the practice will be seen.

One has only to read the history of smallpox and vaccination from
the manuscripts of official records, to learn how the public has been misled by the vaccinator into an absurd panic of fear of smallpox, which can

---

*In our lifetime, we have witnessed the vaccine schedule begin with 6 vaccines to now
16 in total amounting to 68 doses of vaccines administered from birth until adulthood.
Research has never been conducted to evaluate the outcome of the full schedule of vaccines administered to humans. —*Ed.*

be shown to be one of the least things to be feared, as a cause of death by children or adults in our times and climes, and as something no one need worry about whether vaccinated or not, and that lightning in civilized northern lands is about as much to be feared as a cause of death as smallpox.

The common lighting gas in our houses and the vehicles in our streets are ten times more likely to kill us than smallpox ever is. And to prove this, we have only to look at the record of New York City for the past year, where 200 persons were killed by murder, 300 killed by gas and only three died from smallpox in the whole State in the same year.

One has only to read how Leicester, England, prevents smallpox, promotes the general health, and has reduced the death-rate to one of the lowest, without vaccination; and *per contra*, how the Japanese people, one of the best vaccinated in the world, have suffered from the worst recent epidemic of smallpox, from which the most extensive compulsory vaccination failed to protect them. The experience of Japan is one of the strongest object lessons of the century and should have great weight with everyone who would arrive at a correct conclusion on this question.

Our own vaccine virus makers sent to Japan for their so-called *seed virus* which was found to be much more virile and *protective* than our own virus. For, indeed, it seems to be a fact that smallpox infection dies out naturally in our temperate climates if left alone, or is not spread by deliberate propagation or inoculation and neglect of sanitation and isolation. Hence our medical confreres had to send to tropic infected Japan, not for more health but for more and more virile disease. Well, this Japanese virus proved indeed so virile to us that it produced a terrible epidemic of foot and mouth disease among the cattle—the foster mothers and wet nurses of the human race—in the United States, in 1908, which was traced to our vaccine factories and which caused the slaughter of 4,600 farm animals and cost the United States government over $400,000 to suppress and caused our farmers a large additional loss.

Will some medical philosopher kindly find out for a trusting public the great benefits of vaccination in this case, and this is the second epidemic of the kind caused by vaccine virus in this country.

The vaccinators are thus not content to poison the blood of our children, but they have also to poison the blood of our cattle, the wet nurses of our children.

In making this vile stuff, see *25ᵗʰ Report of United States Bureau of Animal Industry*, 1908. It is notorious that many deaths have occurred among school children and other persons under the ban of compulsory vaccination laws, but just how many will never be known. While nearly 100 deaths from vaccination have been reported in the press of the country during the past year, and most of them from lockjaw—yet there is no doubt that the half have not been told.

Any standard medical work upon this subject will admit the more or less frequent presence of the germs of tetanus in vaccine virus.

The death of hogs and cattle by vaccine are recorded, but not the deaths of human; they are carefully concealed in our vital statistics under the head [subheading] of "Tetanus," "Septicemia," "Phlegmen," "Endocarditis," and a dozen other forms of blood poisoning, internal and external suppuration and ulcerative diseases, which afflict humanity; and which are communicated by, or follow after vaccination and the primary cause is continually denied and concealed by our health departments all over the country.

A striking instance of this is exhibited in the *Report of the State Board of Health of Pennsylvania* in which a few cases of smallpox are reported, and no deaths; but, on no account are the large numbers vaccinated and the equally large number of deaths therefrom reported. Why is this? Echo answers, "Why?"

With our health departments all over the country working hand in glove with the manufacturers of vaccine virus, and controlling our vital statistics, this is one of the most shameful medical scandals and outrages of our times and should be corrected at once by our law makers.

In England things are done differently. There the law compels doctors to record vaccination deaths and through this fact we can show by American and English statistics combined that the deaths from vaccination occur at a higher ratio than the deaths from smallpox.*

Great, truly, is vaccination and its prophets, and its profits are truly great, for some people. Millions upon millions are invested in it, and doctors hold the stock.

In order that our position on anti-vaccination may not be misunderstood, we desire to say here that all the reform we wish is this, to let those who believe in vaccination have all they want of it, but they should not be permitted to force it on anyone else; and to truly record and publish all deaths or injuries caused by vaccination, and all fair-minded persons do not wish to force our opinions regarding vaccination upon anyone and are fully determined that they shall not be permitted to force their opinions upon us.

There are too many men in this country with good red blood in their veins who are determined to resist the enforcement of this infamous outrage upon their natural rights, even unto death.

If public health be the plea of vaccination, then there is far more reason that the privilege of public suffrage should depend on vaccination, rather than the privilege of education, since it is an incontrovertible medi-

---

*A January 2015 measles outbreak occurred at Disneyland in California causing a surge in fear and mobilization to promote compulsory vaccination. In the past 10 years, there has been no deaths due to contracting measles and 108 deaths due to receiving the measles vaccines. —Ed.

cal and statistical fact that the school age is actually the least susceptible to smallpox and more susceptible and far more in need of this peculiar law, for the compulsory infliction of disease, if there is any virtue in such a medical and legal barbarism.

Voters, how would you like to have to submit to a certificate to vaccination before you would be allowed to register to vote? And, if it is not needed for you, it certainly is not needed for the most immune age of our population—our school children.

We appeal to you, gentlemen of the Connecticut Legislature of 1911, to fairly weigh the evidence which will be presented to you, from time to time, on this question, and, in casting your vote to decide a matter of such vital importance to our fellow citizens and yourselves; we trust you will do justice to those who have entrusted their welfare to you, by repealing the compulsory vaccination laws and settling the matter right.

Hardly a day passes but sees the announcement of some new vaccine virus for employment against diseases other than smallpox; and could the doctor have his way, there would soon be laws enacted to compel vaccination with all sorts of vaccine for every sort of ailment.

One has only to read the history of smallpox and vaccination from the manuscripts of official records, to learn how the public has been misled by the vaccinator into an absurd panic of fear of smallpox, which can be shown to be one of the least things to be feared, as a cause of death by children or adults in our times and climes, and as something no one need worry about whether vaccinated or not, and that lightning in civilized northern lands is about as much to be feared as a cause of death as smallpox.

For, indeed, it seems to be a fact that smallpox infection dies out naturally in our temperate climates if left alone, or is not spread by deliberate propagation or inoculation and neglect of sanitation and isolation.

With our health departments all over the country working hand in glove with the manufacturers of vaccine virus, and controlling our vital statistics, this is one of the most shameful medical scandals and outrages of our times and should be corrected at once by our law makers.

An Innocent Victim Of That Medical Superstition, Vaccination

by Benedict Lust, N.D.

The Naturopath and the Herald of Health, XVI (5), 312. (1911)

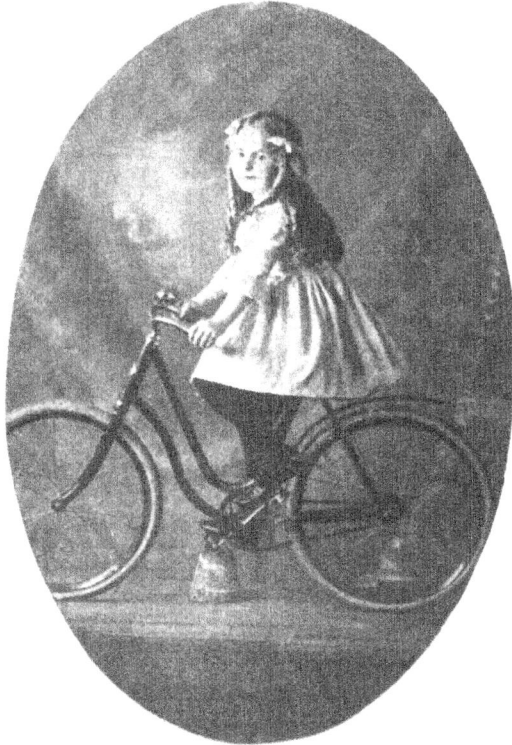

This sweet little girl rides right into the hearts of people from Maine to California wherever her winsome face has become known. She was mourned by her fond parents as the brightest and best of children. She was an only child. Think what that means, you who have lost children, and of what it would mean to you to have lost your only child as the result of forced vaccination.

The father of the child, Homer E. Sturdevant, did all he was able to do to make this costly sacrifice save other children. He placed upon her tombstone the cause of the child's death; he brought suit against the city of Buffalo for $25,000 damages. He has properly given all possible publicity to the case. For these things he has been persecuted and deprived of his situation as a passenger conductor on Lehigh Valley Railroad. He has lost other employment on account of it. But he still adheres to his purpose to make the compulsory vaccination of children a costly thing to the community that permits it, and to do all he can to save other children from such poisoning and possible death.

The circumstances of this child's vaccination and death are as follows:

On May 15, 1902, she was in school 35, Buffalo, N.Y., and two public vaccinators, accompanied by two policemen, visited the school to engraft cow virus into the children at $1 a head. Though Lucille was only six years old she objected, saying she had been vaccinated and that she would go home and be vaccinated if she must. In spite of this the officers threatened and forcibly vaccinated her.

Just thirteen days later, and after ten days of suffering from blood poisoning, she died. This is one of the most pathetic cases on record. The sequel is almost as sad.

The mother lost her reason, and was placed in an asylum. The father, persecuted, broken and discouraged, took to drink.

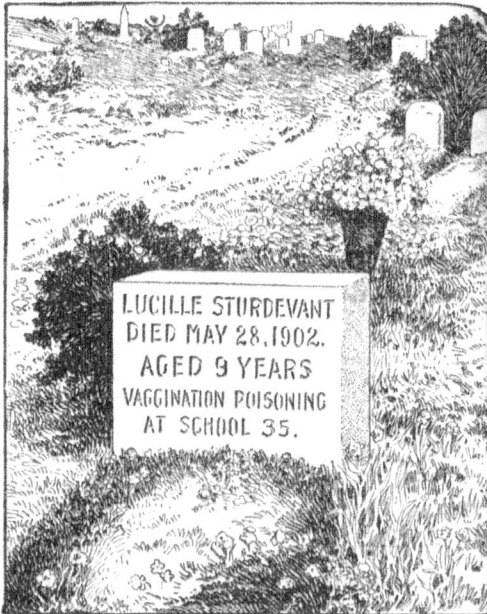

Anti-Vaccination Victory In California

by Dr. F. Antonius

The Naturopath and Herald of Health, XVI (7), 429-430. (1911)

The California Anti-Compulsory Vaccination League, whose headquarters are at Berkeley, California, the other day, celebrated the passage of a law by the recent State Legislature which does away with the compulsory feature of vaccination of school children. Under the new law, children need not be vaccinated, provided the parents sign a certificate that they are opposed to the practice of vaccination, and it is the duty of the school board to furnish every parent with one of these blanks [forms].

The celebrity, in the form of a banquet, was well attended by representative men from various parts of the State, and an enjoyable time was had. It was the sense of the meeting that while a great victory had been won, still the work of educating the people about the abominable dangerous practice of inoculating the blood of fellow beings with deadly vaccine virus must continue until all vaccination and so-called serum-therapy is stopped. A resolution was adopted asking President Taft to revoke the order recently made that all persons going to Alaska must be vaccinated. The protest against this regulation of the public health (?) and marine hospital service relative to vaccination of persons leaving Pacific coast harbors for Alaska has been effective already, and only persons who have been exposed to smallpox need be vaccinated. The vaccination fiends had gone so far that no-one could even buy a ticket to Alaska unless he had been recently vaccinated, and thousands of people were obliged to undergo the dangerous operation and expose themselves to outright blood poisoning during a sea voyage and a trip into an unsettled country, at that.

The price of liberty is eternal vigilance. If we do not watch our rights and liberties, we will lose them, and we will fall into the bondage of our enemies. To enjoy life and liberty means to fight and struggle under the existing conditions of greedy selfishness that ignores the first principles of rights, justice and truth, and put might above right. Until the divine brotherhood of mankind is established, we will have to fight for our rights, and our first right is freedom. *Freedom from all medical oppression* must be our watchword in this great struggle against the medical trust that wants to fasten its nasty clutches on this great country of liberty. Freedom from all compulsory vaccination must be the aim of every lover of health and humanity, just now. Let us go at it systematically, and let us *organize* in every township, in every county, in every state. Without organization nothing will come out of our agitation against the enemy of our rights, *who is well organized.*

The story of the victory in California contains a lesson for all who wish to succeed in this fight for medical freedom and right. The first Anti-Compulsory Vaccination League of California was organized in 1904, at

Berkeley, California, which is the seat of the State University. Due to its efforts, in 1905, an anti-vaccination bill, which was a revision of the Utah law, finally passed the Legislature of California, but was vetoed by the governor, Dr. G. C. Pardee. On account of the veto, the School Board of Berkeley and those favoring vaccination became more arbitrary, and children were forced into vaccination or had to leave school. As a result of this despotism, scores of children left the public schools and were either placed in private schools or kept at home. The League, which was headed by Dr. W. Allen and Dr. E. E. Campbell, kept regular open meetings, and invited anybody especially medical men, to debate the question of compulsory vaccination, but vaccination fiends would not accept the challenge. Finally an *anti-vaccination school* was opened on August 7, 1905, for all the children whose parents were opposed to vaccination. This was the first of its kind ever established in the world, and it had the same number of grades as any public grammar school. The expense of maintaining the school was borne by the parents of the children in attendance and by free contributions of friends of the good cause. During the two years in which the school was maintained, four classes were graduated and numerous socials and entertainments were given by the school.

In the fall of the year 1907 the public school board of Berkeley, seeing the folly of trying to force vaccination upon those opposed to it, and realizing that they had lost some 400 pupils from the public schools in the two years previous, as well as a financial loss of $3,500 a year, decided to give in and accept the disability certificates, and allow the unvaccinated children to attend the public schools. Thus the anti-vaccination school was discontinued.

However, the anti-vaccination spirit was fully alive. In January, 1907, a bill to prevent vaccination being made a condition to admission to the public schools, was introduced in the State Legislature, and was passed, but failed to receive the sanction of the Governor.

But the League of Berkeley, content with nothing short of repeal of the compulsory law, continued its meetings and the distribution of the best literature obtainable for the information about the folly and dangers of vaccination, and it became an important factor in the election of the local School Board in 1909 by supporting only those who were opposed to compulsory vaccination. Since that time but little trouble has been experienced on this question in the Berkeley public schools.

Local conditions in Berkeley having been satisfactorily arranged, the Berkeley League, in conjunction with other organizations in the State in 1910 formed a State League, which now numbers several thousand members. The good work now assumed a state-wide field, and neither time nor expense was spared to have the obnoxious law repealed. Finally the league went before the legislature with another bill, and in the face of a strong opposition on the part of the medical trust, the anti-compulsory bill became a law. Thanks to the efforts of the friends of the good cause who sent petitions of voters from all parts of the State to the legislature and the governor asking for the passage of the bill, and thanks to Governor Hiram Johnson who had backbone and wisdom enough to sign the bill and thereby made it become a law.

A great victory has been won, but the fight must still go on until education will overcome ignorance, superstition and fraud, and vaccination is no more in the fair land of eternal sunshine. As the modified law stands now, only in case of an epidemic of smallpox an unvaccinated child may be barred from attending of public schools and then only during the time of such an epidemic in its own district. Step by step we must fight for our rights and our freedom. The opposition to vaccination comprises the most noted scientists, physicians, statesmen and thinkers of today. And the people are awakening all over the world. Today there are over twenty million people in this country of ours who have no use for drugs and medicine of any form, who could be easily brought into one powerful organization for medical freedom. It takes time, work and sacrifices to accomplish anything in this world. And what the friends of the good cause in California have achieved can be duplicated anywhere else. There is nothing like trying. By following the noble example of the Berkeley league, the same results will follow. Do as they so bravely did, try and try again, in order to succeed. All glory to the victor, and encouragement to the beginners. What others have done, may be done again by others. And we learn things by doing them, since experience is our best teacher. By all means organize. In union there is power. And nothing succeeds like success.

1774 Sutter St., San Francisco, California.

Due to its efforts, in 1905, an anti-vaccination bill, which was a revision of the Utah law, finally passed the Legislature of California, but was vetoed by the governor, Dr. G. C. Pardee.

Finally an anti-vaccination school *was opened on August 7, 1905, for all the children whose parents were opposed to vaccination.*

In the fall of the year 1907 the public school board of Berkeley, seeing the folly of trying to force vaccination upon those opposed to it, and realizing that they had lost some 400 pupils from the public schools in the two years previous, as well as a financial loss of $3,500 a year, decided to give in and accept the disability certificates, and allow the unvaccinated children to attend the public schools.

A DOCTOR'S REASONS FOR OPPOSING VACCINATION

by Unknown Author

The Naturopath and Herald of Health, XVI (7), 449-450. (1911)

In opposing vaccination I am aware that it is a thankless task to brave the abuse and antagonism which everyone who attempts to move forward in the work of medical progress is sure to encounter.

In order that I may not be regarded as prejudiced against the dogma of vaccination, I will preface my remarks with the confession that I was at one time myself a confiding dupe of the "tradition of the dairy maids". While attending medical college I was told that inoculation with cow pox virus was a certain preventative of smallpox, and like most other medical students I accepted with childlike faith and credulity the dictum of my teachers as so much infallible wisdom. After an experience derived from treating a number of cases of post-vaccinal smallpox in patients who gave evidence of having been recently and successfully vaccinated, I awoke to a realization of the unpleasant fact that *protective vaccination* was not all that was claimed for it. I thereupon began a study of the vaccination problem in all its bearings. After several years of reading, observation and experience I became fully convinced that *successful* vaccination not only fails to protect its subjects from smallpox, but that, in reality it renders them more susceptible to this disease by impairing their health and vitality, and by diminishing their power of resistance.

Personally, I know of recently vaccinated patients dying from smallpox while having the plainest foveated vaccine marks upon their bodies, and I have seen other individuals who had never submitted to vaccine inoculation have variola in its mildest and most benign type.

In view of such experience I refused to ignore the evidence of my own senses, and determined to follow the dictates of reason instead of the dogmas of faith, and have, consequently, for the past 15 years refused to pollute the blood of a single person with vaccine virus.

I oppose vaccination because I believe that health is always preferable to disease. The principle and practice of vaccination involves the introduction of the contagion of disease at least twice, and, according to numerous authorities, many times, into the human organism. The disease, conveyed by vaccination causes an undeniable impairment of health and vitality, it being a distinctly morbid process. The morbific matter, miscalled vaccine *lymph*, is taken from a lesion on the body of a diseased beast, and inserted by the vaccinator into the circulation of healthy children. The performance of such an insanitary operation, in the very nature of the case, is a violation of the cardinal principles of hygiene and of sanitary science. ... Moreover, this operation is in direct controversion of the basic principles of aseptic surgery, the legitimate aim of which is to *remove* from the organism the products of disease, but never to *introduce* them.

The prime aim of the modern surgeon is to make every wound aseptic and to keep it so. The careful operator employs every means at his command to clear the field of operations of all bacteria. He utilizes every particle of the marvelously minute and intricate technique of asepsis to prevent the entrance through the wounded tissues of any disease elements before, during or after that operation. He fears sepsis equally with death, and yet, under the blighting and blinding influence of an ancient and venerated myth inherited from his ignorant and superstitious forbears of a pre-scientific age, he will deliberately inoculate the virulent infective products of diseased animal tissues into the circulation of a healthy person. And as if to cap the climax of his stupidity and inconsistency, he performs the operation under *aseptic precautions*.

The poisonous matter which nature wisely eliminates from the body of a diseased calf in an effort to save its life and restore it to health, is seized upon by the vaccinator and implanted into the wholesome body of a helpless child. Think of the unparalleled absurdity of purposely infecting the body of a healthy person in this era of sanitary science with the poison from a diseased beast, under the senseless pretext of protecting the victim of the engrafted disease from the contagion of another disease! Can inconsistency go further?

I oppose the practice of vaccination because it is not known what vaccine virus is, except that it is a mixed contagion of disease. We hear much these days about *pure virus* and *pure calf lymph*. Nothing could be more absurd and meaningless than the flippant talk indulged by vaccinators and the purveyors of vaccine virus about *pure calf lymph*, a hybrid product of diseased animal tissues. *Pure virus* translated into plain English is *pure animal poison*. The phrase *pure calf lymph* as applied to any brand of vaccine virus now in use is a misnomer for two reasons. It is not *pure* and it is not *calf lymph*.

Calf lymph is the normal nutrient fluid which circulates in the lymphatic vessels of the calf. Lymph is described by physiologists as a "transparent, colorless, nutrient alkaline fluid which circulates in the lymphatic vessels and thoracic ducts of animal bodies". Lymph is a physiological product, while the so-called *pure calf lymph* used by vaccinators is a pathological product, derived form a lesion on a diseased calf. The difference between calf lymph and so-called *pure calf lymph* is as great as is the difference between a food and a poison. The vaccine mixture now most generally used by the medical profession is known under the name of *glycerinized vaccine lymph*, but it is not *lymph* at all. It is made by utilizing practically the entire lesion or pock on the heifer when it is in the vesicular stage. Such a lesion is broken open and scraped with a Volkmann spoon until the whole of the tissue is forcibly and roughly curetted away, consisting of pus, morbid serum, epithelium, fibrous tissue of the skin and any foreign matter on or in it, constituting what is called *pulp*. This pulp is then passed between glass rollers for trituration and afterwards mixed with a definite amount of glycerine and distilled water. The complex pathologic product of unknown origin is injected into the wholesome bodies of helpless children under the false but plausible name of *pure calf lymph*.

I oppose the practice of vaccination because under whatever pretext performed the implantation of disease elements into the healthy human organism is irrational and injurious. It is subversive of the fundamental principles of sanitary science, while the attainment of health as a prophylactic measure is rational and in harmony with the ascertained laws of hygiene, and consistent with the canons of common sense. I am firmly convinced that the absurd and unreasonable dogma which assumes to conserve health by propagating disease should receive the open condemnation of every scientific sanitarian. That this health blighting delusion conceived in the ignorance of a past generation should find lodgment in the minds of intelligent people enjoying the light of the world's highest civilization is to my mind inexplicable.

After several years of reading, observation and experience I became fully convinced that successful *vaccination not only fails to protect its subjects from smallpox, but that, in reality it renders them more susceptible to this disease by impairing their health and vitality, and by diminishing their power of resistance.*

The morbific matter, miscalled vaccine lymph, *is taken from a lesion on the body of a diseased beast, and inserted by the vaccinator into the circulation of healthy children. The performance of such an insanitary operation, in the very nature of the case, is a violation of the cardinal principles of hygiene and of sanitary science.*

I oppose the practice of vaccination because under whatever pretext performed the implantation of disease elements into the healthy human organism is irrational and injurious. It is subversive of the fundamental principles of sanitary science, while the attainment of health as a prophylactic measure is rational and in harmony with the ascertained laws of hygiene, and consistent with the canons of common sense.

1912

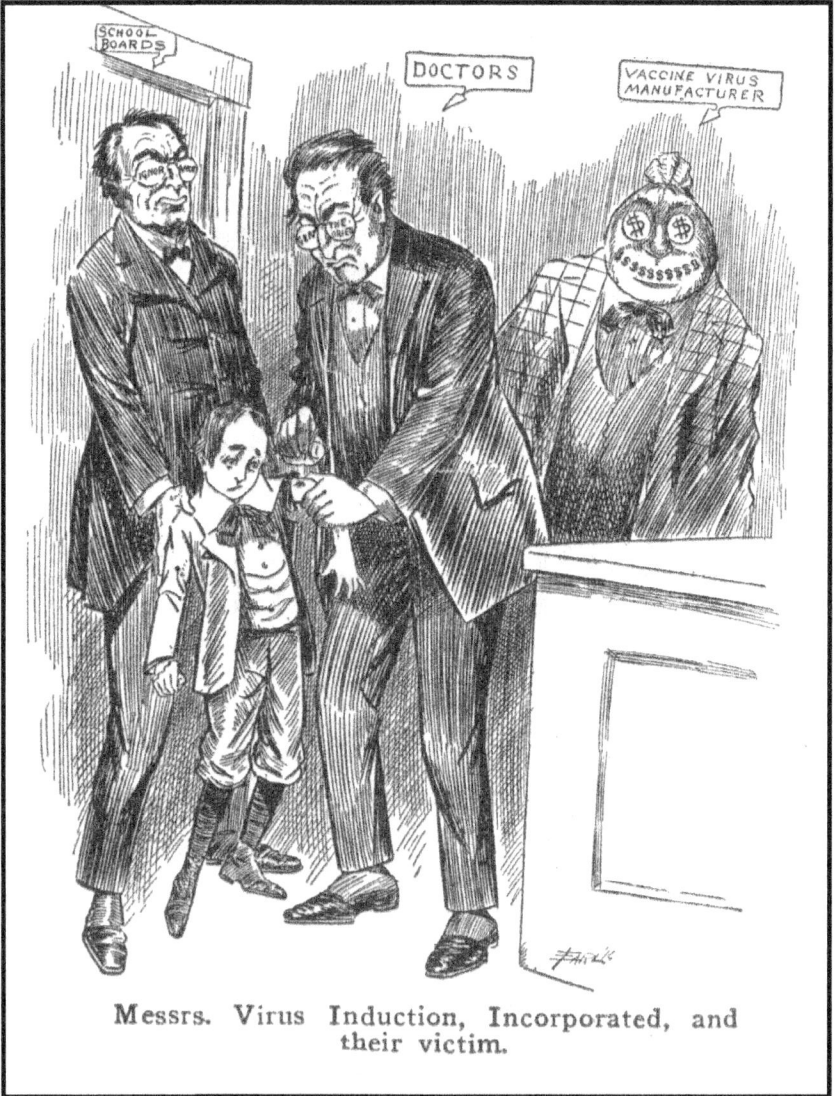

Messrs. Virus Induction, Incorporated, and their victim.

As attested by political cartoons of the era, medical doctors, school boards and vaccine manufacturers colluded to use political force and fear mongering tactics to achieve their goals of compulsory vaccination of school children.

Does Vaccination Prevent Smallpox?

by Charles W. Littlefield, M.D.

The Naturopath and Herald of Health, XVII (1), 12-17. (1912)

There was a debate between Dr. F. S. Bournes, former City Health Officer of Seattle, and Dr. Charles W. Littlefield, Chairman Washington State Branch of the National League for Medical Freedom, on the subject "Does Vaccination Prevent Smallpox?" under the auspices of The Civic Forum, Christensen's Hall, Madison and Broadway, Tuesday evening, August 1, 1911.

As this discussion was held for the sole purpose of arriving at the worldwide results which have followed the practice of vaccination over a period of nearly 200 years, it offered a rare opportunity to hear both sides.

In the following article we reproduce Dr. Littlefield's denial [rebuttal]. —Benedict Lust.

Vaccination represents an honest effort on the part of the medical profession to find a preventive for a simple, yet loathsome disease. This effort, however, like many others of its kind, has not only failed to meet the expectation of its discoverer, but has left in its wake a blighting curse which it will require many generations to remove. Were it not for the fact that vaccination has been enforced by legislation, we would not now be discussing it except as an antiquated medical experiment akin to leeches and blood-letting. But on account of the fact that it has received the sanction of legislation, a moral and scientific support has been accorded it, unlike any other medical prescription involving such vast possibilities for evil. The rite has surrounded itself, therefore, with an artificial respect always accorded to anything sanctioned by law. In every country on earth, popular patronage has always turned towards things upheld by legislation, for the simple reason—people love to be loyal. When, therefore, we remember that the pretension, upon which vaccination originally established itself, was not the beneficent results following its use, but its enforcement by law, we can readily understand why there has been such a universal surrender to its use.

The history of the introduction of vaccination in England, gives us at once a reason for the legislation which was so early enacted in its favor in that country, as well as its unanimous endorsement by the medical profession. As this country affords the most exhaustive and comprehensive survey of this subject, I shall confine my remarks to it, although the practice of inoculation dates from times immemorial in every country on earth.

In 1721, Lady Mary Wortley Montague, the wife of the British Ambassador at Constantinople, writing from that city said: "The smallpox so general and fatal amongst us is here rendered entirely harmless by the invention of 'engrafting' which is the term they give it. There is a set of old women who make it their business to perform this operation." This *operation* consisted in taking the pus from the sore of an infected individual and putting it into the blood of a healthy person.

At the time of its introduction into England from the Empire of the Turks, it was hailed by the medical profession as the greatest of medical discoveries. Why? Because it had proven itself of real value? Not at all. Then why?

In *Spofford's Cyclopedia* we read, "Lady Mary has another claim to remembrance in her courageous adaption of the Turkish practice of inoculation for smallpox, and for her energy in promoting its introduction into England. On her return she resumed her ascendancy in the gay world of wit and fashion."

Do we not see in this a sufficient reason why in 1754 the Royal College of Physicians and Surgeons of London passed the following resolution?

> The college, having been informed that false reports concerning the success of inoculation in England, have been published in foreign countries, think proper to declare their sentiments in the following manner: That the arguments which, at the commencement of this practice were urged against it, have been refuted by experience, that it is now held by the English in greater esteem and practiced among them more than ever it was before, and that the college thinks it to be highly salutary to the human race.

In spite of the influence of Lady Mary, facts could not be ignored. Instead of inoculation proving itself a beneficent invention, it soon became evident that each inoculated person became a new center of contagion, until smallpox had become so prevalent that in 1840, or 119 years after the introduction of inoculation, the British Parliament passed a law branding it a crime, and made the practice punishable by imprisonment.

Does it not seem a little strange that we to-day should be advocating a practice and insisting on legislation in its favor, which in every principle involved, was proven by England during a period of 119 years to be one of the most serious experiments ever indulged in by the medical profession?

About 1776, it having become evident that inoculation, of arm to arm vaccination, was a failure and dangerous, the common belief sprang up among the people that cowpox acquired in milking cows, was a preventative of smallpox. This caused Dr. Edward Jenner to make some inquiry into the subject, and lead to the introduction by him of vaccination in 1796. His method at first met with great opposition from those who had endorsed Lady Mary's method, but was ultimately accepted because, as already stated, it was observed that inoculation from person to person carried with it other diseases more dangerous and loathsome than small-pox.

The question before us to-night is, "Does Vaccination Prevent Small-pox?" In answer to this question, I quote from Dr. Jenner himself, page 8 of his inquiry. He speaks first of direct contagion from the cow:

> Inflamed spots now begin to appear on different parts of the hands of the domestics employed in milking, and sometimes on the wrist, which quickly run on to suppuration, first assuming the appearance of the small vesicles produced by a burn. Most commonly they appear about the joints of the fingers, and at their extremities; but whatever parts are affected, the situation will admit, these superficial suppurations put on a circular form, with their edges more elevated than their center, and of a color distinctly approaching blue. Absorption takes place and tumors appear in each axilla. The system becomes affected—the pulse is quickened; and shivering, with general lassitude and pains about the loins and limbs, with vomiting come on. The head is pain-ful, and the patient is even now and then affected with delirium. These symptoms, varying in their degrees of violence, generally continue from one day to three or four, leaving ulcerated sores about the hands, which, from the sensibility of the parts, are very troublesome, and commonly heal slowly, frequently becom-ing phagedenic, like those from whence they sprung. The lips, nostrils, eyelids, and other parts of the body, are sometimes affect-ed with sores; but these evidently arise from their being needlessly rubbed or scratched with the patient's infected fingers. No erup-tions on the skin have followed the decline of the feverish symp-toms in any instance that has come under my inspection, one only excepted, and in this case a very few appeared on the arms; they were very minute, of a vivid red color, and soon died away without advancing to maturation; so that I cannot determine whether they had any connection with the preceding symptoms.

> Thus the disease makes its progress from the horse to the nipple of the cow, and from the cow to the human subject.

> Morbid matter of various kinds, when absorbed into the system, may produce effects in some degree similar; but what renders the cowpox virus so extremely singular, is, that the person who has thus affected is forever after secure from infection of the small-pox; neither exposure to the various effluvia, nor the insertion of the matter into the skin, producing this distemper.

> In support of so extraordinary a fact, I shall lay before my reader a great number of instances.

> Here is a very accurate description of a well-developed case of small-

pox. The fact that these people were immune, led Jenner to adopt vaccination. He then cites two hundred cases vaccinated with cowpox and shows that they all had the smallpox, some very mild and some severe.

It is evident from this that the purpose of vaccination was not to prevent smallpox but to modify it. Therefore it cannot be said that vaccination prevents smallpox. What is meant by the question is evidently this: Does vaccination grant immunity to smallpox? Jenner began by claiming that vaccination made of a person immune for life, but the facts of observation soon resulted in the term of immunity being shortened to fourteen years, then it was made seven, then two, and in the Spanish-American War, six weeks was the limit of immunity. If six weeks is the period of immunity now, then six weeks must have been the period of immunity when the College of Physicians and Surgeons in London held it as the greatest medical discovery, and a boon to the race. How far wrong was Jenner when he proclaimed immunity for life, while our modern practice grants immunity for only six weeks? Calculating according to the average lifetime this would mean that he was about thirty-three years off. That it does not grant immunity even for six weeks, is proven by the recent official statistics of our Philippine Army. In that army, in the five years from 1898 to 1902, there were 737 cases of smallpox, and 261 deaths. Referring to this great smallpox incident and mortality, Chief Surgeon Lippincott reports, "I can say that no army was ever so thoroughly looked after in the matter of vaccination many times repeated, went on as regularly as the drills at an army post." Thus do the facts not belie the assertion that vaccination grants immunity to smallpox?

It is now admitted by all competent authorities that vaccination during epidemics of smallpox tends to diffuse rather that arrest the disease.

Opposition to the practice of vaccination was brought very prominently before the English people a few years ago, by an article on the subject by the eminent pathologist Dr. Charles Creighton in the *Encyclopedia Britannica*. For the purpose of writing this article, Dr. Creighton, having for many years believed in and practiced vaccination, went into a most exhaustive study of the subject, and it was not long before the conviction forced itself upon him that vaccination was not only useless in preventing smallpox, but dangerous in practice. He so informed the compilers of the *Encyclopedia Britannica*, but they expressed a desire for the unbiased result of his examination, and the result was fifteen columns in that work against vaccination. The facts stated by Dr. Creighton at the beginning of this article, are the outcome of independent and laborious research. This article from so eminent authority so disturbed the pro-vaccinists that, they sought for an equally eminent scientist to reply. It so happened that about the same time the well-known pathologist, Dr. Edgar M. Crookshank, of The Kings College, of London, was devoting himself to pathological research in connection with the diseases communicated from the lower animals to man. The question naturally arose whether his observation supported or refuted the conclusions arrived at by Dr. Creighton as to the result of his historical researches. Dr. Crookshank likewise went into an exhaustive examination of the subject, and the result was two volumes against vaccination. I would like to impress these facts upon you. Here we have two men, most eminent in their profession; both of the regular school; both entered upon the subject for the avowed purpose of supporting it, with no other end in view than to show forth its benefits, and in both cases the result of their research was the same, an absolute condemnation of the practice, not only setting forth the facts that is does not afford immunity against smallpox, but as being actually dangerous and baneful in its results.

Now I ask, in view of these facts, which are open to the investigation of anyone, what authority can an individual like my friend or myself, whose experience and observation have necessarily been limited, what authority, I ask, can my statement or his have in deciding this matter in your mind?

After the publication of Dr. Crookshank's work, the English public became thoroughly aroused, and Royal Commission was appointed, with Lord Herschell as chairman, to investigate the matter. This commission, which was in session for seven years, received the testimony of experts from all parts of the world, and its report, comprised in seven large volumes, constitute what is, perhaps, the most thorough and exhaustive collection of evidence and facts ever made upon the subject. The only feature of this report which especially interests us at the present time is this: "It was no longer contended that vaccination prevented smallpox." After the report was received, one of the last acts of the late Lord Salisbury, at the recommendation of this commission, was the introduction into Parliament of the "Conscience Clause" in the compulsory vaccination law, which was passed unanimously. In 1907, in the Parliamentary election, over one hundred members were returned on an anti-vaccination platform, and there was at that time pending a memorial to the Prime Minister, signed by 174 members of the House of Commons, Petitioning for the entire abolition of the Compulsory Vaccination Act.

Included in the evidence given before this commission, was that of Dr. Gayten, who testified, "Very fleeting, indeed, is the immunity, if any, rendered by vaccination. I have seen in fourteen years 1,306 vaccinated cases of smallpox."

Dr. Bridewood testified that after two years in a hospital ship, he had seen 12,000 cases, and when asked by the commission if vaccination could be relied on as an absolute protection or as of any advantage whatever, replied, "I say no."

This is certainly sufficient, my friends, upon the question of immunity granted by vaccination.

There is, however, a phase of this subject in which we are more interested than the question of immunity, and this is the question of risk, which has by far the larger claim on our attention. For, if the operation were merely useless, we might regard it with indifference, or even with philosophic amusement, and allow the experimenters to continue their foolish practice, and permit our State Legislatures, if they will, to enforce it upon us. But in this aspect, however, the subject is really too serious for satire.

It is no longer a question in the mind of any person whether vaccination is dangerous, the only question is, how dangerous? It is not open to question that there have been cases in which injuries and deaths have resulted from vaccination. It is established beyond question that vaccination lymph contains organisms many of which, under certain conditions, produce the most loathsome disease with which the human family has ever been afflicted, and it is proven beyond a doubt that vaccination does serves as an exciting cause for the outbreak of diseases lying latent and dormant within the system. All of these things should be taken into serious consideration by the man who would inject this disease-bearing substance into the blood of a healthy and innocent person.

It was these dangers especially, which, after seven years of investigation, resulting in such damaging admission, impelled the Royal Commission to advise unanimously the relaxation of the compulsory vaccination law. The majority of the commissioners, while admitting the risk, suggested that it may be reasonable to disregard this risk for the benefit of the community. They cited the fact that while it had been shown that there were more than 14,000 deaths from vaccination, yet railway fatalities furnished a like number. But we must remember that railway fatalities are the result of accidents not imposed by legislation or a risk accepted to prevent a disease. In that report more than forty different diseases are enumerated as having been communicated by vaccination. Among them, are enumerated some diseases that this presence forbids me mentioning; but others I may mention, as 126 cases of erysipelas, 64 eczema, 222 cancer, 9 of scrofula, with convulsions, blindness, abscesses, boils, tuberculosis, paralysis, meningitis, and many others. Such returns, however, represent only cases where the mischief followed directly and obviously on vaccination, and they can form only a small proportion of the whole evil that must have been rife during the 119 years that inoculation and vaccination were practiced in England prior to the report of this commission.

I must, therefore, before leaving this part of the question, invite your attention to two thoughts that should give us great concern: The first is the manifest increases of tuberculosis following vaccination. We are making many sacrifices to stamp out what is known as the *white plague*, and yet through this practice of vaccination we are, without a question, spreading it. Tuberculosis is a disease to which the cow is especially liable, and its presence in the animal, as experiments have proved, can often be determined by a postmortem examination.

According to Dr. Perron, in an article in a French Medical Journal, tuberculosis, which was once an exceptional thing, has in the last 100 years been steadily extending its ravages in spite of the general advancement in hygiene, until to-day it has attained the rank of a pestilence. He finds himself compelled to the conviction that the causative factor is vaccination, since this is the only practice which has advanced step by step with tuberculosis. Herein we find an explanation of the extraordinary devastation wrought in the European armies, where revaccination is the order of the day, and where tuberculosis is by far the largest cause of mortality.

With this clue we find significance in the figures recently published, showing the deaths from tuberculosis in Germany, where vaccination is now so much at home, as thrice more common and numerous than in England, where vaccination is no longer compulsory.

The second thought to which I would invite your attention is that of the alarming increases in cancer in Germany. In spite of the weird and wonderful causes of cancer, which range in the medical mind from tomatoes to common salt, in the twenty years ending in 1907, the yearly fatality has gone, steadily forward from 17,506 to 31,754 per year.

Even at home we find a corresponding increase of both tuberculosis and cancer with vaccination.

The question asked, "Does Vaccination Prevent Smallpox?" may be answered NO.

1. Who are the leading opponents of vaccination? A host of honored physicians of world-wide reputation who have practiced vaccination, have seen the evil effects of it, and have had the courage and honesty to bear testimony to them such medical men as Creighton, Crookshank, Hadwin and Wilkinson, of England; Hodge, Winterburn, Oswald, Ross and Leverson, of this country; Foster of Germany, and Ricord of France; such eminent scientists as Herbert Spencer, William Tebb, Alfred Russel Wallace, Professor Ruata, of Italy; Professor Vogt, of Switzerland, and others too numerous to mention, all of who have based their opposition upon facts brought to light and viewed without prejudice. Certainly this is good company.

2. It is not intended, it is not necessary, to bring a railing accusation against doctors in general, or question the high standing of personal worth and honor which rule in the medical profession. It is only necessary to assume that they like other people, suffer from human nature; and, this being so, it is imperative to remind the public that its patient and passive acquiescence in medical tyranny exposes it to dangers of the most alarming kind. Apart from the various inducements into intellectual error already adverted to, there is, in the present instance,

a very special liability conscious or unconscious to personal bias. It is emphatically good in a personal sense to support vaccination; it is bad to question it.

3. But a policy which insists upon polluting repeatedly, the blood of every human being, however healthy or healthily circumstanced with a virus obtained by squeezing the filth from sores raised on a calf's belly. A virus of whose nature and pedigree there is no scientific knowledge, but which has proved capable of causing loathsome and moral diseases, and all this for the purpose of obtaining an admittedly qualified, temporary and doubtful protection from one only of the many thousand diseases to which flesh is heir. A disease, moreover, which grows so rare that even in in so-called epidemics fatality is surpassed many times by half a dozen other diseases, about which no artificial panic has been induced; a disease which has been proved both preventable, and mitigated by hygienic means, a disease of which the risk, except in slums, is practically negligible, and which rational treatment has now robbed of its most dreaded feature—such a policy need only to be clearly stated to be seen for what it is, a monstrous and indefensible outrage upon the common sense and sacred personal rights of every human being. An unbearable tyranny, it has roused, and justly roused, an exasperation so intense that it is impossible to give it satisfying expression without breach of the properties of debate. There is a determined insurgence at work, and it will not subside till vaccination has been finally relegated to the shells of that well stocked scientific museum where the dishonored fetishes and perished fallacies of medicine remain on view for the warning and instruction of mankind.

Vaccination represents an honest effort on the part of the medical profession to find a preventive for a simple, yet loathsome disease. This effort, however, like many others of its kind, has not only failed to meet the expectation of its discoverer, but has left in its wake, a blighting curse which it will require many generations to remove. Were it not for the fact that vaccination has been enforced by legislation, we would not now be discussing it except as an antiquated medical experiment akin to leeches and blood-letting.

In every country on earth, popular patronage has always turned towards things upheld by legislation, for the simple reason—people love to be loyal. When, therefore, we remember that the pretension, upon which vaccination originally established itself, was not the beneficent results following its use, but its enforcement by law, we can readily understand why there has been such a universal surrender to its use.

Instead of inoculation proving itself a beneficent invention, it soon became evident that each inoculated person became a new center of contagion, until smallpox had become so prevalent that in 1840, or 119 years after the introduction of inoculation, the British Parliament passed a law branding it a crime, and made the practice punishable by imprisonment.

Jenner began by claiming that vaccination made of a person immune for life, but the facts of observation soon resulted in the term of immunity being shortened to fourteen years, then it was made seven, then two, and in the Spanish-American War, six weeks was the limit of immunity.

It is no longer a question in the mind of any person whether vaccination is dangerous, the only question is, how dangerous?

In that report more than forty different diseases are enumerated as having been communicated by vaccination. Among them, are enumerated some diseases that this presence forbids me mentioning; but others I may mention, as 126 cases of erysipelas, 64 eczema, 222 cancer, 9 of scrofula, with convulsions, blindness, abscesses, boils, tuberculosis, paralysis, meningitis, and many others.

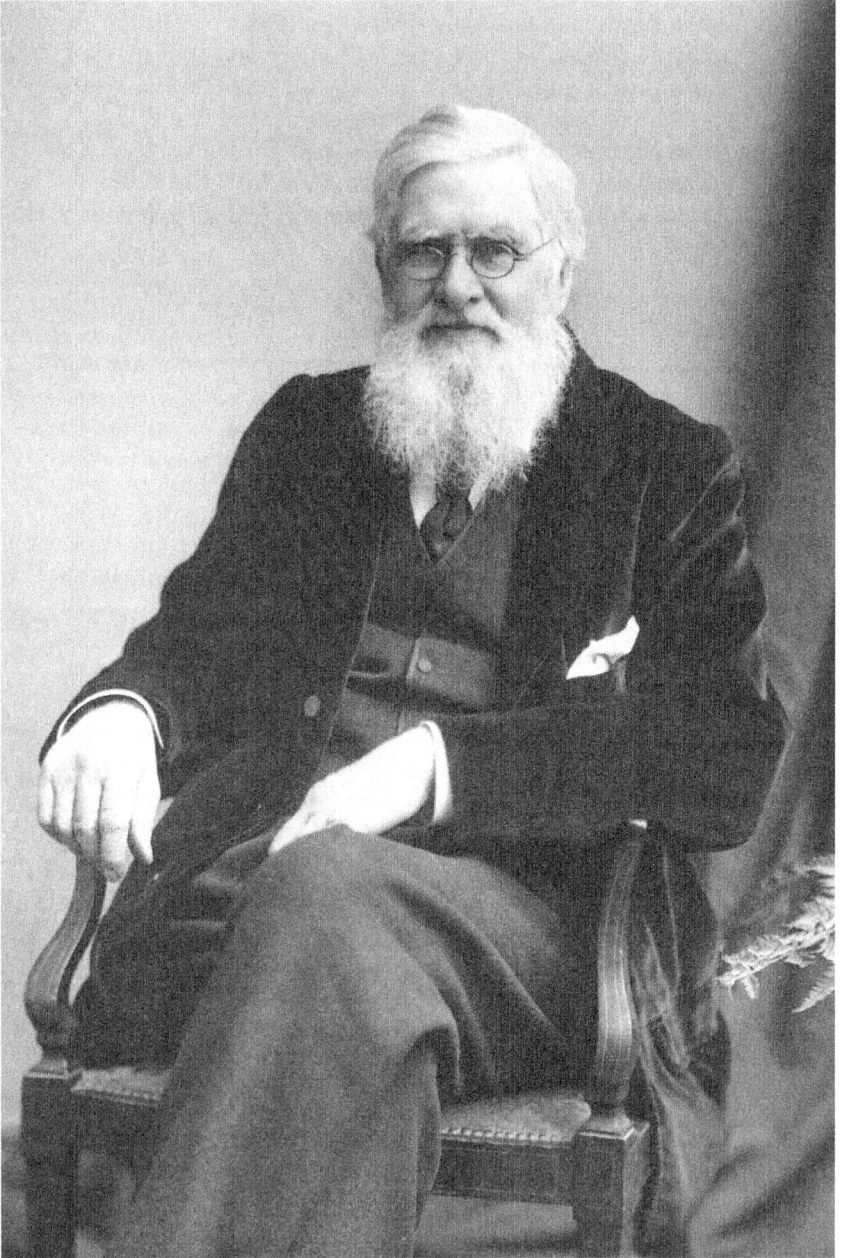

Alfred Russel Wallace [1823-1913].

Alfred Russel Wallace And The Vaccination Question

by Alfred Russel Wallace

The Naturopath and Herald of Health, XVII (1), 41-42. (1912)

I will here say a few words about another subject in which I take a great interest, and upon which I have ventured to express views contrary to those held by the orthodox authorities.

I was brought up to believe that vaccination was a scientific procedure, and that Jenner was one of the great benefactors of mankind. I was vaccinated in infancy, and before going to the Amazon I was persuaded to be vaccinated again. My children were duly vaccinated, and I never had the slightest doubt of the value of the operation—taking everything on trust without any inquiry whatever—till about 1875-80, when I first heard that there are anti-vaccinators, and read some articles on the subject. These did not much impress me, as I could not believe so many eminent men could be mistaken on such an important matter. But a little later I met Mr. William Tebb, and through him was introduced to some of the more important statistical facts bearing upon the subject. Some of these I was able to test by reference to the original authorities, and also to the various *Reports of the Registrar-General*, Dr. Farr's evidence as to the diminution of smallpox before Jenner's time, and the extraordinary misstatements of the supporters of vaccination. Mr. Tebb supplied me with a good deal of anti-vaccination literature, especially with *Pearce's Vital Statistics,* claims for vaccination was enormously exaggerated, if not altogether fallacious. I also now learnt for the first time that vaccination itself produced a disease which was often injurious to health and sometimes fatal to life, and I also found to my astonishment that even Herbert Spencer had long ago pointed out that the first Compulsory Vaccination Act had led to an increase of smallpox. I then began to study the *Reports of the Registrar-General* myself, and to draw out curves of smallpox mortality, and of other zymotic diseases (the only way of showing the general course of a disease as well as its annual inequalities) and then found that the course of the former disease ran so generally parallel to that of the latter as to disprove altogether any special protective effect of vaccination.

As I could find no short and clear statement of the main statistical facts adverse to vaccination, I wrote a short pamphlet of thirty-eight pages, entitled *Forty-five Years of Registration Statistics, proving Vaccination to be both Useless and Dangerous.* This was published in 1885 at Mr. W. Tebb's expense, and it had the effect of convincing many persons, among whom were some of my personal friends.

A few years later, when the Royal Commission on Vaccination was appointed, I was invited to become a member of it, but declined, as I could not give up the necessary time, but chiefly because I thought I could do more good as a witness. I accordingly prepared a number of large diagrams, and stated the arguments drawn from them, and in the 1890 gave my evidence during part of three days. As about half the Commissioners were doctors, most of the others gave way to them. I told them, at the beginning of my evidence, that I knew nothing of medicine, but that, following the principle laid down by Sir John Simon and Dr. Guy, that "the evidence for the benefits of vaccination must now be statistical," I was prepared to show the bearing of the best statistics only. Yet they insisted on putting medical arguments and alleged medical facts to me, asking me how I explained this, how I accounted for that; and though I stated again and again that there were plenty of medical witnesses who would deal with those points, they continually recurred to them; and when I said I had no answer to give, not having inquired into those alleged facts, they seemed to think they had got the best of it. Yet they were so ignorant of statistics and statistical methods that one great doctor held out a diagram, showing the same facts as one of mine, and asked me almost triumphantly how it was that mine was so different. After comparing the two diagrams for a few moments, I replied that they were drawn on different scales, but that with that exception I could see no substantial difference between them. The other diagram was on a greatly exaggerated vertical scale, so that the line showing each year's death-rate went up and down with tremendous peaks and chasms, while mine approximated more to a very irregular curve. But my questioner could not see this simple point; and later he referred to it a second time, and asked me if I really meant to tell them that those two diagrams were both accurate, and when I said again that though on different scales both represented the same facts, he looked up at the ceiling with an air which plainly said, "If you will say that you will say anything."

The Commission lingered on for six years, and did not issue its final report till 1896, while the evidence, statistics, and diagrams occupied numerous bulky blue-books. The most valuable parts of it were the appendices, containing the tables and diagrams presented by the chief witnesses, together with a large number of official tables and statistics, both of our own and foreign countries, affording a mass of material never before brought together. This enabled me to present the general statistical argument more completely and forcibly than I had done before, and I devoted several months of very hard work to doing this, and brought it out in pamphlet form in January, 1898, in order that a copy might be sent to every member of the House of Commons before the new Vaccination Act came up for discussion. This was done by the National Anti-Vaccination League, and I wrote to the half-dozen members I knew personally, begging them to give one evening to its careful perusal. But so far as any of their speeches showed, not one of the six hundred and seventy members gave even that amount of their time to obtain information on a subject involving the health, life, and personal freedom of their constituents. Yet I *know* that in no work I have written have I presented so clear and so conclusive a demonstration of the fallacy of a popular belief as is given in this work, which was entitled *Vaccination a Delusion: Its Penal Enforcement a Crime, Proved by the Official Evidence in the Reports of the Royal Commission.* This was included in the second part of my *Wonderful Century*, published in June, 1898, and was also published separately in the pamphlet form as it continues to be; and I feel sure that the time is not far distant when this will be held to be one of the most important and most truly scientific of my works.

Mr. Tebb supplied me with a good deal of anti-vaccination literature, especially with Pearce's Vital Statistics, *claims for vaccination was enormously exaggerated, if not altogether fallacious. I also now learnt for the first time that vaccination itself produced a disease which was often injurious to health and sometimes fatal to life, and I also found to my astonishment that even Herbert Spencer had long ago pointed out that the first Compulsory Vaccination Act had led to an increase of small-pox.*

Yet they were so ignorant of statistics and statistical methods that one great doctor held out a diagram, showing the same facts as one of mine, and asked me almost triumphantly how it was that mine was so different. After comparing the two diagrams for a few moments, I replied that they were drawn on different scales, but that with that exception I could see no substantial difference between them.

What Is Their Real Purpose?

by Honorable Charles W. Miller,

Member of the Iowa State Legislature

The Naturopath and Herald of Health, XVII (2), 84-86. (1912)

Henry M. Hyde recently contributed to the *Saturday Evening Post* a cleverly written and prettily illustrated story purporting to set forth the great benefits that have resulted from medical inspection in the public schools. Therein is found a paragraph the analysis of which illumines the whole subject so well that I adopt it as my text. It is as follows:

> It was the doctors who first gave the alarm. And here let it be remarked, to the honor of the brotherhood of Aesculapius, the physicians are the only class of men in the world whose hardest and most zealous work is devoted to the destruction of the prospects of their own business.

The first of the above statements will be given ready acquiescence. The *political-doctors* were not only the first to give the alarm, but there have been few alarms since the first was sounded which they have not been directly or indirectly responsible for. Ever since organized medicine became established on a commercial basis, it has maintained a well-equipped alarm-sounding department, which establishment, by the way, was never in such fine working order as at the present time. The alarms sounded by this department during recent years pertain not merely to the awful havoc disease is causing in the public schools for lack of expert medical inspection, but encompass the wider scope of endeavoring to convince people generally that death and disease are lurking in every nook and cranny of our homes and every-day surroundings, and in promoting the fiction that their only hope of a healthful existence and serene old age lies in the medical surveillance and censorship that the physicians, out of the goodness of their hearts, are insistently offering them.

And this brings me to the second part of my quotation from Mr. Hyde's story. That the medical profession has so completely eliminated from itself the element of human selfishness that it is gladly offering its material prospects on the altar of public weal, is not only incredible, but arrogantly, flagrantly and ridiculously untrue. In support of the farfetched assumption there is but the brazen suggestion of the *political-doctors* and those who speak for them. In denial of it there is the existence of the great American Medical Association, embracing a vast number of *regular* physicians, the major purpose of which is to make the doctor business more profitable, and through whose inspiration and suggestion its subsidiary organizations adopt outrageous fee bills and cruel blacklist agreements and send lobbies to state legislatures to strive for laws calculated to tighten their monopoly and compel medical attendance upon people who do not want it and would rather be without it.

The medical inspection of schools propaganda had its birth some twenty years ago, about the time various drugless systems of healing began to gain respectable standing and win many patients from the *regular* physicians. The *regular* doctors noted with irritation the ever-increasing number of homes being closed to them, and out of this irritation was born the idea of reaching the children of such homes through the public schools.

Medical inspection in the public schools, like all propaganda born of medical greed, is glossed thick with the gilt of philanthropy. Moreover, it has a sentimental side that readily appeals to the unthinking. That which pertains to the welfare of the boys and girls finds ready response in the breast of all loyal citizens. Their welfare is of vast importance, and unless we understand what is lurking in the back of the minds of the members of the American Medical Association, we are apt to let them have their way and applaud them for their magnanimous interest in the children's welfare.

But ere we do so again, let us consider the case of Chicago. In the fall of 1908 representatives of the local medical society waited upon the school board in that city and offered to inaugurate and carry on a system of medical inspection of the schools at so low a figure that it seemed almost like giving away money. The offer at once attracted the notice of the newspapers and many expressions were printed complimentary to the gentlemen making it. The offer was eventually accepted and the inspection began. A couple of weeks later, after it had progressed through enough of the schools to permit a fair estimate as to the whole, the papers were able to announce, in glaring headlines, "SIXTY THOUSAND CHICAGO SCHOOL CHILDREN REQUIRE MEDICAL ATTENDANCE."

Did that mean anything to the noble disciplines of Aesculapius who, we are asked to believe, are urging medical inspection of schools at the expense of destroying the prospects of their own business?

Possibly. Let us see. It goes without saying that when the inspection was completed approximately sixty thousand boys and girls were packed home to their parents bearing letters describing the more or less awful things that had been found to be the matter with them.

How many devoted mothers, rendered frantic by the intelligence the letter brought, seized their children by the hand and hurried off with them to a doctor to receive a week's, a month's, or perchance even a year's treatment? How many children marked by the medical inspector had their tonsils removed or were operated upon for adenoids? (For such operations the doctor's trust fee bill designates a fee of from $10.00 to

$50.00) How many were *fitted* with spectacles and perhaps wrongfully condemned to be encumbered with them to the end of their existence? We can but conjecture. But a very great number of those sixty thousand children, it is safe to assume, did not get back into school without the payment of some sort of a fee to a doctor, and when we consider that the sixty thousand children were the grist of the first inspection, and that it was followed by other grists at monthly intervals, and consider it in the light of the figures in a doctor's trust fee bill, no wild flight of the imagination is necessary to transport us quickly from the realm of noble philanthropy where the *political-doctors* would have us dwell as we contemplate their undertakings, into a realm of high finance where sordidness seems all the meaner for the cloak of benevolence with which it garbs itself.

And what of the sixty thousand children that were marked for medical treatment at the first gleaning and of the thousands who were marked afterward? Were they benefited by the treatment persuaded or forced upon them?

That is for the reader to answer. If he believes that a child's health can be benefited by the taking into his system of mineral poisons, by the pollution of his blood with virus taken from diseased animals, or the laceration or removal of the organs with which an all-wise God equipped his children when he gave them to the world, then in all conscience you may answer "yes". But if you hold a contrary opinion—if you believe that the theories and methods of the dominant school of medicine, which invariably takes charge of school inspection wherever it is established, have been superseded by others more efficacious, then, with equal sincerity you may answer "no". If, however, you assume to have control over the persons of your minor offspring, whether at school or at home, and would resent the persuasion or compulsion upon them of a medical treatment in your eyes useless or dangerous, then you must concede that same privilege to others even though they are but a small minority.

This brings us to the crux of the whole subject: Our public schools are free and should be kept free. Supported by all citizens alike, all should have an equal enjoyment of their privileges. Because religion is necessarily sectarian (but no more so than medicine), religion has been kept out of them. Religion has only to do with the conscience and the mind, but if we insist that our children at school be safeguarded from religious instruction of a kind that we do not approve, how much more important is it that we insist that their bodies be protected from medical treatment that we do not approve? The introduction of a disease into the blood of our children is a matter too often beyond remedy.

This is a subject that strikes not only at the very vitals of our free public school system, but involves most intimately the whole question of human rights. It is a grave subject and one entitled to the very gravest consideration.

The alarms sounded by this department during recent years pertain not merely to the awful havoc disease is causing in the public schools for lack of expert medical inspection, but encompass the wider scope of endeavoring to convince people generally that death and disease are lurking in every nook and cranny of our homes and every-day surroundings, and in promoting the fiction that their only hope of a healthful existence and serene old age lies in the medical surveillance and censorship that the physicians, out of the goodness of their hearts, are insistently offering them.

Medical inspection in the public schools, like all propaganda born of medical greed, is glossed thick with the gilt of philanthropy.

ANENT* THE MICROBE MANIA

by John W. Hodge, M.D.

The Naturopath and Herald of Health, XVII (3), 173-174. (1912)

It is touchingly pitiful to note the hold which the superstition about germs and their destruction has obtained over the minds of certain sensational and credulous newspaper editors who implicitly follow faith instead of reason.

The *Niagara Falls Gazette,* following in the wake of yellow journalism, devoted nearly a column of its editorial page yesterday to the exploitation of the vague speculations of an official germ theorist on "House Flies and Disease". So much has been written in the sensational press about disease germs and the efforts of health departments to protect the dear people against the assaults of these microscopic enemies, which official doctors tell us swarm in the air we breathe, in the water we drink and in the food we eat, lurk on the lips of lovers of millions, billions, trillions, quadrillions, quintillions, sextillions, and so on ad infinitum, that one is led to inquire where will this craze about germs end?

Every day some hitherto unheard of bacteriologist, whose sheepskin still has a fresh smell, promulgates through the yellow newspapers the alleged discovery of some new form of microbe with a long name. Every day some germ crazed theorist points to a new form of alleged danger hidden under some familiar guise, and anxiously asks how it is to be met. Nearly every day fresh horror is to be added to the existence of credulous people by the announcement of some alarming discovery purporting to bear the hallmark of science. All the actions of daily life, our down sitting, and our uprising, our letters, our books, our money, our clothes, our dwellings, the cab, the trolley car, the waiting room, the train, the theatre, the drinking cup, our every bite and sup, our work and our play, all are fraught with the most hideous perils, if we are to believe what these "bugologists" tell us. Senator Gallinger of New Hampshire, who is an eminent physician, is reported as having said anent [concerning} this subject, in a recent speech in the United States Senate: "If we believed one-half of it we should not dare to breathe, eat or drink, but would want to get into glass cases, but would be hermetically sealed up." Like Senator Gallinger, no sensible physician believes one-half of what the microbe cranks and Health Board doctors say about the alleged ravages of these minute organisms. The disease producing germ is myth, a creation of the imagination. It is really very strange that supposedly intelligent people will allow themselves to be repeatedly deluded by such sensationalists as the bacteriologists have proven themselves to be. Why not believe in ghosts, hobgoblins, fairies, werewolves and all the other superstitious inventions of senseless visionists?

---

* Anent: about, concerning. A term out of contemporary common usage. —*Ed.*

The superstitious fear engendered by bacteriologists, aided by shallow and sensational newspaper writers is developing into an instrument of power and possible oppression which Health Boards, being political bodies, know but too well how to manipulate to their own advantage. Absurd and irrational as are the claims of the microbe cranks, if no one rises to challenge or contradict their assertions, they will increase and spread until the profession and the people have been snared into a web so light, so fine, and yet so strong that it will require no mean effort to throw it off. The *Buffalo Courier* of yesterday, under the headline, "War Against the Agile Germ," says: "Fighting germs and preventing the adulteration of foods, costs the people of Buffalo over $15,900 a year." How much better are the people off now than they were before all of this useless expenditure of capital? The disease germ is a product of German imagination, which has been successfully manipulated as speculative capital both in Europe and America to an extent that is almost as fabulous as the theory on which this fad is based.

When Robert Koch announced his germ theory and imitators caught, cultivated and identified innumerable varieties of microbes, he added a new and heavy burden to the many with which man was already afflicted. A few years ago the world was in blissful ignorance of any kind of microbes save those "small deer" which the microscope discovered in the drop of water for the amusement or the terror of children. Now the microbe is here, there and everywhere. Thus do the microbe hunters rapidly increase the area of human despair and make of life an apprehensive possibility and a galling suspicion. There can henceforth be no rest for the man who believes in this disease germ and its universality. A new anxiety has been added to his life, and the anxiety is all the more burdensome because the object of it is unseen, and he cannot tell at what instant he may be exposing himself to its insidious attacks. There may be happiness in Patagonia and other remote parts of the earth where the microbe is unknown, just as there used to be happiness everywhere before it was found.

The views here presented are shared by some of the most eminent scientists and are advocated by some of the leading medical journals of all schools of medicine, as I could show if space were at my disposal for that purpose.

But I hear someone say, "Do you deny the existence of germs?" I answer "No." The germ is a fact, a fact of great interest to the biologist, but in which the pathologist has no portion. It is a physical fact and the attempt to consign the germ to the domain of pathology is a libel on these tiny creatures which swarm in all vital air, in all sparkling and potable water, in all wholesome food, and in every healthful tissue of our bodies.

But someone asks: Do we not find germs in diseased as well as in healthy tissues? I answer Yes. They are there as scavengers, as friends to the patient and as foes to the disease. To charge them with being the cause of the disease would be as unjust to them as it would be unfair to the street scavenger to charge him with having produced the filth which he is engaged in removing. The so-called cholera bacillus has frequently been found in the saliva of people who were enjoying the best of health. Prof. Petenkoffer and Prof. Esmarch, each in his own person, demonstrated the non-pathogenic character of the cholera bacillus by swallowing cultures containing hundreds of millions of these bacilli as prepared by Prof. Koch for the occasion. Metchnikoff, a renowned authority, holds that same view regarding the typhoid bacillus. He says he has found the typhoid bacilli profusely distributed in localities in which typhoid fever had never been known to occur among the inhabitants and in hospitals in which for many years there has been no case of typhoid fever. The Klebs-Loeffler bacilli, which are supposed to cause diphtheria, have been found in many healthy throats and are not capable of producing the disease even when swallowed in large numbers, as has been repeatedly demonstrated by actual experiment. Metchnikoff found, as recorded in a recent issue of the *Medical Brief*, that the cholera bacillus was widely diffused in water in many places which have been and are actually free from cholera. So much for the autopsy of a decaying medical theory. Its friends should solemnly intern the remains.

From the *Cataract Journal* of June 24, 1902.

Senator Gallinger of New Hampshire, who is an eminent physician, is reported as having said anent this subject, in a recent speech in the United States Senate: "If we believed one-half of it we should not dare to breathe, eat or drink, but would want to get into glass cases, but would be hermetically sealed up."

The superstitious fear engendered by bacteriologists, aided by shallow and sensational newspaper writers is developing into an instrument of power and possible oppression which Health Boards, being political bodies, know but too well how to manipulate to their own advantage.

But someone asks: Do we not find germs in diseased as well as in healthy tissues? I answer Yes. They are there as scavengers, as friends to the patient and as foes to the disease. To charge them with being the cause of the disease would be as unjust to them as it would be unfair to the street scavenger to charge him with having produced the filth which he is engaged in removing.

A Physician's Reasons For Having Renounced Vaccination

by John W. Hodge, M.D.

The Naturopath and Herald of Health, XVII (4), 223-226. (1912)

How I Became An Anti-Vaccinist

Before presenting to the reader my reasons for having at first accepted, then doubted, and finally repudiated vaccination, I desire to preliminate a few words in explanation of the way in which I was at first brought under the influence of the Jennerian delusion and how I was subsequently held there; and how I was afterwards enabled to throw off the hypnotic spell which the credulous dupes of disastrous medical delusion had imposed upon me at a time when I was unable to think or reason for myself. From childhood up to adolescence I had been trained to look upon vaccination as an absolute and qualified preventive of smallpox infection. I was confidently assured by my parents and teachers that everybody who had been once vaccinated was thereby rendered forever afterward proof [safe] against smallpox infection. From my earliest recollection I had confided in the Jennerian rite more implicitly than in my clerical tenet or religious creed. I never entertained the slightest doubt as to the alleged value of the vaccine operations, taking everything on trust without any inquiry whatever. The numerous and obvious failures of vaccination to protect its duly vaccinated subjects from smallpox infection or even from death by that *dread disease*, did not shake my cherished faith in the Jennerian dogma. I had been taught to ascribe all those obvious failures and disasters either to the carelessness or incompetence of the vaccinator to the inertness, or to the badness of the *lymph*, or else, to explain them away on the assumption that the operation had not been *properly done* that the protection had *run out* or had become exhausted and needed renewing. Later in life, when I came under the care of my medical *Alma Mater*, I was most emphatically re-assured after the most arbitrary and dogmatic fashion by my medical preceptors that inoculation with *cowpox-lymph* was a safe and certain protection against smallpox infection. I was told that vaccination rendered its subjects smallpox proof. Like the average student of medicine, I accepted with blind unreasoning faith the preposterous Jennerian doctrine at the arbitrary dictum of my medical instructors, whom I looked up to as omniscient and well-nigh infallible in matters pertaining to medical lore. In short I accepted vaccination on trust.

How I Happened To Lose My Faith In Jennerism

We frequently learn by accident and surprise what of ourselves we should never have expected.

After having been held for many years under the spell of the Jennerian delusion, I, fortuitously, became disillusioned under the following described circumstances:

My long cherished faith in the Jennerian scheme of salvation from smallpox through the *saving grace* of inoculated *cowpox*, which faith had been imbibed from my nurses and confirmed by my medical preceptors remained serenely undisturbed until the year 1882, during which time I was engaged in the general practice of medicine in the City of Lockport, N. Y. During that year a single case of smallpox "broke out in that municipality, which case was promptly seized upon by the Health Board doctor as material for *working up* a smallpox *scare* which, being interpreted into medical parlance, means *a vaccination-harvest* for the doctors. The announcement of that first case of the *dread disease* was advertised in the sensational newspaper-press under big scare-headlines, whereby the credulous gaping, gullible public were gravely warned of the alleged dire danger which threatened their lives unless they promptly fed from *the wrath to come* by getting vaccinated (diseased). Through the combined efforts of the Health Board and the sensational newspapers the masses of the people became panic stricken and in their frenzy gasped: "What shall we do to be saved from the loathsome smallpox." At this juncture, the Health Board, *hell bent* in their consuming zeal for the salvation of the *dear public* got busy, drew forth a copy of a musty vaccination law from its dusty pigeon hole and on the strength thereof gravely promulgated an official edict that general vaccination of the city's entire population must be resorted to without delay, as the only available means of averting an impending epidemic of the dread smallpox which it was declared threatened to decimate the city. The order to vaccinate everybody who had not been *recently* vaccinated went forth. Health Boards in those days were medico-political organizations, just as they are in these days. The qualifications or fitness of any candidate for a position on said Board was a political *pull.* A candidate's chances of securing an appointment to any position on the Health Board depended wholly and solely upon the strength of his *pull* with the political party then in power.

Wholesale vaccination having been ordered by the health-authorities of the city meant that some political *plums* in the shape of appointments of doctors to do the vaccinations at the city's expense would be handed out. At that time I was a newly fledged doctor, just turned loose from medical college. My sheep-skin had a decidedly fresh smell and its proud owner was sorely in need of clients and funds. The political *plums* in sight quickly attracted my attention and, resolving to secure some of the coveted fruit, I *got busy.* Through the influence of a friend of mine who was a prominent politician and kindly interceded in my behalf, I was enabled to land the appointment of official vaccinator or disease dispenser. Having secured the much coveted *plum*, I was duly commissioned to arm myself with lancet and *lymph* and go forth from house to house and jab with the vaccine lancet every mother's son and daughter too, whom I could lay hands upon who did not present satisfactory evidence in the shape of good *marks* showing that *recent and successful* vaccination had been performed. All previously vaccinated subjects whose *marks* were adjudged, *atypical*, indistinct, or otherwise unsatisfactory, were assumed to be *unvaccinated* and were peremptorily treated to a compulsory dose of diseased calf-skin at the taxpayers' expense. This was called *gratuitous* vaccination. The vaccine substance which is employed at the time referred to had been purchased direct from the Department of Health of the City of New York and was considered impeccable in quality and unsurpassed in efficiency as an antidote to smallpox. After having inserted the quintessence of diseased veal, now a days, mendaciously branded, *pure calf lymph* into the blood of some 3,200 presumably healthy children and adults. I was, to my great astonishment confronted with sundry cases of smallpox which had *broken out*, here and there, in daily *protected* subjects upon whom I had recently operated with *pure lymph* and *good takes*. My astonishment, however, reached its climax when a number of those cases of post-vaccinal smallpox which I had diagnosed *varioloid* developed into the confluent variety of the *dread disease* and several of those cases resulted fatally in spite of the *mitigative* effects of recent and *successful* vaccination with *pure lymph* at my own hands.

Still another surprise confronted me.

Following the wake of the public vaccinators in that vigorously conducted vaccination crusade smallpox of a severe type spread throughout the city of Lockport like wild fire on a prairie until the city was in the throes of a raging epidemic of the *dread disease*, while it lasted for many months, cost the city thousands of dollars and left a number of deaths to its record. Notwithstanding the fact that general vaccination was ordered and carried out shortly after the appearance of the first case of smallpox which occurred in the city, the disease spread with great rapidity. A barrel of ignited turpentine could not have flared up with more startling effect than did the epidemic of smallpox in the face of the vicious vaccination crusade. The vaccine virus seemed to add fuel to the flame, or that the vaccinators were openly charged by parents with having inoculated the smallpox into their children's blood, the vaccine lancet. I was myself charged with that offence and although I stoutly denied the charge at the time it was made, I am not now so sure that it was not well founded and true. However, that may be [why] I have never vaccinated another victim since that memorable event.

The astounding revelations above referred to were so contrary to my preconceived notions concerning the alleged efficacy of the essence of diseased calf-skin as an anti-variolous agent that they rudely jarred my sleepy faith in Dr. Jenner's prophylactic. Having been thus rudely roused from my utopian dreams, my eyes were opened to the unwelcome and grim suspicion that *vaccinal prophylaxy* might not be all that it was presumed by its interested advocates to be. Thus was my child-like faith in a long-cherished and previously unquestioned medical creed rudely shaken, then shattered and ultimately demolished by the united testimony of my own personal experience, observation, and reason, which combined to disillusion me and which in the end left no sort of doubt in my mind as to the utter baselessness of the vaccine theory and the worse than uselessness of the vaccine practice as an alleged prophylactic against smallpox in the duly vaccinated subject. After having been thus reluctantly forced by the stern logic of stubborn facts to surrender my long-cherished faith in the alleged efficacy of *vaccinal prophylaxy*. I next tried to persuade myself that while vaccination had failed to prevent smallpox, it at least must have rendered the *dread disease* milder and less fatal in vaccinated subjects. But subsequent experience drove that delusion out of my mind. The Lockport experience was an eye-opener to me. From that time on I studied the subject of vaccination as I should have studied it before and as every physician should study it, with a mind open to conviction; and I became actually appalled on discovering how fearfully and how wonderfully I had been deceived and how grossly I had deluded my trustful clients by inflicting this ruinous rite upon them. Subsequent experience in the treatment of cases of post-vaccinal smallpox and painstaking observations of the effects of vaccination, extending over a period of nearly thirty years have served only to confirm my settled convictions that so-called *preventive vaccination* is a snare and delusion, a sham and a fraud upon human credulity.

I am now fully and firmly convinced that vaccination not only utterly fails to protect its subjects from smallpox infection for any namable period of time, but that, on the contrary, it renders them more liable to attack by that disease, as well as by other diseases, by impairing their health and diminishing the vigor of their vital powers of resistance.

In support of my unavoidable convictions that vaccination tends rather to *increase* than to diminish the liability to variolous infection, I may cite the recorded testimony of the distinguished vaccinologist and epidemiologist, Dr. Charles Creighton, A.M., M.D., Emeritus Professor of Cambridge University, London, England. In his classical work on *History of Epidemics in Britain,* Dr. Creighton tells us that in all the great epidemics of smallpox, which have scourged civilized nations since the adoption and establishment of vaccination, it has been the *vaccinated, not the unvaccinated*, who were first seized by smallpox, which disease subsequently spread from them, as foci of infection, to the unvaccinated.

As an illustrative instance of this sort—of which there are hundreds—
I may here cite the case of the smallpox epidemic which invaded Leicester,
England, in 1902-1903. That epidemic started with a vaccinated and
previously smallpoxed, i .e., doubly protected tramp. In the official report
of said epidemic by Dr. C. K. Millard, the medical officer of health, for
Leicester, it is recorded that the variolous infection was spread through
that borough almost wholly by vaccinated subjects who were the first
to contract smallpox and subsequently to communicate it to the unvaccinated.

In his article on vaccination in the ninth English edition of the *Encyclopedia Britannica*, Dr. Charles Creighton tells us that the first unvaccinated person attacked in the smallpox epidemic in Liegnitz in 1871, was
the 225th in order of time. This means that 224 vaccinated persons were
seized by smallpox before one unvaccinated person was attacked.

At Cologne, Dr. Creighton tells us that in the epidemic of smallpox
in 1870, the first unvaccinated person attacked was the 174th Query! If
vaccination affords any protection at all against smallpox infection, why
does the *dread disease* always attack the vaccinated first in variolous epidemics?

Will some High Priest of Jennerism please arise and explain?

I next present the testimony of another distinguished advocate and
ardent supporter of the Jennerism doctrine. His name is Dr. W. A. Guy,
M.D., F.R.C.P., an allopathic pro-vaccinal authority of unquestioned vaccinal orthodoxy. "It is now admitted," writes Dr. Guy, "by all competent
authorities that vaccination during epidemics of smallpox tends to diffuse,
rather than to arrest the disease" (smallpox). Since smallpox contagion
is now known to constitute the basis of all strains of vaccine substances,
at present in general use by vaccinators, common sense should enable one
to understand clearly the meaning of all this. Common sense, however,
is so very *uncommon* with vaccinators that any physician who makes use
of it is denounced as a *crank or a fanatic* by the biased upholders of the
unclean rite.

In the face of these damaging testimonies from the pens of two of
the world's most distinguished high priests of the Jennerian cult, Health
Boards all over the world frantically insist upon the compulsory enforcement of general vaccination during the prevalence of epidemics of smallpox under the lying and hypocritical pretense that vaccination *stamps
out* smallpox. Health Board officials egged on by a motley crowd of
impecunious fee-hungry, self-serving doctors force the people of an infected community to have their sound skins broken open at a time when
an epidemic of smallpox prevails and during the prevalence of which an
infected atmosphere is heavily charged with the variolous infection in its
most active and concentrated form. The antics of the Jenner fanatics in

this frantically persisting in their efforts to vaccinate everybody during the prevalence of an epidemic of smallpox are paralleled only by a lunatic, who, by pouring petroleum upon a flame to extinguish the fire brought on a conflagration.

Considering the affirmation of facts more trustworthy guides than the assertions of doctors, I have during the past quarter of a century refused to pollute the blood of a single person with *pure calf-lymph* or with any other infective animal poison. In consequence I have been frequently taken to task by the promoters of the vaccine industry for presuming to question the infallibility of an ancient medical dogma, which the rank and file of the allopathic medical profession has implicitly accepted for more than one hundred years.

My critics argue that *I* must be *wrong* and that vaccination must be *right* because they say, "The great majority of the members of the medical profession all over the world sanction and uphold it." My reply to this *ad captandum* argument is: On the same theory and with just as much logic and show of reason it might be argued by distillers, liquor dealers and saloonists, that the habitual use of alcoholic beverages is right and wholesome on the analogous plea that it is sanctioned and upheld by the vast majority of saloon keepers all over the world.

I tell my critics that votes should be weighed as well as counted and that he who would estimate the value of vaccination by the votes of the ignorant and prejudiced majorities who have vested interests in the filthy practice has no right to take part in the discussion of this question, because he has shown himself incompetent to do so.

Like the average student of medicine, I accepted with blind unreasoning faith the preposterous Jennerian doctrine at the arbitrary dictum of my medical instructors, whom I looked up to as omniscient and well-nigh infallible in matters pertaining to medical lore. In short I accepted vaccination on trust.

Having secured the much coveted plum, *I was duly commissioned to arm myself with lancet and* lymph *and go forth from house to house and jab with the vaccine lancet every mother's son and daughter too, whom I could lay hands upon who did not present satisfactory evidence in the shape of good marks showing that* recent *and* successful *vaccination had been performed.*

A barrel of ignited turpentine could not have flared up with more startling effect than did the epidemic of smallpox in the face of the vicious vaccination crusade.

I am now fully and firmly convinced that vaccination not only utterly fails to protect its subjects from smallpox infection for any namable period of time, but that, on the contrary, it renders them more liable to attack by that disease, as well as by other diseases, by impairing their health and diminishing the vigor of their vital powers of resistance.

In his classical work on History of Epidemics in Britain *Dr. Creighton tells us that in all the great epidemics of smallpox, which have scourged civilized nations since the adoption and establishment of vaccination, it has been the* vaccinated, not the unvaccinated, *who were first seized by smallpox, which disease subsequently spread from them, as foci of infection, to the unvaccinated.*

If vaccination affords any protection at all against smallpox infection, why does the dread disease *always attack the vaccinated first in variolous epidemics?*

SMALLPOX, THE MUMBO JUMBO OF THE MEDICAL PROFESSION

by Helen Sayr Gray, N.D.*

The Naturopath and Herald of Health, XVII (6), 381-383. (1912)

There are other diseases quite as bad or worse and more fatal than smallpox, but they do not occasion the alarm that smallpox creates. For years smallpox has been the Mumbo Jumbo of the medical profession, a bogie with which to create a panic.

Since there is such a growing distrust of medical statistics showing the efficacy of vaccination, it would be well for everyone who is sufficiently interested to collect some statistics on the subject for himself—to ask his friends and acquaintances what their personal experiences have been. If he is thorough in his investigation and careful to verify reports he will secure statistics that he will not distrust. Then let him decide whether vaccination is beneficial or pernicious and whether it really prevents smallpox.

Recently I asked some of my friends and acquaintances to tell their personal experiences as to the results of vaccination and what has come to their notice among their neighbors. Several testified that a member of their family or an acquaintance had been killed by it. A Denver woman was vaccinated on the leg and the lower half of her body was paralyzed as a result of the inoculation. A number of cases were reported of those who had been made very sick or who had never been well afterward. Three who had been vaccinated had smallpox, notwithstanding, a few weeks or months later. One had black smallpox, another had so severe a case of confluent smallpox that he was given up to die. A boy was crippled for life by vaccination, a man was crippled for seven years and is still helpless, and a woman was so crippled by it that she had to go on crutches for three years afterward, and still uses a cane. The disastrous outcome in her case was said to have resulted because "her blood was impure". If it was impure, was it not bad enough that it was already full of the poison of auto-intoxication without igniting the fuse by injecting some more poison? A number of persons, including a nurse and a girl who formerly worked in a doctor's office, testified that they had not been disabled by vaccination themselves nor had they seen any very bad results from it. One woman nursed eight or ten cases of smallpox that broke out in the family of one of her friends and stayed quarantined with them for sixteen days. Subsequently she nursed two cases in the family of a relative.

---

*Dr. Helen Sayr Gray was a Naturopath who practiced in Portland, Oregon. She was outspoken against vaccinations and published a very witty pamphlet, "In defense of Thomas and Tabby" which was published in the Lust journals and can be found in *Philosophy of Naturopathic Medicine*, pp 218-224. —Ed.

She had been vaccinated nearly thirty years before. She did not contract the disease in either instance. She attributed her immunity to her good habits and consequent good health and to the absence of fear.

In Montreal, where I am told there are frequent outbreaks of smallpox, I once visited a church belonging to one of the monastic orders there. The admission of some new candidates into the order had drawn a large crowd to see the ceremonies. The place smelt like a stable. From the stench of unwashed bodies it was very evident that few of the congregation gave any concern to bathing and ventilation. After that experience I was not surprised to hear that smallpox is frequently rampant in the town.

Doctors, like various other people, are very proficient in appropriating credit and transferring blame. When death or impaired health results from vaccination, its advocates have a number of scapegoats that they put the blame on. When a vaccinated person contracts smallpox, the doctors say that he was not vaccinated successfully or not recently enough or not prior to exposure, or they reassure and console him by telling him that he would have had a severer or perhaps a fatal case, if he had not been vaccinated. I recall an instance in which a woman who had been vaccinated fifty-five years before had an attack of smallpox. The secretary of the Oregon State Board of Health attributed her escape from death to vaccination. It had not prevented her from getting the disease. How can he prove that it saved her from death? If the patient dies from vaccination or his health is seriously affected by it, the doctors charge that the virus was not pure, or the needle must have been dirty, or *the technique of the operation was faulty* in some other respect or death ensued because it was a very malignant case.

Dr. Edward Ashley recently died in New York of cerebro-spinal-meningitis, in spite of the fact that Flexner's celebrated serum was administered. It was powerless to save his life. The explanation given was that *it was a very malignant case.* If a person was vaccinated several decades ago, he is told that it is not safe to rely on it as a safeguard after so long an interval, that protection ceases in seven years, or five, or less; but, if he is exposed to smallpox and does not contract it, the doctors give vaccination the credit for his escape, no matter how long before the vaccination occurred. It is even contended by some of its partisans that, if an unvaccinated child does not have smallpox after having been exposed, it is immune because its ancestors were vaccinated! Health Board officials when confronted with such a case say that *two, or three generations of vaccinated parentage will produce in many instances immunized progeny!* When antitoxin is administered to prevent or save a case of diphtheria and the patient contracts the disease or dies from it notwithstanding, this dire result, the doctors declare, occurred, not because antitoxin is powerless to prevent or cure the disease, but because it was not used in time or not enough of it was used.

It frequently happens that one of a family of children who have been living under like conditions and have all been exposed to scarlet fever contracts that disease and the rest do not. Vaccination has not yet been introduced for scarlet fever. It cannot be said that the children who escape owe their immunity to any such measure. Some other explanation has to be made. So, too, it frequently happens that unvaccinated persons are exposed to smallpox without contracting the disease. Are they not immune from smallpox for the same reason the children just spoken of were immune from scarlet fever?

A distinguished physician, Dr. J. H. Tilden, who is an opponent of vaccination, says: "Health is the only immunity against disease. If there is any state that man can be put into that will cause him to be less liable to come under disease producing influences than full health, then law and order are not supreme and the world must be the victim of caprice, haphazard and chance."

Real immunity is overlooked and lost sight of in the mad chase after imaginary ones, such as serums, antitoxins, and vaccines. The use of these measures to cure or prevent disease diverts attention from genuine immunity, from the means that ought to be employed to secure such immunity. Several centuries ago little attention was paid to domestic and municipal sanitation in Europe. Whenever filthy surroundings and autotoxemia from food poisoning and other bad habits caused an outbreak of plague, it was believed that the Jews had poisoned the wells. Of course, it followed that people thought if they could only get rid of the Jews, there would be no epidemics. The savage relies on a fetish to save him from plagues and other misfortunes. His attention is riveted on not losing his precious possession. If he could be shown that it is ineffectual, then he would cast about to find out what he must do to be saved. So long as people are led to believe that vaccination is a safeguard, they will not look for any other. A large number will continue to live in filthy surroundings and to have gross habits of eating—eating too much, eating carelessly and ignorantly cooked food and bolting it, and eating incompatible foods at a meal—and other injurious habits and will place their dependence for physical salvation on a rabbit's foot, vaccination or some other superstition. The medical profession complains that patients will not heed advice about their habits. But, if the profession did not offer *vicarious atonement*, through drugs, operations, and serums and the patients realized that there is no alternative, they would give more attention to correcting their habits:

Anti-vaccinationists hold that smallpox is less prevalent than formerly, not because vaccination has checked its ravages, but because sanitary conditions have improved, that it is the general adoption of such protective measures as the installation of municipal sewer and pure water systems, the consequent bathing facilities, street cleaning, the enforced sanitary disposal of garbage, drainage of the soil, etc., that has wiped out altogether some pestilence that formerly scourged the nations and has diminished the virulence and prevalence of others. It seems to me that what is needed is more sanitation engineers to continue and promote such commendable work and thereby protect the public health, instead of Boards of Health to inject serums and viruses.

Box 692, Portland, Oregon

A distinguished physician, Dr. J. H. Tilden, who is an opponent of vaccination, says: "Health is the only immunity against disease... ."

Real immunity is overlooked and lost sight of in the mad chase after imaginary ones, such as serums, antitoxins, and vaccines. The use of these measures to cure or prevent disease diverts attention from genuine immunity, from the means that ought to be employed to secure such immunity.

So long as people are led to believe that vaccination is a safeguard, they will not look for any other. A large number will continue to live in filthy surroundings and to have gross habits of eating—eating too much, eating carelessly and ignorantly cooked food and bolting it, and eating incompatible foods at a meal—and other injurious habits and will place their dependence for physical salvation on a rabbit's foot, vaccination or some other superstition.

Anti-vaccinationists hold that smallpox is less prevalent than formerly, not because vaccination has checked its ravages, but because sanitary conditions have improved, that it is the general adoption of such protective measures as the installation of municipal sewer and pure water systems, the consequent bathing facilities, street cleaning, the enforced sanitary disposal of garbage, drainage of the soil, etc., that has wiped out altogether some pestilence that formerly scourged the nations and has diminished the virulence and prevalence of others.

HOW VACCINE VIRUS IS MADE

by Anti-Vaccination League of America

The Naturopath and Herald of Health, XVII (10), 614. (1912)

The calf is tied down to an operating table, the stomach is shaved for twelve to fifteen inches square, and about one hundred incisions are made. Into these incisions, one drop of glycerinated lymph (a culture of smallpox passed through a solution of glycerine) is allowed to drop and is thoroughly rubbed in. Fever sets in, and the animal becomes exceedingly sick. In a few days the vesicles appear, the scabs form, and the elimination of impurities of various kinds from the blood of the calf begins, in the form of PUS, which is thrown out of the blood into the vesicles. At the end of six days, the process of elimination has proceeded so far that the vesicles contain a quantity of pus, putrid cells, etc., and a scab has formed over the reservoir of disease. The calf is once more bound and laid upon the operating table. The inoculated area is washed with warm water, and each vesicle is clasped with clamps, separately. The crust is carefully scraped with the edge of a steel instrument and the dead skin cells [and] matter that is exuded from the small blood vessels, etc., is transferred to a small crucible.

To this horrible mass of putrid matter is added an equal measure of glycerine. The mass is then thoroughly stirred and mixed by a small electric motor. As soon as it is rendered homogeneous, it is placed in another crucible and passed through a very fine sieve, in order to remove the course pieces of ROTTEN FLESH, HAIR, etc., then the mixture is again beaten up and thoroughly mixed and transferred to tubes and distributed throughout the country as PURE CALF LYMPH when in reality there is no such thing as PURE LYMPH. It is this rotten stuff that our HEALTH BOARDS, SCHOOL BOARDS and family physicians insist upon having introduced directly into the circulation of the blood of millions of school children every year.

The results of vaccination are disease, constitutional debility and DEATH. Many a sufferer from debility and blood deterioration can trace that condition to vaccination, and many other like sufferers from vaccination are not aware of the REAL CAUSE of their condition. The cause of such sickness and death from lockjaw, etc., after vaccination is too often concealed UNDER ANOTHER NAME. Vaccination sows the seeds of Erysipelas, Scrofula, Cancers, Leprosy, Consumption, Eczema, and other loathsome diseases.

Medical authorities in this country and in Europe to-day claim, those inoculations are degenerating the human race which is being serumized, and thousands of dollars are invested in SERUM PLANTS in this country. Many physicians are shareholders in these 'alleged benefits' to mankind, although their names do not appear on the list of stockholders.

1913

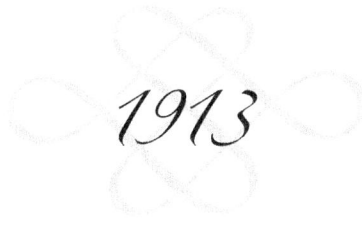

MEDICAL LAWS VS RIGHTS AND CONSTITUTION
AUGUST ANDREW ERZ, N.D., D.C.

THE MEDICAL QUESTION

The Truth About Official Medicine and Why We Must Have Medical Freedom

Medical Laws vs. Human Rights and Constitution. The Great Need of the Hour. What Constitutes the True Science and Art of Healing

By A. A. ERZ, N. D., D. C.

HERE is a book that cheers one like a draught of ozone after having breathed the mephitic vapors of the philosophy of official medicine, that exploits the immorality of vivisection, and swears by the unscientific and useless products of the torture trough.

It consists of 600 pages, written by the trenchant pen of one who is master of his subject. It embodies the revolt of the latest and most efficient school of medical healing against the tyranny and ignorance of the drug doctors, who, while attacking symptoms, fail to understand the need of the higher practice of treating the causes of disease instead. The charlatanry and inefficiency of official medicine has reason to be envious of the successes of the natural school whose philosophic practices are here fully manifested.

Dr. Erz makes very clear his position in the art of healing. He is an enthusiastic Naturopath. He believes that when a man becomes ill, he should employ the natural forces of hydropathy, diet, exercise, sunshine, electricity, mechano-therapy, massage, and all the healing agencies that have proven their worth as prophylactics, and their ability to arouse the inherent restorative power for health that resides in every organism. His information is illuminating in the highest degree.

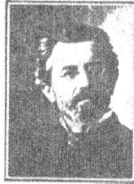

He is the sworn enemy of the "scientific medicine" of the allopaths, that consists of poisonous drugs on the one hand, and the equally poisonous and wholly dangerous serums, inoculations and vaccines on the other, that form a body of medical superstition that is propagating disease rather than curing it. He discusses, one by one, the most loudly-praised products of medical research, and proves them either to be utterly useless, or of deadly danger to the duped and unsuspecting patient.

In support of his statements, he quotes the opinions of the greatest exponents of official medicine who confess that allopathic medicine has produced more misery and premature death than famine, pestilence and war combined. As Billroth says, "Our progress is over mountains of corpses."

He proves that the American Medical Association, and the various State and County Associations affiliated therewith, form one vast engine of oppression, armed with legal power to harass, crush, and if possible destroy, the true saviors of mankind, the exponents of natural healing, whose activities naturally discredit official medicine. By legally securing a monopoly of practising medicine, THEY ARE ABLE TO MAKE IT MORE OF A CRIME TO CURE A PERSON THAN TO KILL HIM.

He shows how easy it is to understand why the unthinking legislator favors official medicine to the exclusion of the natural school of therapy. The psychological pressure of an institution, no matter how despotic its use of power may be, or how false and deadly its products are, that has its roots deeply rooted in history, is vastly greater on the unenlightened mind, than a true and noble institution that was born but yesterday—where man does not know conservatism rules.

Dr. Erz fully proves that the so-called remedies of medical research are violations of every law of nature, of health, of life, and a disregard of every principle of physiology, biology and therapeutics.

The people were never consulted about these laws, and never asked for them

They are the product of medical feudalism, which means intolerance, injustice and brutality, instead of charity, justice and dignity. The people should rise in their might and stay the infamous activities of these medical malefactors.

It is a startling indictment of humanity that its saviors are never recognized until the advance guard, and many of the main army, are killed, or trodden underfoot, and official medicine in America, the glorious Land of Freedom, is busy at this moment, as it has been for many years past, in hunting down the drugless' practitioner, whose only fault is the fact that he cures patients by natural methods, where the vendors of rotten pus have signally failed. He is arrested, and heavily fined, or thrown into jail for the offense of practising medicine without a pus-vendor's license.

Dr. Erz rightly advocates the urgent need of a great Academy of Natural Healing to convince the thinking masses of the superiority of the Natural Healing System, and to protect it against all misrepresentations and abuses, and assure its efficiency and permanent success. Medical Freedom is the great need of the hour to prove that Nature's constructive laws overshadow all ignorance, superstition and ambition. As the exponent of a standard of drugless healing, and as a monitor, mentor, and defence of humanity from rapacity and superstition, such an institution would be of enormous value to mankind.

Dr. Erz's work is a standard contribution to the great propaganda of Drugless Therapy that is sweeping over the land. No drugless practitioner can afford to be without its inspiring companionship. It marks an epoch in the history of the grand science and art of Natural Healing.

Price, in cloth, postpaid, $5.00; paper cover, $4.00.

THE NATURE CURE PUBLISHING CO., BUTLER, N. J.

Medical Laws vs Human Rights and Constitution was written by August Andrew Erz, N.D., D.C., voicing concerns of the tyrannical activities of the A.M.A.

Medical Laws vs Rights And Constitution (Excerpt)

by August Andrew Erz, N.D., D.C.

Copyright, 1913, by A. A. Erz

The Naturopath and Herald of Health, XVIII (12), 834-836. (1913)

There Is No Harmony Of Opinion On Vaccination

There is no harmony of opinion on vaccination even among the friends of this most unnatural of all medical treatments, except in the matter of fee, of course, which they all claim. And there is a great difference of opinion in regard to the technique. Some recommend cutting, others use puncturing; some advocate very little scarring, others claim that the larger the wound the greater the protection. There are those who insist upon vaccination immediately after birth, and those who wish to impart protection in utero by vaccinating the mothers. Others rather wait until the infant is

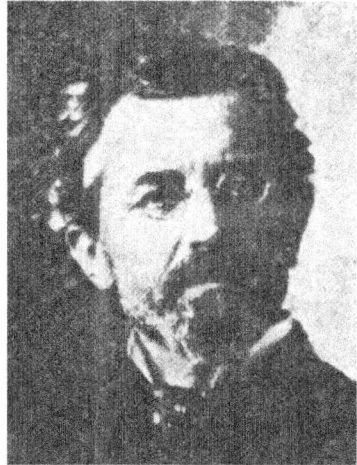

August Andrew Erz, N.D., D.C.

developed and vigorous. This very difference of opinion on matters pertaining to vaccination is certainly proof for the uncertainty, worthlessness and untenableness of the whole proposition.

The great variety of diseases and the considerable number of deaths directly or indirectly resulting from vaccination constitute a special chapter in the history of vaccination not very agreeable to its advocates. Before the introduction of inoculation and vaccination, through which the disease tended to spread, smallpox used to be a disease of children only; now it is common to all ages. We have already mentioned that syphilis, scrofula and tuberculosis have been transmitted through vaccination to great masses of people. One of the most common after-effects of vaccination is a certain form of erysipelas which is very dangerous and often ends fatal. There are also various very painful and extensive skin diseases resulting from vaccination that are causing their victims great sufferings for months. Intense inflammations of the axillary and cervical glands with weakening pus formation are a frequent aftermath of vaccination. Not infrequently follow inflammation and necrosis of the joints of the elbow leaving a permanent lameness of the upper extremities. Deforming swellings often cover the scars of vaccination. A direct effect of the vaccine poison is a frequent inflammation of the nerves of the arm or a paralysis with permanent lameness. These and other diseases such as lockjaw, resulting from vaccination often lead to a fatal end. Frequently death follows within a few days after vaccination, as a sequence of general blood poisoning to which danger every vaccinated person is exposed. This list of suffering following vaccination by no means comprises everything of which the history of vaccination tells us; we had to confine ourselves to the more common after-effects which ought to be sufficient to show the dangers of vaccination. All medical authorities have been unable to disprove the various detrimental effects of vaccination, and their attempts to explain matters usually end in plain contradictions and failures.

The mitigation theory is but another subterfuge, and actually implies another confession that vaccination does not protect. If the prevention theory were true, then no person could possibly ever have smallpox in any form after vaccination. Thus one subterfuge after another was resorted to by Jenner and the profession to explain away the failures. Facts unfavorable to the scheme were often suppressed or minimized, and are to this day. Even Jenner had to admit "that smallpox might succeed perfect vaccination, but could account for the great number of failures that occurred only by supposing that some circumstances interrupted the proper influence of vaccination on the system". Thus by the inventor of the scheme himself the efficacy of vaccination is made to rest on a baseless supposition, where, in fact, it always did rest.

The fact remains that all vaccination is a poisoning of the blood, and that there is in this process the production of a real contagious disease, acting by zymosis in the blood, thus endangering the organism, and making the system certainly not proof against the disease. And besides, there is the possibility of inoculating other diseases, thus producing a complication of trouble difficult to be overcome.

At first, official medicine entirely forgot the fact that the cows had also diseases of the udder. Then they went on vaccinating from arm to arm. If it had been a poisoning even with the very best real cowpox, it now became a poisoning of nearly all children with the most horrible diseases; many even were murdered, and an infinite number poisoned for life. After all, smallpox epidemics appeared under the title of varioloid, the cleverly invented name to cover the failure of vaccination.

THE VARIOLOID SUBTERFUGE

Varioloid is a term invented by the profession to conceal the failures of vaccination, and means "smallpox-like." How much like it? Nobody knows. According to the vaccination law no person can rightly have smallpox after vaccination, because vaccination prevents smallpox; but he may have, by kind permission of the profession, varioloid—which is in plain language, smallpox that occurs after vaccination, no more and no less, if you please.

If you consult *Dungleson's Medical Dictionary*, a standard work, you are informed that, "to smallpox, which may occur in a modified form after vaccination, the term varioloid has been given." Again he says: "VARIOLOID IS TRUE SMALLPOX, though mild, and a person suffering from it may communicate any form, even the malignant." In the edition of 1874, he still states the generally admitted fact that "smallpox occurs, at times, as an epidemic after vaccination". So there cannot be any doubt that varioloid is genuine smallpox—but it sounds like another thing under this masquerade hiding the real thing, and the fact that vaccination is not a preventive at all. That reminds one of the old saw, *Tricks in all trades*. In order to save the boasted "discovery of Jenner" from ignoble and total perdition, they invented this bogus term. Microscopic examination of varioloid and vaccine show that both contain the elements of common pus and their origin is the same, according to reliable observations, implying that vaccination produces that much dreaded disease, pyaemia.

According to some medical authorities, vaccination is equivalent to an attack of smallpox. Thus, instead of being a preventive and protection against smallpox, it is producing same. Dr. Martin, of Boston, Mass., tells us that the Boston epidemic of 1872 and 1873 was the most malignant and destructive in living memory; more malignant and contagious than in 1721; and what was true of Boston was true of every city and large town in Europe and America during the dread visitation. And this occurred in Boston, after eighteen years of compulsory vaccination! They sowed the seed of disease by vaccination and reaped a bountiful harvest of death. In the Boston epidemic, 3187 cases of smallpox were reported, of which 1045 died. And these victims had nearly all been vaccinated. It is estimated that about 90 percent were vaccinated.

Over 1400 vaccinated persons died of smallpox in Montreal from April, 1885, to January, 1886. In England and Wales during the first ten years following compulsory vaccination, over 33,000 died of smallpox, and during the second decade the number exceeded 70,000.

Dr. Baron, the eulogist of Jenner, in his life of the latter—where he also advised his professional brethren to suppress facts about the failures of vaccination, which hint they have not been slow to take ever—furnishes evidence that already during Jenner's life-time bad results following vaccination were observed by many: "It seems that a greater number of children now die of measles than formerly." "Scrofula, for example, in all its forms, was certainly very often excited, and in particular, pulmonary consumption." Jenner himself, those last days were rendered very unhappy by the sad consequences of his own work, lamented: "What dreadful strides pulmonary consumption seems to be making over every part of our island (England). I have lately been deprived of the aid of my secretary. He was cut off by that dreadful disease (consumption) which I fear will shortly take from me my son." In spite of these terrible lessons he persisted in his awful error!

Before the introduction of inoculation and vaccination, through which the disease tended to spread, smallpox used to be a disease of children only; now it is common to all ages. We have already mentioned that syphilis, scrofula and tuberculosis have been transmitted through vaccination to great masses of people.

All medical authorities have been unable to disprove the various detrimental effects of vaccination, and their attempts to explain matters usually end in plain contradictions and failures.

After all, smallpox epidemics appeared under the title of varioloid, the cleverly invented name to cover the failure of vaccination.

Thus one subterfuge after another was resorted to by Jenner and the profession to explain away the failures.

According to the vaccination law no person can rightly have smallpox after vaccination, because vaccination prevents smallpox; but he may have, by kind permission of the profession, varioloid—which is in plain language, smallpox that occurs after vaccination, no more and no less, if you please.

So there cannot be any doubt that varioloid is genuine smallpox—but it sounds like another thing under this masquerade hiding the real thing, and the fact that vaccination is not a preventive at all.

1914

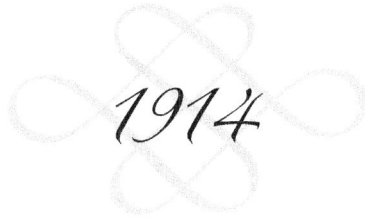

Vaccination And The Law
Honorable Harry Weinberger

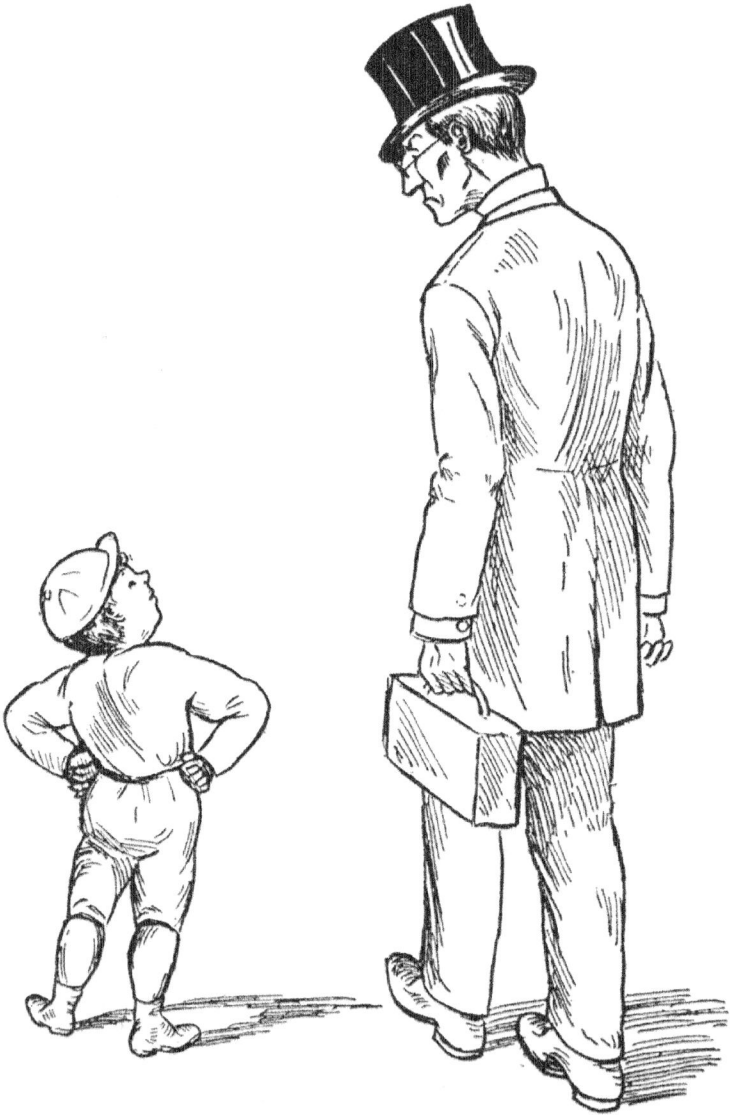

"Say, Doc! Does that M. D. you sign after your name stand for **much dope?**"

Vaccination And The Law

by Honorable Harry Weinberger, of the New York Bar

The Naturopath and Herald of Health, XIX (6), 393-395. (1914)

Lawyers do not know the law—at the best they only know where to find it. Most lawyers are under the impression that the Board of Health, under the so-called Police Power, has the right to vaccinate even against your wishes.

When the doctor of the Board of Health comes to your house, with his big protecting policeman, to vaccinate you and your family, what are your rights under the law? Of course, if you are in favor of vaccination, you let him vaccinate. But assuming that from your study, reading and observation you have come to the conclusion that you do not want to be vaccinated, and do not want your family vaccinated, because it does not protect from smallpox, and every time one is vaccinated he takes the risk of tetanus (lockjaw), syphilis, cancer and other diseases and even death— because all vaccine virus contains bacterial taint—what should you do, and what may you do?

Blackstone in his Commentaries said: "No laws are binding on the human subject which assault the body or violate the conscience. The right of personal security consists in a person's legal and uninterrupted enjoyment of his life, his limbs, and his reputation. Both the life and the limbs of a human subject are of such high value in the estimation of the law that it pardons even homicide if committed in defense of them or in order to preserve them."

Vaccination An Assault

New York State is typical of practically all the States of the Union in reference to vaccination. The only law in New York on the statute books in reference to vaccination is that, in order to go to school—that is, public school—a child must be vaccinated. You will immediately note that there is nothing about children who go to private school, or who are above school age, and there is nothing about adults. Boards of Health may have rules about vaccination in epidemics and at other times, but they are only rules without the force of law.

In the case of Smith versus Health Commissioner Emery, the question of compulsory vaccination in New York was given its deathblow. Smith had been quarantined because he refused to allow himself to be vaccinated. He applied to the Supreme Court for a writ of *habeas corpus*, setting forth that he was imprisoned and restrained of his liberty at his house in the said City of Brooklyn by the direction and order of the Commissioner of Health; that he had been exposed to no contagion and was not afflicted with any contagious disease.

The Commissioner, in his answer, stated that for several months smallpox had been epidemic in the city; that as he was informed and believes, before being detained in quarantine, he (Smith) was engaged in the prosecution of the express delivery business in said city, and in its worst-infected districts; that the business includes the carrying of house-hold furniture and other articles which may come from infected centers and be infected with the germ of smallpox; and that Smith was unusually exposed to such contagion and it was of special importance that he should be vaccinated at once, and that he was detained in quarantine because of his refusal to be vaccinated. The Court held that though every local Board of Health is required to guard against the introduction of conta-gious and infectious disease, and to require the isolation of all persons infected with and exposed to such disease yet to justify such isolation the fact must exist that the persons are infected with the contagious disease or have been exposed to it. No authority is given by said laws to said health commissioner to quarantine any person simply because he refuses to be vaccinated and to continue him in quarantine until he consents to such vaccination.

The Court further held that though Smith went through the districts where smallpox was, still that could not be considered exposure to small-pox, and the fear that he might carry infected articles is not enough; and, further, that there was no right of compelling any one to be vaccinated.

One case in the Supreme Court of New York held that vaccination against your wishes is an assault—in other words, in the same category with the use of brass knuckles and the sling-shot.

That Compulsory Vaccination Law

The Thorpe case had a good many interesting features to anti-vacci-nationists. Herbert A. Thorpe, of Princess Bay, Staten Island, sent his two children to school with a letter in part as follows: "I am sending you my two children, both in perfect health, for schooling. Children have been vaccinated without the parents' consent and often without their knowl-edge. My children must not be vaccinated, and I will shoot dead any man who vaccinates them. As you are the principal I will also hold you respon-sible." Needless to say, inasmuch as the children were not vaccinated, they were sent home. Later, the Board of Education, upon making inquiry of Thorpe, were informed that he was not giving them the exact education required by the law, nor the exact amount of time—in fact, a good deal less. The Board thereupon requested him to have his children vaccinated, and that he would be allowed then to send them to school. Upon Thorpe refusing, he was served with a summons from the police court, under the Compulsory Education Law.

The following argument was made before the Court: "All children are healthy or unhealthy—both sides can agree on that. If the Court and the Board of Education claim that the Thorpe children are healthy, though unvaccinated, then Thorpe complied with the law by sending healthy children to school in the first place, and the Board of Education was at fault in not taking them. But if the Court and the Board of Education say the Thorpe children are unhealthy, because unvaccinated, then Thorpe did not have to comply with the law, because the law distinctly says that children in proper physical condition must be sent to school." The Court and the Board of Education were asked to take either horn of the dilemma. Thorpe was dismissed and the Board of Education woefully failed.

THE ATTITUDE OF THE COURTS

The pro-vaccinationists contend that the courts have upheld vaccination, and yet when we examine the records what do we find? In the Viemeister case, decided by the New York Court of Appeals, and which is the leading case in the United States, and typical of almost all of the cases which have got into the courts, and in which the pro-vaccinationists claim victory, we find that Viemeister asked that the Board of Education be compelled by *mandamus* to take his child into school, even though unvaccinated. The Court held that public education, even though guaranteed in the constitution of the State of New York, was only a privilege and not a right, and that, therefore, the State had a right to prescribe rules for the admission of children into schools. Without quibbling as to whether the Court was correct in deciding that education was a privilege and not a right, and without going into the question of whether there really is any difference between the two, the Court yet refuses to pass on vaccination, except that it is a rule that the State can pass, the majority of the people believing in it, and with which you must therefore comply before your children can go to school. Judge Woodward of the Appellate Division in the same case, said: "It may be conceded right to compel any person to submit to vaccination."

THE SITUATION IN MASSACHUSETTS

The United States Supreme Court in Jacobson versus Massachusetts held: That where there was an epidemic of smallpox and the law prescribed that everyone should be vaccinated, and anyone who refused should be fined five dollars*, that that did not infringe upon the constitutional rights of the individual. The Court also seemed to hold that a State could pass a law that everyone should be vaccinated. Yet, that not being the real issue before the Court, it is only *obiter dictum*. And furthermore, the decision

---

*A five dollar fine imposed in 1914 was a huge burden on families, equivalent to several days' pay in many cases —Ed.

is not final, because it is not decided according to principle. It stands with the Dred Scott decision—involving the slavery of the black man—and which would not stay settled because not settled right. If any State passed a law compelling vaccination, and you resisted, I believe the United States Supreme Court would protect you, and declare the law unconstitutional. It must be noted in the Jacobson case that there was an epidemic, and the penalty for refusing to be vaccinated was a five-dollar fine, a sort of bribe to be vaccinated. The Court may have also been influenced by the fact that the Massachusetts law was like the old English Compulsory Vaccination Law, where if you refused to be vaccinated you were fined. In England to-day, if you file a certificate that you have conscientious objections against vaccination, you and your family are free from the fine and your children can remain unvaccinated.

Vaccination stands today in the position of any medical operation, and requires the consent of the person to be operated upon, and in the case of the infant requires the consent of the parents. No medical prescription, even though written into law, at the request of the politico-medicos, can be really enforced. They may attempt to bulldoze by fines in some States—bribe by public-school education for children in others—but you can apply your reason to the question of vaccination and decide for yourself whether you want to be vaccinated or not.

In the words of Alfred Russel Wallace, the great scientist, "Vaccination is a delusion—its penal enforcement a crime."

> "No laws are binding on the human subject which assault the body or violate the conscience. The right of personal security consists in a person's legal and uninterrupted enjoyment of his life, his limbs, and his reputation... ."
>
> Vaccination stands today in the position of any medical operation, and requires the consent of the person to be operated upon, and in the case of the infant requires the consent of the parents.

1915

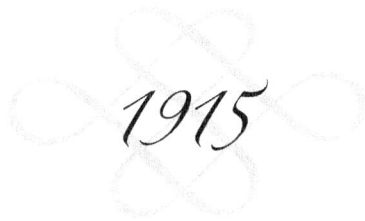

Dangers Of Contagion
Dr. Katz

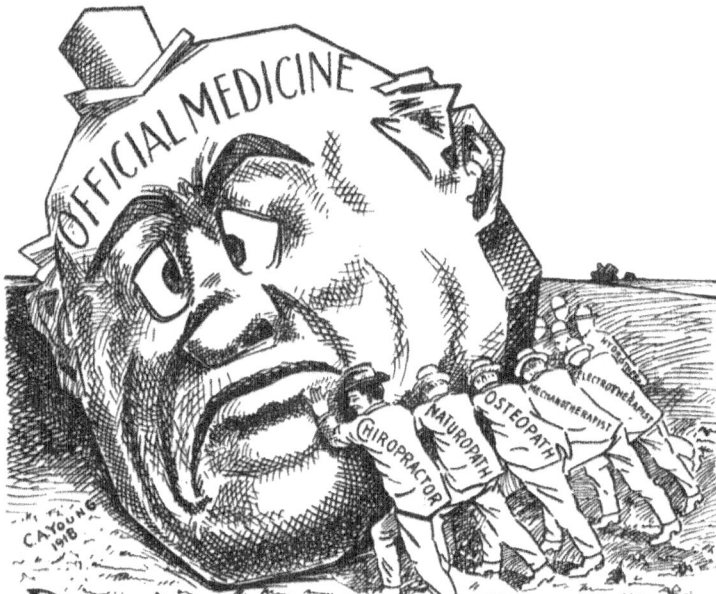

DRUGLESS FIELD

IN ORDER TO GET THE BEST OUT OF A PIECE OF LAND IT MUST BE FIRST CLEARED OF ALL OBSTRUCTIONS THIS SAME RULE APPLIES TO THE DRUGLESS FIELD BUT IT IS TOO MUCH FOR ONE ALONE. THE DRUGLESS DOCTORS MUST WORK TOGETHER AS THE OLD GANG "REGULARS" AND OFFICIAL MEDICINE DOES

Dangers Of Contagion

by Dr. Katz, Surgeon General in the German Army

The Naturopath and Herald of Health, XX (7), 427-428. (1915)

Nowadays many diseases are believed to be contagious, which causes not only a general fear among people, but also suffering on the side of the patients. Some people think [it] to be dangerous to enter a room, where a sick person is, and avoid therefore to have anything to do with patients. They fear that every sick person might endanger their health, although the question of contagiousness by no means has been resolved.

Some diseases, which once were believed to be harmless and not contagious, are supposed to be now-a-days, with the development of the bacteriology, very contagious. Bacteria are believed to be carriers of dis-

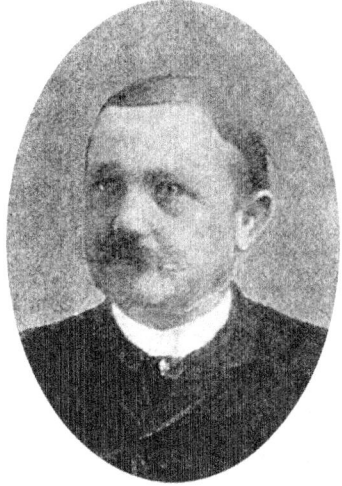

Dr. Katz

ease, and yet in no ways it has been scientifically proved that they are the real cause of disease.

Let us look at the most ravaging disease of the present time, consumption, which science affirms to be very contagious: the daily experience teaches us that this opinion is not supported by an objective observation. There are many instances of marriages in which one of the parties got this disease and was nursed till the end by the other party, without this or any other member of the family being attacked by the feared disease. And the same experience has been made even in families, living in the most unfavorable sanitary conditions.

In the sanatoria, in which only suspected or positive consumptives are treated, and where therefore the danger of contagion should be very great, the daily experience teaches us that doctors and nurses do not suffer from contagion and that only seldom are they attacked by the disease. The means, but which these good results are reached, are great cleanliness, natural and moderate habits, and fresh air. Furthermore it is important to notice that in places like Davos, the Riviera, etc., where thousands of consumptives come together, hoping to cure themselves, it has never been noticed an increase of cases of consumption, among the resident people, but rather the opposite.

Let us look at another disease, just as much feared, among the so-called contagious diseases, diphtheria and we shall see that this disease almost never appears in an epidemic form, but always attacks a house or a family.

It can be observed that one or more members of a family are attacked by this disease and that some of the cases might even be followed by death, without causing any ill effect on the people of the other families, living in the same house. And we know that the bacterium, designated as specific of this disease, is also often found, and in great quantity in the organisms of healthy people, without producing any disturbance. There are families, in which children and other members often are attacked by diphtheria, without any contagiousness on the other members of the same family.

Therefore we can affirm, with logical certainty, that a patient of diphtheria, if under strict observance of hygienic rules, is not dangerous for those around him and that it is cruel to take him away from the care of his family, to send him to a hospital. In many cases, this fact has done more harm to the patient than the disease for itself.

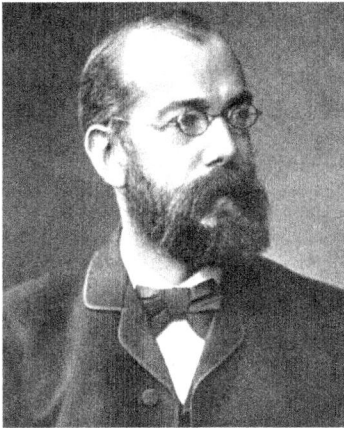

Prof. Robert Koch

Cholera, which most of the people believe to be specially contagious and which on this account is so much feared, is not thought so in India, its place of origin, where it never completely dies out. In Europe also, where it often appeared in the past centuries, it was not considered contagious. It was only after the discovery of the comma bacillus [*Vibrio cholera*] that the fear of contagion came, although this bacillus has been found also in healthy organisms, without any disturbance of their welfare. An absolute proof of the harmlessness of the comma bacillus has been given in Munich (Germany) by Profs. Pettenkofer and Emmerich, for each of them, with the digestive apparatus in perfect order, swallowed a considerable quantity of bacilli cultures, supplied by Prof. Koch himself, without the slightest disturbance in their health.

Similar are the conditions of the other contagious diseases, scarlet fever, measles, smallpox, typhus, influenza, etc. Their contagiousness is generally accepted and believed, though not yet proved.

The frequent and epidemic-like appearance of a disease is by no means a proof of its contagious nature, because in all epidemics it can be observed that healthy persons are protected against these diseases and that the victims are generally persons living in unfavorable circumstances and which on this account were already in poor health.

But also fear of contagion causes a diminution of the power of resistance, so that people who fear run a greater chance of falling victims of the disease, while those who have courage will keep in good health.

In literature we find instances of pusillanimous people who, without any other cause than their own fear, became sick and died.

Never has the belief in contagion been so widespread as at the present time so that many people avoid, so much as possible, the contact with sick persons, in order to protect their own dear selves. They ask a great number of disposition from the State and the Police for the protection of health, while they continue in their unhealthy habits, without thinking the necessity of leading a healthful life.

Only personal sanitary cares can protect us from diseases, whether believed to be contagious or not, while all what the State can do is to bring dangerous patients in hospitals and to isolate those afflicted with a contagious disease. But this isolation is often more dangerous than the disease itself, for children and adolescents; for nothing can substitute the mother's care. Nobody will deny that some of these little patients perish just on account of those dispositions, while they would perhaps recover, by remaining in the habitual conditions, under the loving care of their mother.

Instructions, for the protection of the other members of the family, would surely avoid the danger of a spreading of the disease. In no time, it is more necessary to be moderate and sober, and to improve the power of resistance of the body, through cleanliness and fresh air, than in epidemics. Hippocrates advised to be moderate in working, eating, drinking, sleeping and love, in such time, for a sober life gives the best protection against the so-called contagious diseases; and it is very possible that with a general moderation and sobriety, not only the contagious diseases, but also all others might tend to disappear.

It would be much more useful for the humanity, if there would be less talk about the contagiousness of the diseases and more about the precautions to be taken to avoid disease; thereby the fear of contagion would cease to exist and people would live instead a healthful and happy life.

And we know that the bacterium, designated as specific of this disease, is also often found, and in great quantity in the organisms of healthy people, without producing any disturbance.

An absolute proof of the harmlessness of the comma bacillus has been given in Munich (Germany) by Profs. Pettenkofer and Emmerich, for each of them, with the digestive apparatus in perfect order, swallowed a considerable quantity of bacilli cultures, supplied by Prof. Koch himself, without the slightest disturbance in their health.

Never the belief in contagion has been so widespread as at the present time so that many people avoid, so much as possible, the contact with sick persons, in order to protect their own dear selves.

The frequent and epidemic-like appearance of a disease is by no means a proof of its contagious nature, because in all epidemics it can be observed that healthy persons are protected against these diseases and that the victims are generally persons living in unfavorable circumstances and which on this account were already in poor health.

In no time, it is more necessary to be moderate and sober, and to improve the power of resistance of the body, through cleanliness and fresh air, than in epidemics.

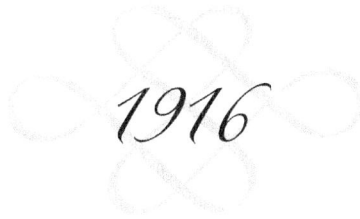

1916

THE PASSING OF THE SERUM CRAZE

CHARLES ZURMUHLEN, M.D.

Listerine ads appeared in the earliest issues of *The Naturopath and Herald of Health.* Listerine was invented by Dr. Joseph Lawrence and Jordan Lambert as an antiseptic with four essential oils: eucalyptol, mental, thymol, methyl salicylate.

THE PASSING OF THE SERUM CRAZE

by Charles Zurmuhlen, M.D.

Herald of Health and Naturopath, XXI (8), 537-541. (1916)

During this study hour we will temporarily depart from our scientific and philosophic study of medicine and analyze and criticize some current events in medicine.

As the falling leaves of autumn are an infallible sign that the end of summer has come, so the frequent failures of the serum treatment of disease are a sure indication that the end of this unnatural, irrational, ungodly treatment is fast approaching. Why is the serum treatment of disease unnatural, irrational and ungodly? **Nature is the material and dynamic manifestation of the operation of God's will.** He made all things and beings in the universe for a definite purpose. He made animals and men immune against disease.

So long as the skin and mucous membrane are intact men and animals are immune against bacteria. Immunity and health are Divine gifts bestowed upon men and animals by an all-knowing Creator. Now ignorant ungodly men make animals diseased by a violent and unnatural method. They fill a large hypodermic syringe with an enormous quantity of bacteria, the quantity is always so large that it is sure to overcome the immunity of the animal, and then they puncture the natural barrier, the skin, and inject the bacteria into the blood. By this unnatural and inhuman method they cultivate disease in animals. When the poor, defenseless animal is thoroughly diseased, the serum from the diseased blood is advertised as a sure cure for all disease. **It is important to remember that the serum from the blood of animals that suffer from disease that is due to natural causes, has no healing power; only the serum produced by artificial and unnatural methods is praised as a specific for disease.** The serum doctors get as far away from nature and natural methods as possible. Why is the serum from the blood of horses suffering from natural diphtheria not a specific for diphtheria? Diphtheria is not a natural disease in horses; it must be produced by the artificial and unnatural method of injecting the bacillus of diphtheria into them. Only the serums produced by irrational, unnatural, ungodly methods is advertised as a specific for disease.

The serum treatment is irrational for it shows the entire absence of logical reasoning. A rational creature is one who is endowed with the power of reasoning and is capable of exercising that power. If we have the power of reasoning and exercise it we soon see that bacteria are not the cause of disease. We have already seen that God made men and animals immune against them. As rational beings we must carry on our inquiry until we have found the universal dynamic and moral cause of all forms of

disease. We find that the cause of disease is the ignorant or willful violation of natural laws. Now what do we do when we assert that bacteria
are the cause of disease? Come! Let us reason together and see what we
do. It is our duty to discover the true cause of disease; God has given us
intelligence and the power to reason, for this very purpose. When we
assert that bacteria are the cause of disease, we accuse God, who made
bacteria, of being malicious, hateful Creator of disease. What do we do
when we assert that the serums made from the blood of diseased animals
are a sure cure for disease, and denounce the natural drugs as worthless?
First we accuse God of maliciously creating disease that he may derive
pleasure from the helpless suffering of men and animals. The bacterial
theory of disease is simply a revival of the pagan theory which attributes
all disease to the influence of demons or evil spirits. When we assert that
serums made by men are the only cure for disease and denounce natural
drugs as worthless, we accuse God of ignorance and incompetence. For
unknown thousands of years men have had to suffer from disease without
relief for God did not possess the necessary knowledge and power to provide means that can mitigate the suffering of men and heal disease. We
begin to see where the bacterial and serum theory is leading us. When
we claim that serums are superior to natural drugs, we assert that men
are wiser and more potent than God. Men can do what God cannot do.
The serum doctors claims that they can defy the natural laws, thwart the
will of God, make men immune against disease with vaccine and serums.
Charges: ten dollars per shot.

The serum treatment is ungodly for it is a stupid, irrational violation
of the Divine plan and will. God made plants and stored them with healing power long before he made men, for in His infinite wisdom he knew
that men would disobey Him and suffer for this disobedience. So, in His
infinite goodness and mercy He gave men natural drugs and methods to
relieve their suffering and it is His will that we shall see them.

Now we have carried the theory that bacteria are the cause of diseases; that serums are the only cure for disease, to its logical conclusion, and
we are shocked at our discovery. We now understand why the irrational,
unnatural and ungodly serum craze is dying.

The rational and logical analysis of the theory of bacteria and serums
has taught us an exceedingly valuable lesson. Man must learn through
mistakes and failures. Our greatest failures frequently teach us a more
valuable lesson and bring us nearer to the truth, then our most brilliant
successes. We must learn through bitter experience what is false, injurious and useless before we can know what is true, good and helpful.
The failure of vaccines and serums has taught us that God still rules the
universe, that His will is still universal law; that He has made natural
drugs, methods and laws that we may relieve our suffering when we have
violated His will.

To every action there is an equal reaction. This is a universal law. The medical profession is now recovering from the mild delirium of the serum craze and returning to the use of natural drugs and natural methods. The natural drugs are the plants of the fields and forest, the metals and minerals in the earth. The natural methods are Massage, Osteopathy, Chiropractic or Naturopathy, that includes all branches of natural healing.

But philosophic and logical reasoning does not satisfy us; we want practical proof that our reasoning is true. The following article in the *Scientific American Supplement* No. 2013, April 22, 1916, page 259, is practical proof that our logic is true:

GARLIC JUICE IN THE TREATMENT OF WOUNDS

At the beginning of the campaign, anti-septic treatment of wounds and injuries in civil life had fallen into much disfavor—almost into disrepute—and some authorities has openly stated that the antiseptic method was practically dead. Many measures have been suggested and tried; among these not the least successful has been the employment of hydrogen peroxide. But the substance that has proved its worth is garlic juice.

In the *Medical Press and Circular*, November, 17th, 1915, Dr. A. D. Serrell Cook writes concerning this method. The way in which the juice was used is as follows:

After sufficient drainage has been established, the infected wound is washed carefully twice daily with a lotion of garlic juice and distilled water in a strength of one to three or one to four. After this treatment in a large number of cases a noticeable improvement in 24 hours and a decided improvement in 48 hours. The kind of wounds treated were recent dirty wounds in which suppuration had not yet occurred, foul, lacerated wounds of the face, scalp, thigh, etc.; extensive superficial burns of the face, scalp, chest, limbs, and abdomen in children; suppurating burns about the knees; cases of emphysema, foul ulcers of the leg: infected and suppurating wounds in connection with compound fractures; carbuncle; one particularly interesting case of moist spreading gangrene of the leg in an old woman 71 years, etc. The good effects of the garlic are ascribed to the active principles contained in the essential oil derived from it; and oleum alic [sic] is stated to contain allyl sulphide, in addition to certain volatile terpenes. The red-skinned variety of Allium sativa are said to contain more of the essential oil than the white skinned; the juice of the former has been chiefly employed.

The report of the healing action of garlic juice deserves careful analysis, for it proves several important facts.

First, bacteria are not the cause of disease.

Second, leading authorities have denounced the antiseptic treatment of disease as worthless.

Third, the return to natural drugs in the treatment of wounds, ulcers, carbuncles, burns, gangrene and **cancer.**

The passing of the antiseptic treatment of wounds, burns and ulcers is the knell of bacteriology. We have seen that men and animals are immune against bacteria so long as the skin and mucous membrane are not injured. Now eminent authorities state that the destruction of bacteria in wounds is useless, therefore, we come to the logical conclusion that bacteria are not the cause of disease.

I have always held that the antiseptic treatment of wounds with bichloride of mercury was unnatural, irrational and unscientific. The strong poisons used to kill the bacteria in the wounds also exerted a devitalizing action on the growing cells that nature is putting forth to repair the injury and close the wound. It actually retarded the healing process of wounds, burns and ulcers. The garlic juice that is so highly praised has but slight antiseptic action, but it has great healing virtues. The report seems to value peroxide of hydrogen as a cleansing agent. Even the peroxide is unnecessary. I have used a solution of one teaspoonful of salt, and one teaspoonful of baking soda dissolved in one quart of boiling water. This alkaline solution has about the same alkalinity as the normal blood. It readily dissolves blood, mucus and pus and is an excellent solution to cleanse wounds, burns, ulcers, gangrene and cancer. It also nourished the cells of the diseased tissues, increases their vitality and promotes healing.

The following cases are practical proof that the use of natural drugs gives much better results in the treatment of wounds and septicemia than antiseptics and serums.

I was called one afternoon to treat a man suffering from severe blood-poisoning. He was employed in a fertilizer works where dead animals were skinned and reduced to fertilizer. While skinning a horse he cut himself across the shin. It was only a slight wound about one inch long and one fourth inch deep. The cadaveric poison was introduced through this incision and soon produced a thorough poisoning of the blood. When I saw him he had a temperature of 105° F/41° C, a bounding pulse, face flushed, hot and covered with hot perspiration. The leg was greatly swollen, red and very hot. These symptoms called for belladonna. I put 30 drops of a 1:100 alcoholic dilution of the tincture of belladonna into one glass of water; of this I gave him one teaspoonful every half hour. I wrapped the leg in absorbent cotton. Then I prepared a solution of carbolic acid, one teaspoonful to one quart of water, over it. This gives us a solution of one part carbolic acid to 256 parts of water. The cotton was kept wet with this solution. I saw him again about nine a.m. next day. He was free from fever, and the inflammation of the leg was almost gone.

What healing action did the belladonna and carbolic acid exert in this severe case of septicemia? The belladonna controlled the fever and inflammation, the carbolic acid antidoted the cadaveric poison. No bacteriologist will claim the carbolic acid in a 1:256 solution is an antiseptic that kills bacteria. The acid exerted a dynamic healing action.

One New Year's night as the bells were ringing in the year, I was called to attend a young man who had been badly cut during a drinking bout. I found the young man lying on the floor in a pool of blood and in a drunken stupor. There was a deep cut running from the ball of the thumb to the outer edge of right hand and a transverse cut running from the root of the middle finger down the wrist. Both cuts were deep and had severed the large arteries in the hand. To make matters worse he had vomited over the wound. I had to work quickly. I cleansed the wound with dirty Ohio River water in which I had dissolved salt and baking soda. The alkaline solution cleansed the wound thoroughly, which was then closed with fifteen deep, silk sutures. There was never the slightest sign of suppuration and the wound healed rapidly. Now this is no uncommon experience for country doctors are often compelled to work under similar conditions without the use of antiseptics.

The healing virtues of garlic juice were not discovered by the staff of the Rockefeller Institute that is equipped with the latest and best apparatus for research work. The work is carried on by corps of eminent specialists. But these men are only serum and vaccine experts. They have no knowledge of natural drugs and natural laws. Their work has not increased our knowledge of the healing virtues of natural drugs as much as the stroke of the "t" or the dot of the "i". The Indian Medicine Men have done far more to increase our knowledge of natural drugs than the staff of the Rockefeller Institute ever can. Why have the Indians done more than the Rockefeller Institute? The Indians are godly men who believe in the Great Spirit; they study the healing powers that He has stored in the plants.

The Indians have given us such precious drugs as Echinacea, Hydrastis, Poke, Plantain or ribwort, Sanguinaria or blood-root, Sarsaparilla and a great number of other equally valuable plants that cure cancer, boils, gangrene and heal poisoned wounds. The staff of the Institute is ignorant of these drugs.

Every penny spent by the staff of the Rockefeller Institute is wasted; all their time and labor is thrown away. Some ten years ago several members of the staff of the Institute experimented with snake venoms. They worked under the most favorable conditions they could desire, in laboratories equipped with every apparatus that science and mechanical skill can construct. What did they discover? Nothing new; they simply verified the well-known fact that snake poisons destroy the coagulability of the blood and paralyze the heart and muscles of respiration.

The Indians, on the other hand have long known that Echinacea, Plantago and Cimicifuga will promptly cure snake bite.

I experimented with snake venoms about ten years ago. I used the dried venom of the moccasin snake, the cobra and Russell's viper. I was guided by the **natural law of harmony** in my research work. I studied the symptoms and effects produced and these led me to the natural drugs that antidote the action of the venoms with which I experimented. I found Arnica to be the true antidote to the venom of the moccasin snake. I had no splendid laboratory in which to carry on my research work. The work was done in my office during odd hours. I had no apparatus but a balance sensitive to one-tenth milligram and a hypodermic syringe. I dissolved the dried venom in distilled water.

The combined labors of the Rockefeller Institute and all other allopathic schools and universities have done less to increase our knowledge of the medical treatment of cancer than the Indians, who have given us Hydrastis, Phytolacca, and Sanguinaria that cure cancer. This is more than the Allopaths have given us.

Has the Rockefeller Institute accomplished nothing? Are all the energy and money wasted?

The law of conservation of energy teaches us that whenever energy is expended there is an amount of work done that is equal to the energy expended. Now the staff of the Institute has expended an enormous amount of energy. We have shown that it has done no good, so it must have done evil, no other conclusion is possible. It has not contributed to the knowledge, intellectual, moral or spiritual advancement of humanity. On the other hand, it has advanced the moral and spiritual degradation of humanity for it has led men away from natural drugs, natural laws, and the will of God. It teaches men that they can sin with perfect impunity for the serums manufactured under the methods of the Institute render men immune against disease. Their theory destroys faith in God, for it teaches men can thwart the will of God with vaccines and serums.

Our analysis has shown us why the serum craze has failed. It is unnatural, irrational and ungodly.

Why is the serum from the blood of horses suffering from natural diphtheria not a specific for diphtheria? Diphtheria is not a natural disease in horses; it must be produced by the artificial and unnatural method of injecting the bacillus of diphtheria into them.

We find that the cause of disease is the ignorant or willful violation of natural laws.

When we claim that serums are superior to natural drugs, we assert that men are wiser and more potent than God. Men can do what God cannot do. The serum doctors claims that they can defy the natural laws, thwart the will of God, make men immune against disease with vaccine and serums.

The serum doctors claims that they can defy the natural laws, thwart the will of God, make men immune against disease with vaccine and serums. Charges: ten dollars per shot.

To every action there is an equal reaction. This is a universal law. The medical profession is now recovering from the mild delirium of the serum craze and returning to the use of natural drugs and natural methods.

The healing virtues of garlic juice were not discovered by the staff of the Rockefeller Institute that is equipped with the latest and best apparatus for research work.

It teaches men that they can sin with perfect impunity for the serums manufactured under the methods of the Institute render men immune against disease. Their theory destroys faith in God, for it teaches men can thwart the will of God with vaccines and serums.

1917

The Crime Of The Century

Dr. E. D. Titus

Lecture By Prof. Wm. R. Bradshaw
At The 21st Annual Convention Of The American Naturopathic Association

William R. Bradshaw

Vaccination And Serum Treatment

Dr. Gilbert Bowman

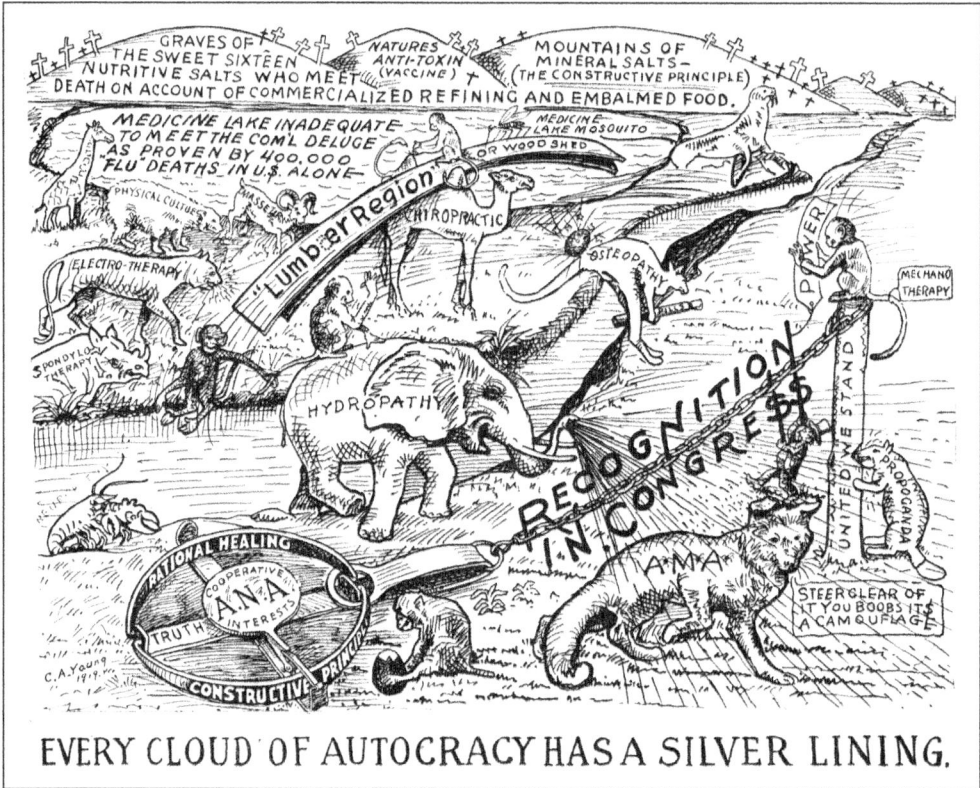

EVERY CLOUD OF AUTOCRACY HAS A SILVER LINING.

THE CRIME OF THE CENTURY

by Dr. E. D. Titus

Herald of Health and Naturopath, XXII (3), 129-133. (1917)

QUARTER OF A MILLION OF HUMAN LIVES PERISH ANNUALLY TO SATISFY THE INCOMPETENCE AND GREED OF THE MEDICAL MAFIA*

SANITATION

During a period of eighteen years, the fumes of pitch from the pine tree; certain derivatives from coal tar and an alkali have constantly permeated the building of a Minneapolis manufacturing plant that puts out disinfectants, sanitary soaps, animal dips and other sanitary specialties. During the first twelve years of that period, the second floor was occupied by four tenement living flats, people moving out and in as is usual with all buildings. The ceiling was [not] plastered; hence the fumes named permeated the whole building.

During all these eighteen years, no one connected with the plant has ever experienced an hour's sickness and no physician has ever been called in to treat a contagious disease or any disease of a germ origin. If every public building and dwelling could be as well protected, who can say that human life cannot be prolonged to 100 years?

It has been claimed that no one ever contracted tuberculosis who slept in a pine forest and that tuberculosis is rarely ever contracted in a coal mine and the dearth of tuberculosis in the alkali country of the West is well known. Here is an effect, covering a period of eighteen years and when we search for the cause, the combined fumes of the pine forest, the coal mines and the alkali regions of the West are the answer.

It is an answer based upon sound pathological reasoning, requiring too much space to explain in this brief work. If it is true that the inhaling of these fumes prevents disease (they cost almost nothing), we are constrained to ask, why our health officers everywhere disregard their far reaching power for good, not only as applied to man, but also animals? It is because it is not the mission of a political doctor to **Prevent Disease.**

FALLACY OF MEDICAL INSPECTION

One of the peculiarities of humanity is an overpowering desire on the part of many people, to dominate the acts and conduct of others. It may be noticed that those crying the loudest for medical inspection in our

---

*Guylaine Lancot, M.D., a doctor practicing in Quebec, Canada had become disillusioned with the practice of medicine and wrote *Medical Mafia* 90 years later in 1994 and consequently lost her medical license. —Ed.

schools have no children of their own to be inspected at public expense and along with these are found emissaries of the medical trust, working in the interest of the political doctor who wants a job.

You are taken sick with stretching limbs, flushed fever, headache, sore throat, loss of appetite and various other symptoms, but the doctor is slow to express an opinion. Because these primary symptoms are so nearly alike in a majority of diseases of a germ origin, it sometimes requires from two to three days to diagnose the disease to a certainty. Now the medical inspector in a school comes only in contact with the primary symptoms and has no way of knowing what the disease really is and consequently can perform no service other than to send the pupil home, which the teacher can do without the services of a doctor.

The only way to prevent disease is to remove the cause through sanitary conditions, exercise and good wholesome food, but these things the political doctor secretly fights. As applied to schools, in addition to sanitation a penny lunch would be of more help to the pupil where food is scarce at home than all the doctors, and in addition to complete the requisites, include a well-equipped playground. Think of a school system where all these are disregarded and in their place, a hoard of doctors prying into the bodily conditions of pupils. It is depriving a parent of the sacred right to look after the bodily condition of a child, and with certainty beyond dispute is gradually Russianizing America.

PURE FOOD

The human body is composed of 15 of nature's elements as follows: viz., oxygen, hydrogen, nitrogen, chlorine, fluorine, phosphorous, lime, potassium, iron, sodium, magnesium, silicon, carbon, sulphur and manganese.

A grain of wheat comes nearer to supplying these elements, in the proportions required, than any other known cereal, providing every portion of the kernel is used, including the shell, which, notwithstanding its value for building up bone, muscular and nerve tissue, is usually discarded and fed to animals. The wheat flour in general use on this account, contains little else than gluten and starch. In order to obtain the full benefits of this cereal therefore, what is known as *Whole Wheat Flour* is coming into general use.

Next to wheat comes rice, the staff of life, of nearly two-thirds of the population of the earth. Its efficiency as a food, however, is greatly diminished by the polishing process of late years to bleach it white, which as in wheat, removes some of the most valuable elements required for food, called rice polish, which is exported to Europe to feed stock. This objection is being overcome by the use of *Hulled and Unpolished Rice*, which is making its appearance on the market.

Milk is the primary food for all mammals including man, but the nutritive properties in milk, required to build up bone and muscular tissue is found in the skimmed milk and buttermilk, the cream consisting mainly of oils and fats.

In the husks of wheat and rice, in skimmed milk and buttermilk, the phosphate of lime found forms bone and teeth and is a constituent mainly of muscular, nerve and brain tissue. Silica forms the enamel of the bone, teeth, and nails and is constituent of the hair and other parts of a physical organism. Iron is necessary to the red blood cells, the carriers and distributors of oxygen from the lungs and with it vitality and vigor. It also gives the coloring matter to the eyes and hair.

It will be seen that for children or mothers nursing infants, the use of these primary foods in their natural state, such as *Whole Wheat Flour* or *Hulled and Unpolished Rice* is of the greatest importance.

Nature in providing milk for food, also took care that it should not deteriorate with age, but would undergo changes of a beneficial nature. The farmer uses sour milk to grow and fatten his calves and pigs and the housewife keeps a pan of sour milk in the poultry yard to make her hens lay. No sooner is milk produced than bacteria forms, one kind feeding upon another, but the record of the ages shows that all are wholesome food for man and beast. If this bacteria laden sour milk will cause a calf, pig or other suckling to grow and take on flesh, it is evident it will do the same for a baby. It has been demonstrated that bacterial milk will relieve pain and suffering in certain stomach and intestinal troubles where other known remedial agents have failed. It is held that buttermilk bacillus has a destructive effect upon what is termed senile bacillus found along the alimentary canal, the germ that is said to destroy certain cellular tissue and causing premature old age.

It is of historical record that men have occasionally lived to 300 years of age. As we ponder, there comes to us, something more than a belief, that if men through education could better understand primary conditions and observe their requirements, his span of life would embrace five score years and while living experience greater happiness.

If these things are true and the record of the ages affirms their truth, why does a pure food officer seize and confiscate milk because of the presence of bacteria found? The answer is that the political doctor wants a job. As an illustration, some time ago the government seized and confiscated a car of beef shipped from Chicago to Pennsylvania upon the grounds that it contained a preservative, but no evidence was produced that such a preservative was harmful.

Another car was shipped and was seized and confiscated upon the grounds that bacteria was found, and again no evidence was produced that such bacteria was harmful. Finally a shipment of 145 cases of frozen eggs was seized for confiscation, upon the grounds of bacteria being found and the parties contested the case in court.

On trial, the so-called government experts were forced to admit that it had never been demonstrated that bacteria in food stuff like eggs, milk and meat were harmful and the case was thrown out of court.

One does not have far to look for the cause of the high cost of living.

Bacteria is animated matter and as varied in its form as the life we see about us, embracing the fungus or it is the presence of bacteria that gives the delicate flavor to a large percent of foods and beverages.

In nearly every community are found men or concerns who make a specialty of securing and selling these primary articles of food so essential to the health and growth of infants and children and especially for mothers nursing infants, in response to the growing demand for such articles.

PURE FOOD LAWS

When heat, moisture and organic matter come together, decomposition follows. It is a process of nature to reduce compounds to their original elements, in order to utilize them in building up new forms of life. Were it not for this, there would be no flowers in the spring or life to greet their appearance. Cook meat and place it in a sealed vessel and if kept in a cool place, it will keep for an indefinite period. Expose it to the heat of the sun in a grocer's window, for instance, or in a warm room and through natural causes, decomposition will take place and poisons will be generated, unless preservatives are used in packing, and those eating it will be made sick.

A political doctor is called. He looks wise and discourses about the meat packers putting up rotten meat and declares that congress should pass more stringent food laws and make larger appropriations to stop it.

Who put the poison in the meat? Why, that very doctor, because he has been working with tooth and nail, through the Medical Trust to prevent preservatives being used in packing food stuff. Why does he do it? Because he knows that if preservatives are not incorporated, decomposition will follow and poisons will be generated and sickness will follow, creating business for the doctors.

The constitution confers upon Congress the power to regulate commerce between the States, but reason ought to tell any person that the framers of their constitution never dreamed that under that clause a police supervision as withering as that of Russia would be over commerce and in the interest of a vicious trust.

HIGH COST OF LIVING

The aspiration of the political doctor is to control everything—sort of a power that creates and rules kings. The only way for him to secure this control is to advocate government control of everything in sight, upon the theory that if once the craze is started, a doctor would be employed in every department of government, except perhaps the products of wood and iron.

He has succeeded and the land has been filled with detectives, inspectors and special agents spying upon commerce and interfering with business. To pay these, the appropriations of the general government have been doubled in the last few years.

The plains and canyons of the West were bleached with the bones of animals destroyed by the villainous methods of the political doctors in the Bureau of Animal Industry of the general government until finally the power for evil was at last broken after a five years' fight.

Commerce has suffered losses of similar magnitude through the abuse of power exercised in enforcing the pure food law and needlessly. This incompetency and maladministration have kindled counter combinations.

The producer says to the consumer: "If you want the luxury of government interfering with business you can have it, but you must pay for it. These ruthless acts cause losses, and losses increase the cost of production, which the consumer must pay in the form of higher prices." These laws have been secured through the rankest and most villainous fabrications inspired by the medical trust this country has ever seen.

WHO ARE THE POLITICAL DOCTORS?

The Allopathic School of Medicine has evolved from the Dark Ages, when the doctors boiled human hair, snake's eyes, and gizzards with herbs and bark and called it medicine. About 117 years ago a certain Dr. Jenner introduced the scabs taken from cowpox and called it vaccine. Seventy-five years ago these doctors were bleeding people to death until finally the Eclectics and Homeopaths came along and drove them out of it. Forty years ago they were filling humanity with mercury (quicksilver), opium and quinine, but soon after the germ theory was evolved and revolutionized all preconceived theories as to cause and cure of disease, but the inherited inclination of these doctors to use gruesome animal matter as medicine prompted the evolution of antitoxin, lymph and serum, the products of disease germs.

They are becoming ashamed of their past record and are seeking to be known as Regulars, instead of Allopaths, with the double view of having all others known as Irregulars. About fifteen years ago the American Medical Society (Allopathic) is said to have numbered not over 5,000 members and was looked upon as sort of a school of science, an honor to be a member of. About this time a craze was on for trusts and combinations and the promoters were abroad in the land. The American Medical Society took the craze and the organizers became active, until now the trust is said to embrace upwards of 100,000 members. They dominate the appointment of every sanitary or medical officer in the land, seating and unseating governors, senators, congressman, and state and city officials even down to alderman and school directors. They embrace only about one-tenth of one percent of the population of the country, but are so potent a factor, embracing their allied forces, the politician hesitates to question their acts.

If a move is started to conserve human life, they jump in the lead and by misleading destroy it. To sanctify their acts they have the temerity to ask the clergy to set aside a Sabbath or prayer to bless their efforts.

ALL DOCTORS NOT MEMBERS OF THE MAFIA

While the medical trust has its origin in the Allopathic School, a few Eclectics and Homeopaths were induced to join, but the ranks of the trust are being split as the better class turn with disgust from the acts of the mafia and are seeking to free themselves from the stigma of being a member.

The only way to prevent disease, is to remove the cause through sanitary conditions, exercise and good wholesome food, but these things the political doctor secretly fights. As applied to schools, in addition to sanitation, a penny lunch would be of more help to the pupil where food is scarce at home than all the doctors, and in addition to complete the requisites, include a well-equipped playground.

No sooner is milk produced, than bacteria forms, one kind feeding upon another, but the record of the ages shows that all are wholesome food for man and beast. If this bacteria laden sour milk will cause a calf, pig, or other suckling to grow and take on flesh, it is evident it will do the same for a baby.

They dominate the appointment of every sanitary or medical officer in the land, seating and unseating governors, senators, congressman, and state and city officials even down to alderman and school directors. They embrace only about one-tenth of one percent of the population of the country, but are so potent a factor, embracing their allied forces, the politician hesitates to question their acts.

Lecture By Prof. Wm. R. Bradshaw At The 21ST Annual Convention Of The American Naturopathic Association

by Prof. William R. Bradshaw

Herald of Health and Naturopath, XXII (6), 327-329. (1917)

I have been honored by a request from your worthy president to address you on the subject of Vivisection. As the lecturer for the New York Anti-Vivisection Society, I am very glad, indeed, to respond to such an invitation.

Vivisection is an immoral and unscientific practice. After describing its moral and scientific significance, I shall show you a number of pictures which will give you a good idea of what is being done with animals in the medical laboratories.

First of all, vivisection is an immoral pursuit. This universe is not merely controlled by material

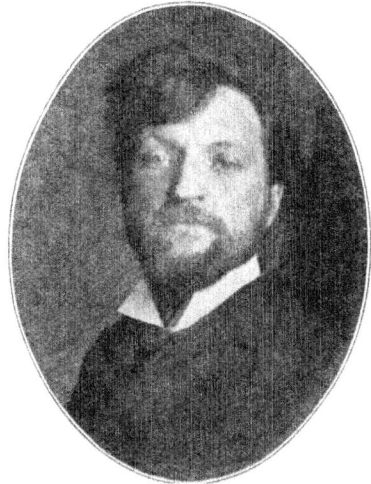

Prof. William R. Bradshaw

forces, but also by moral law, by the laws of order, truth, justice, humanity and temperance. To live under allegiance to moral law is the only thing that distinguishes man from the brutes. In fact, many so-called brutes are more moral in their conduct than some men. Man in the mass is an animal that has arrived at so imperfect a stage in moral development that he is ever ready for selfish reasons to prostitute his allegiance to morality.

The science of vivisection highly offends moral law, and the vivisectors say that they curse animals that they may bless mankind with such curses. They do this because they are morally insane. Two thousand years ago, man threw his own offspring into the flaming furnaces of Moloch to obtain the favor of a false god. He slowly evolved from this insanity, but a thousand years later we find him burning his neighbors as heretics, to merit, as he thought, the favor of heaven. He has evolved from this barbarity, and a thousand years later, that is today, the measure of his civilization is that he now burns the dog. Moral evolution is an awfully slow process.

The theory of the vivisectors is that they may rightfully trample on moral law, and not only escape the consequences, but gain honor and happiness by so doing. They say, "Let us draw a line between ourselves and the animals, and beyond that line we will cut, crush, choke, freeze, boil, burn, and otherwise destroy animal life in the most fiendish manner, so that by so doing we may lift ourselves and humanity to higher planes of health and happiness, love and tenderness, honor and renown." Did you ever hear of so diabolical a doctrine as that?

When I say that this is the conception and deed of the finite mind of man, I explain everything. The Bible, regarded simply as a repository of wisdom, gives us startling glimpses of how the Infinite Mind regards vivisection as one of those practices that tramples on righteousness. St. Paul, as the amanuensis of Infinite Truth, makes use of this pregnant statement. "Beware of those who spoil you with philosophy and vain decent, after the traditions of men, after the rudiments of the world, and not after the wisdom of Christ. For the rudiments of the world are weak and beggarly."

Stupendous words, stupendous meaning! The *rudiments of the world* are the products of man's reason trampling on moral law. Man riots in rebellion against moral authority where his selfish interests are concerned, for of him it is said, "My thoughts are not your thoughts, nor are your ways my ways."

Mark the conclusion of the Divine argument. It is not that nothing results from moral insanity, but that all results are of necessity *weak and beggarly.*

This statement was corroborated by a vivisector, Dr. Woglom, of Columbia University, the head of a cancer research laboratory, who in a lecture last winter in the Academy of Music, Brooklyn, on the subject of Cancer and Experimental Research, stated that "over two million animals had been destroyed under circumstances of great cruelty, to find the cause and cure for cancer, but nothing of the kind had ever been discovered, and if anyone said that he had found a cure for cancer through animal experimentation, that man was a liar."

There is no reason for vivisection, which means the performance of cruel experiments on animals and many humans, not for the benefit of the organism experimented upon, but for some ulterior purpose, chiefly that in the very multitude of experiments something may be discovered that will give the discoverer fame and fortune.

In the multitudinous everyday operations in surgery and in the endless experiments with drugs on the human organism in the attempts to cure disease, fields of unlimited extent are provided for every possible medical discovery that can benefit mankind. Both surgeons and practicing physicians, under the plea of healing their patients, continually and habitually experiment with their patients, even where the chances are "heads I win, tails you lose."

The human brain will never understand the inner self-regulated processes of life; no mortal mind will ever understand what life is, and yet these men who can never possess the mental equipment to understand these problems, hope by unlimited holocausts of animal life to create out of the frightful agony of God's creatures those brain cells that will enable them to understand the innermost secrets of life and disease, and, unless stopped by the arm of the law, will go on vivisecting until the Day of Judgment.

Of the utter foolishness of vivisection as a means of finding cures for disease, I am going to give you a concrete example. I will pass over the hundreds of failures, such as Koch's tuberculin and Friedman's turtle cure for tuberculosis, and give you a still later example.

Dr. Simon Flexner of the Rockefeller Institute lectured last winter in the Academy of Music, Brooklyn, on the subject of Infantile Paralysis, which I heard.* Dr. Flexner dilated on his experiments on live monkeys to find a cure for a disease that in most localities has a fatality of 100 percent, but not less, on an average, than 25 percent, with an additional 25 percent of supervening paralysis, a most distressing complication. He admitted that, notwithstanding many former claims, some of them emanating from the Rockefeller Institute itself, that a serum had been discovered that would cure the disease; no serum yet on the market would absolutely cure poliomyelitis. He further stated that after the most diligent search, no germ or microbe of the disease had yet been discovered. He showed upon the screen several microscopic granulations, which he asserted were the *virus* of the disease, a term used to conceal the ignorance of the medical profession as to the real cause of the ailment. The *virus* was in reality the microscopic granulations of Béchamp, that may, or may not evolve into microbes, the wherefore of such conduct being still an unknown quantity.

This is the same Dr. Flexner who loudly proclaimed some ten years ago that he had discovered a serum that would cure epidemic meningitis, and claimed that its use had brought down the death rate in that dread disease from 95 percent to 20 percent.

I have made a study of Dr. Flexner's statements as to the merits of his serum, and know that the death rate has remained around 95 percent ever since the Flexner serum has been available, and that no such amelioration of the disease as claimed has been affected anywhere.

At the termination of the lecture, I rose and asked Dr. Flexner the following question: "In view of the fact, Dr. Flexner, that during the summer of 1916, in the city of New York, there were 9,000 cases of infantile paralysis, of which 2,300 died, and as many more were crippled in spite

---

*Simon Flexner was appointed by J. D. Rockefeller as the director of the Rockefeller Institute, dedicated to medical research. His brother was Abraham Flexner, the architect of the 1910 Flexner Report that transformed medical education and also the medical landscape forever. —Ed.

of all the advances of medical science; and in view of the further fact that your own serum for epidemic meningitis is of no value in the cure of that disease, and in view of the further failure of a multitude of so-called remedies that are the product of vivisection, how can you pretend that any benefit can obtain to medical science by a method of research that combines knowledge with the powers of hell?"

Dr. Flexner sat transfixed to his chair while a ghastly smile overspread his features. He uttered not a word. A number of his medical friends who sat in the first two rows of seats, taking their cue from the discomfited lecturer, affected to smile hugely, like the chorus in a Greek play, to save their leader's face; but not one of them ventured to argue the question. They evidently knew that I knew the truth about the serum referred to. My statement as to its utter uselessness is corroborated by the fact that during the first three or four years when Dr. Flexner's serum was in use, the death rate in New York, as testified to by the Department of Health of New York City, rose from 82 percent to 97 percent. This fact is proved by the bulletins issued in the case.

How does Dr. Flexner arrive at his claimed reduction to 20 percent of fatalities? Let me speak in round numbers to avoid the confusion of fig-ures attending his repeated eliminations of fatal cases, while doctoring his statistics. Suppose he treats 100 children during a month with his serum. So fatal is the disease that 90 of them will die in spite of the remedy. This leaves ten cases—hand-picked cases, as it were—to consider. Of these ten, two more will die. Two out of ten is twenty percent!

Again at an address delivered by me on Vivisection in the Y.M.C.A. of Utica, N.Y., in February, 1912, the president of the Board of Health of Utica, who attended the meeting, rose and contradicted my statement that the Flexner serum was of no value in meningitis and stated that "the doc-tors in Utica had pulled the death rate in that disease down to 20 percent by the use of the same." Not being able to contradict that statement at the moment, I went the next day to the office of the Board of Health, to find, if possible, the truth about the meningitis statistics. The record in that office stated that there were 24 cases of cerebro-spinal meningitis in Utica in 1911, and of these there were 24 deaths. The deaths were 100 percent.

I consequently asked the editors of the local papers to correct their statements quoting the president of the Board of Health, as to the merits of the Flexner serum, by publishing his official report, made by him on his office records. They refused to do so. They said that the discussion would have to cease. They said that the doctors were good fellows, and that they had to live with them, and that some of them were the friends of their advertisers, and that they were going to favor Utica first, last, and all the time. Thus is the dear public doped and duped by the vivisectors.

Once more I will introduce a witness that Dr. Flexner cannot contradict, and that witness is Dr. Flexner himself. In his initial report of his experiences with his serum he thus appraises its value, in an outburst of despair intended exclusively for the eyes of the medical profession.

He says: "No one can be less convinced of the future fact of its value than we are."

After ten years of effort to improve this serum, it has become of less value than ever before. Thus does the Surgeon-General of the United States corroborate Dr. Flexner's avowal of its utter uselessness? He states in a report dated August 24, 1917, that in three-fourths of the principal cities in the United States in 1916, the death rate in cerebro-spinal meningitis was 100 percent!

Truly, the combination of science with the powers of hell is "weak and beggarly."

Prof. Bradshaw, at the close of his lecture, gave a fine exhibition of laboratory scenes by means of a stereopticon. They were a revelation of what devils in the shape of men will do.

They say, "Let us draw a line between ourselves and the animals, and beyond that line we will cut, crush, choke, freeze, boil, burn, and otherwise destroy animal life in the most fiendish manner, so that by so doing we may lift ourselves and humanity to higher planes of health and happiness, love and tenderness, honor and renown."

This is the same Dr. Flexner who loudly proclaimed some ten years ago that he had discovered a serum that would cure epidemic meningitis, and claimed that its use had brought down the death rate in that dread disease from 95 percent to 20 percent.

The record in that office stated that there were 24 cases of cerebro-spinal meningitis in Utica in 1911, and of these there were 24 deaths. The deaths were 100 percent.

VACCINATION AND SERUM TREATMENT

by Dr. Gilbert Bowman

Herald of Health and Naturopath, XXII (6), 372-377. (1917)

Department of Medical Freedom

This Department has been established to defend the rights of every citizen and resident of the United States to medical freedom without interference from medical dictation of any kind, and that no individual in the army, navy or in civil life should be compelled to submit to any form of medical treatment against his will.

Address all communications for this department to its editor

Dr. GILBERT BOWMAN, 1708 Warren Avenue, Chicago, Ill.

Dr. Gilbert Bowman, the editor of this Department, is Director of the United Schools of Physical Culture in Chicago, Ill. He also conducts a course of physical culture for home practice, which is in use all over the United States, with a membership running into the thousands. Dr. Bowman prescribes specific remedial exercises, corrective diet, and general suggestions for the proper care of the body in individual cases. He has had exceptionally fine success in promoting the health, development and general fitness of all classes of men and women. He possesses a world of information on the subject of medical freedom, which he will exploit in successive articles in this department. He is a fearless advocate for the medical rights of our citizens, and is always seeking to defend the people from the tyranny of the medical trust that has already succeeded in trampling upon the rights of the very defenders of the country in the present war.—Editor-in-chief.

INTRODUCTION

Perhaps a few words in explanation of the circumstances leading to the birth of this Department of Medical Freedom will not be amiss. A couple of months ago I launched a campaign for the repeal of the compulsory vaccination and serum-treatment laws of the army and namely, so as to give the American fighting boys the privilege now enjoyed by their British brothers, namely, the right to serve their country without serum or vaccine treatment of any kind, if opposed to these measures.

One of my first moves was to write to all of the leading health magazines and publications, calling attention to the present unjust regulations of the army and navy, and urging the co-operation of these magazines in the movement to give freedom to our fighting lads. Dr. Lust, of course, was among those to whom I wrote, and I am pleased to say that he offered his unreserved co-operation at once. In addition to taking the matter up actively himself, he suggested that we create a Department of Medical Freedom in the *Herald of Health*, so as to have an active medium for bringing these matters to the attention of the public until all forms of medical oppression have been overthrown. It is with great pleasure and keen appreciation that I have accepted his invitation to become a co-editor of this magazine and conduct this Department.

---

*Interesting to note that in the following year, a flu originating in the US within the American military ranks spread to the battlefields in Europe and brought WWI to an abrupt end. Known as the Spanish Flu, an estimated 35-50 million people died in 1918-1919. —Ed.

The Herald of Health is one of the most powerful and influential of the many publications devoted to health and right living, and no better medium for promulgating the facts of medical oppression and monopoly could be asked. This department, therefore, will appear regularly as long as there may be need for it and will persistently combat any and all attempts to abridge the rights of the people in medical and health matters.

The Constitution of the United States of America guarantees to every citizen and resident of this country the right to think for himself or herself and to live and conduct himself according to the dictates of his own reason and conscience, as long as he does not interfere with the similar privileges of his fellow citizens. America stands for liberty and freedom above everything else. And yet we harbor, tolerate and even submit to the most vicious tyranny and oppression in medical matters. We are less free in this respect than many of the European nations. I contend that each individual is the absolute owner of his or her own body and should have the final and deciding vote in regard to its proper treatment and care. No body of men, however well-meaning they may be, has any right to violate the constitutional rights of any citizen or resident and compel him to submit to any form of medical treatment against his will. This is being done constantly throughout the United States, however, and, especially, in the fighting service of Uncle Sam. It is the duty of every true American to take an active interest in these matters and I want every reader of the *Herald of Health* to consider carefully the facts I am about to set forth, and to then exert his or her best effort towards promoting the realization of absolute freedom in medical matters, in the army, in the navy and in civil life.

The phase of medical oppression and mismanagement that is of the greatest importance to the American people at the present time is the compulsory vaccination and serum treatment regulations of the army and navy, and to those, we shall, therefore, give consideration in this issue. The facts and figures that I give are authentic and reliable, and can be verified by anyone wishing to do so.

First. Let it be understood that the army and navy, indeed the entire government, is dominated absolutely in medical affairs by the Allopathic school, in other words, by the American Medical Association, a huge medico-political machine, boss-ridden, autocratic and wholly un-American in its aims and methods, that has well-earned for itself the sobriquet "The Medical Trust". It is a trust, in fact and in effect. No other school of practice, no matter how successful, is able to secure any representation in the government or in the army or navy. The views, beliefs and principles of drugless schools and physicians, or of Christian Scientists, are given absolutely no consideration or respect by the powers in control of army and navy affairs. This in spite of the fact that one-third of the

American people are actively opposed to Allopathy, and favor the drugless or natural form of treatment, and that this one-third is being augmented daily by long-suffering people who are forced to turn from Allopathy to more rational forms of treatment for relief from their ills and suffering. And by far, the majority of the remaining two-thirds of the population are opposed to most of the methods of the Medical Trust. If that were not so, it would not be necessary for the Medical Trust to seek the aid of the law in enforcing its nostrums, serums and methods.

Second. Let it be understood that, because of the absolute control of the military and naval affairs by the Medical Trust, every soldier, sailor, marine or airman, is required to submit to vaccination and to an injection of anti-typhus serum as soon as he enlists or is called to service, and as often thereafter as the medical officers may decree. This applies to those men coming from the one-third of the people that is actively opposed to the use of such measures, their objections to the treatment notwithstanding.

Should any soldier, sailor, airman or marine refuse to submit to the treatment, he is promptly court-martialed for insubordination, the punishment for which is a prison term of probably one or two years. That is not all. Here comes the "joker." When he arrives at military prison, he finds that the rules there also require that he take the treatment, and should he again refuse, of course, it means more punishment. As near as I can determine, this sort of thing may be kept up indefinitely, until the poor fellow is either badgered into taking the treatment or the medicos tire of their persecution. If I am wrong in this, I shall be glad to find it out and to correct the error in the next issue of this magazine. I think I have not exaggerated the facts, however. Senator Works, in his excellent speech to the Senate, opposing the Owen Bill,* brought out a case similar to this, the man in question being a Christian Scientist serving in the navy, and conscientiously opposed to vaccination and serum-therapy. The man was court-martialed, sentenced to two years' imprisonment, which was reduced to one year at the intercession of Senator Works, and he finally was obliged to submit to the prison rules and take the treatment. Perhaps he would have been in jail yet, if he had not done so. It is almost inconceivable that such things can happen in our free America is it not? The narration of this case, given by Senator Works, sounds more like a page from the history of the Spanish Inquisition, than an account of the treatment accorded our heroic fighting men!

From the way in which this alleged prophylaxis is forced upon our

---

*Senator Robert Owen introduced a bill in 1910 to create a cabinet level department to coordinate medical interests that included vaccination and medical inspection of school children. The bill did not pass but it successfully galvanized the drugless practitioners. —Ed.

fighting men, it might be reasonably supposed that it actually possesses some merit, and has actually proven itself to be a potent factor in preserving the health and efficiency of our fighters, and of mankind in general. We shall see. We shall also see how capable (?) the Medical Trust has proven itself to be in caring for the health of our fighting men—how worthy (?) it has been of the great faith and unlimited power reposed in it by our government.

Going back to our Philippine army, we have one of the best arguments obtainable against vaccination. The troops were vaccinated and re-vaccinated time after time, yet smallpox prevailed. There were some 260 deaths from this disease during the years 1898 to 1902. In his report to the War Department, Chief Surgeon Lippincott reported "I can say that no army was ever so thoroughly looked after in the matter of vaccination as ours. Vaccination and revaccination, many times repeated, went on as systematically as the drills at a well-regulated post." Why, then these 260 odd deaths, if vaccination has any protective powers at all?

General Otis, in his report to the War Department from Manila, January 31, 1899, gave the names of 14 of our soldiers who had died from smallpox. Up to February 4, 1899, he reported 43 cases of smallpox, although the entire command had been vaccinated several times. On March 6, 1899, Lieutenant-Colonel Henry Lippincott, Chief Surgeon at Manila, reported that up to January 16, there had been 124 admissions to the smallpox hospital, and 33 deaths. The entire command had been vaccinated four times since the arrival of the troops in the Philippines.

The official records show that we still have cases of both smallpox and typhoid in the army and navy, and also paratyphoid, which was unknown prior to the introduction of anti-typhus inoculation. We have also a multitude of other diseases which opponents of serum-therapy and vaccination contend, with good cause, are due entirely to the use of these alleged prophylactic measures. Here are some figures on soldiers' health, prepared from government statistics. These figures cover the period from 1905 to 1914, inclusive:

In these ten years we have an average annual enlisted strength of the army of 69,741.5; total reported sick during such period, 68,089.9 or 976 men reported as sick for each 1000 of enlisted strength; days lost per case, 13.58. During such ten-year period there were 3,657 deaths, and 11,926 discharged on surgeons' certificates of disability, or a total loss to the army of 15,583.

In the same period we have an average annual enlisted strength for the navy and marine corps of 55,396.6; average annual sick, 43,950.7, or 800.86 per 1000 enlisted strength; days lost per case, 12.80. During the ten-year period there were 2,732 deaths and 14,125 discharged on surgeons' certificates of disability, or a total loss of 16,587 men.

Striking a grand average for the military and naval forces of the United States, we have an average enlisted strength of 12,138.1 per year for the ten years; total reported sick per year, 11,040.6 or 888.38 per each 1000 of enlisted strength; days lost per case amounted to an average of 13.19. For all the forces, we have for the ten years, 6,389 deaths and 26,051 discharges on surgeons' certificates. To quite appreciate the loss on account of deaths and disability discharge, if the army, navy and marine corps had remained stationary, with no enlistments, at an annual average of 125,138.1, the loss from such causes would have amounted to more than one-fourth the total force. It is well to remember also that the death figures quoted do not include those who died subsequent to discharge, because of their disabilities. A large number of these die annually.

These figures, in time of peace, are little short of appalling, especially when we keep in mind the fact that our army, navy and marine corps are made up of picked men; men who have been obliged to pass a rigid test of physical fitness before they could gain admittance to the service, and that they have all of the advantages of modern sanitation, good clothing and the best of allopathic care. Certainly it seems that the medical treatment and care given these men is, to say the least, inadequate and inefficient. There is nothing about this record to warrant a continuance of allopathic domination of the fighting forces to the exclusion of all other schools of healing. Let us have medical freedom; let us cease sowing disease in the blood of our men on the fool notion that it prevents disease; let us welcome the Osteopath, the Chiropractor, the Naprapath and the other drugless schools of healing into the Government service and give them an opportunity to demonstrate their ability to cope with the situation and keep the disease, disability and death figures of the army and navy within reasonable bounds!

In passing, it may be of interest to note that during the period quoted, in the two services, every adult disease on the medical calendar was represented, including typhoid and smallpox, also a number of diseases commonly associated with childhood, as mumps, measles, scarlet fever, etc. It will be of further interest to state that the Chicago papers quite recently came out with the headline, "Pershing's men yield to Mumps and Measles." Why? Why should these picked men, after entering the army and being vaccinated, "yield to mumps and measles?" Is it coincidence, or cause and effect?

Vaccination has been a total failure in every country where it has been made compulsory. Perhaps the best modern illustrations of its inadequacy are furnished by the experience of Germany and Japan. These two nations have been held up by the allopathic fraternity the world over as the most completely vaccinated of all nations. Germany has been overrun with smallpox since the beginning of this year. In a speech by Herr Hoffman, "minority" member of the Prussian Diet [Assembly], delivered in March of this year, the honorable gentleman stated that "In North Germany, the Vienna papers reported there had already been 30,000 cases of smallpox. It was owing to underfeeding that smallpox has been able to find such fertile soil. **Inoculation in such a case was of no use.**" So Germany has just found out that vaccination is no good unless the vaccinee is well nourished! We are told also by Dr. W. A. Guy, F.R.S., allopathic pro-vaccinal authority of unquestioned vaccinal orthodoxy and ardent supporter and advocate of the Jennerian doctrine, that "It is now admitted by all competent authorities that vaccination during epidemics of smallpox tends to diffuse rather than to arrest the disease." Hence it is no good during epidemics! And the eminent English authority on vaccination, Dr. Millard, tells us in effect that vaccination is no good except in an epidemic or unless frequently repeated. We have also been told by various authorities, who have found it necessary to make excuses quite often for the failure of vaccination that it is no good unless done in the right way with the right lymph in the right number of places (the right ways and right number of places being still in dispute). In view of all this jumble of asinine contradictions, would it not be well to completely do away with all vaccination until such time as the numerous *authorities* can get together on the subject and prove to the entire satisfaction of the thinking world under just what circumstances vaccination may be relied upon to do its duty?

Consider for a moment the case of the other *best* vaccinated country, Japan. Let us take the figures of one of Japan's foremost pro-vaccinal authorities, S. Kitasato, M.D., Director of the Japanese Institute for Research in Infectious Diseases, and see what an excellent case he makes out **against** vaccination, while really trying to make out a case **for** it: "In 1874 the first (Japanese) vaccination law was enacted, and in 1876 the regulations for the prevention of smallpox were promulgated, which provided for compulsory vaccination. In 1885 a revised law concerning vaccination was enacted. It provided that every baby should be vaccinated within the first year of its age and re-vaccinated every 5 to 7 years.

It was in the same year (1885), just after the enactment of these regulations, that one of the greatest epidemics of smallpox during the last 40 years broke out, and lasted 3 years, with 125,315 cases and 31,960 deaths. The epidemic began to decline in 1888. It reappeared in 1892 and again lasted 3 years. During this second outbreak 88,095 cases were recorded, of which 23,603 patients died. The third outbreak extended over two years (1896-1897), with 52,650 cases and 15,664 deaths. In 1907 the disease reappeared at Kobi. **This caused an uncommonly severe epidemic, which spread all through the empire.** It began to die out in the spring 1908. During the fourth epidemic 19,101 cases and 6,273 deaths were reported. Ever since the promulgation of the first vaccination law in 1874 and that of the second in 1876, when compulsory measures were first adopted, Japan has suffered from epidemics from time to time."

Dr. Kitasato further states: "The average death rate of smallpox is estimated at from 20 to 40 percent in European literature. In Japan, it shows a higher standard, ranging from 25 to 69 percent, even during the small epidemics. During the epidemic of 1896-97, it averaged 55.08 percent, and that of the years 1907-8 reached the high standard of 69.4. When the virulence reaches this point, higher than has been encountered in European or American epidemics, **even individuals previously attacked, as well as those vaccinated, contract the disease.**" The emphasis in this case is ours. You will note that Dr. Kitasato admits the inability of vaccination to protect when the epidemic of smallpox amounts to much.

Note also that these mortalities are all far ahead of those from smallpox in the days before vaccination was ever heard of, and that completely vaccinated, hence *protected* (?) Japan, has a much higher mortality than Europe or America, where the practice of vaccination is not at all completely carried out! Will some pro-vaccinist please explain this incongruity?

Every country where compulsory vaccination has been tried has had the same distressing experience. I might go on and enumerate page after page of official statistics to prove not only the utter worthlessness of vaccination as a preventive of smallpox, but its positively injurious effect upon the health of the people thus treated. Space will not permit, however. Enough facts have already been cited to convince any open-minded, thinking person that there is no need for vaccination at all, much less compulsory vaccination. Before leaving the subject, however, I shall submit the opinions of a few famous physicians and scientists on this question of timely importance.

Dr. Charles Creighton, famous English writer and author of the article on vaccination in the ninth edition of the *Encyclopedia Britannica*, wrote: "It is difficult to conceive what will be the excuse made for a century of cowpoxing; but it cannot be doubted that the practice will appear in as absurd a light to the common sense of the twentieth century as bloodletting now does to us."

Dr. George Gregory, Director of the Smallpox Hospital, London, for 50 years said: "Smallpox does invade the vaccinated, and the extirpation of that dire disorder is as distant as when it was first heedlessly, and, in my humble judgment, most presumptuously anticipated by Jenner. The idea of extinguishing smallpox by vaccination is as absurd as it is chimerical; it is as irrational as it is presumptuous."

Prof. Alfred Russel Wallace, dean of English scientists, wrote: "I affirm that vaccination is a gigantic delusion; that it has never saved a single life; but that it has been the cause of so much disease, so many deaths, such a vast amount of utterly needless and altogether undeserved suffering, that it will be classed by coming generations among the greatest errors of an ignorant and prejudiced age, and its penal enforcement as the foulest blot on the generally beneficent course of legislation during our century."

Herbert Spencer said: "Compulsory vaccination I detest, and voluntary vaccination I disapprove."

That anti-typhus serum is no more effective than vaccination, has been demonstrated in the British armies in the present war. In Mesopotamia and the Dardanelles, where the troops were all inoculated with anti-typhus serum, and where the sanitary conditions were very bad, typhoid fever blazed up precisely as in the days before serum therapy. In the Boer War, the British troops were thoroughly inoculated, Sir Almroth Wright bestowing 400,000 doses of his anti-typhoid serum on them. Nevertheless, there were nearly 60,000 cases of typhoid admitted to hospital, and 8,227 deaths.

In spite of the claims and false statistics of the allopathic fraternity, the fact remains that wherever the sanitary conditions are bad, typhoid and smallpox will likely develop, irrespective of serums and vaccines; and that wherever the sanitary conditions are good, individuals who have not been treated with vaccination or serums, are not bothered by smallpox or typhoid any more than those who have been thus treated, and their general health, fitness and happiness is decidedly greater. Clean living is the key to health. To pollute the blood by serums and vaccination is the height of folly. It lowers the vital resistance of the person thus treated and predisposes to malignant diseases such as cancer, tuberculosis, cerebro-spinal meningitis, lock-jaw, etc. To compel such pollution is criminal.

Now, you fighters, you who believe that this glorious country of ours should continue to be "the land of the free and the home of the brave", get into action and do your bit for the men who are going to France. It is within the power of every man and woman to wage as valiant a fight here at home in behalf of our soldiers and sailors. Give the boys a chance to free themselves of this curse. In every military camp in this country the men will tell you that they suffer misery from the introduction of filth into their blood by means of the hypodermic needle; that many of them are sick and in hospital for weeks as a result of this mistreatment. In the name of justice, how long are we going to stand for this? How long are **you** going to let it go on?

You have enough facts here for a starter. Get in touch with your Congressman and urge him to help put a stop to this. Induce your friends to do the same. Take it up with your city or country newspapers. Get up a petition and secure the signatures of all the people in your town and locality who believe in liberty and justice, and send the petition to your Congressmen, so that they may have something to work upon; some tangible support. This department will gladly co-operate with you and will welcome any facts or material you may have to send. Get into the fight for justice! Don't be discouraged by rebuffs, but keep fighting persistently until the object of absolute medical freedom is achieved.

Let it be understood that the army and navy, indeed the entire government, is dominated absolutely in medical affairs by the Allopathic school, in other words, by the American Medical Association, a huge medico-political machine, boss-ridden, autocratic and wholly un-American in its aims and methods, that has well-earned for itself the sobriquet "The Medical Trust."

Let it be understood that, because of the absolute control of the military and naval affairs by the Medical Trust, every soldier, sailor, marine or airman, is required to submit to vaccination and to an injection of anti-typhus serum as soon as he enlists or is called to service, and as often thereafter as the medical officers may decree.

Should any soldier, sailor, airman or marine, refuse to submit to the treatment, he is promptly court-martialed for insubordination, the punishment for which is a prison term of probably one or two years.

In his report to the War Department, Chief Surgeon Lippincott reported "I can say that no army was ever so thoroughly looked after in the matter of vaccination as ours. Vaccination and revaccination, many times repeated, went on as systematically as the drills at a well-regulated post." Why, then these 260 odd deaths, if vaccination has any protective powers at all?

These figures, in time of peace, are little short of appalling, especially when we keep in mind the fact that our army, navy and marine corps are made up of picked men; men who have been obliged to pass a rigid test of physical fitness before they could gain admittance to the service, and that they have all of the advantages of modern sanitation, good clothing and the best of allopathic care.

(cont'd)

Why? Why should these picked men, after entering the army and being vaccinated, "yield to mumps and measles?" Is it coincidence, or cause and effect?

Dr. Charles Creighton, famous English writer and author of the article on vaccination in the ninth edition of the Encyclopedia Britannica, *wrote: "It is difficult to conceive what will be the excuse made for a century of cowpoxing; but it cannot be doubted that the practice will appear in as absurd a light to the common sense of the twentieth century as blood-letting now does to us."*

To pollute the blood by serums and vaccination is the height of folly. It lowers the vital resistance of the person thus treated and predisposes to malignant diseases such as cancer, tuberculosis, cerebro-spinal meningitis, lock-jaw, etc. To compel such pollution is criminal.

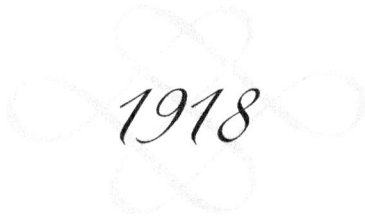

1918

VACCINATION
C. OSCAR BEASLEY

EDITORIAL, INFLUENZA, IMMUNIZATION
WILLIAM FREEMAN HAVARD, N.D.

The Vicious Circle

By William Freeman Havard

From initial cause to ultimate effect is a circle.

A good act starts a beneficial cycle of events.

A careless or mischievous act starts a vicious circle of disturbance that works destruction.

I remember a play that depicted the story of a small lie that caused the death of an entire family and many outsiders years after its telling.

A vicious circle once started is difficult to break.

Philosophy, religion and common sense tell us to acknowledge the original fault, make a confession and then set to work to remedy all damage that has resulted.

Fear prompts us to cover up our sinful acts, to hide our faults, to shift responsibility and to seek immunity from consequences. But how many escape?

Disease surely works in a vicious circle from which there can be but one escape.

Acknowledge your fault. Confess to yourself your violations of natural law. Assume your responsibility for them and the gates of regeneration will be open to you.

William Freeman Havard contributed many poems and articles to Benedict Lust's publications.

Vaccination

by C. Oscar Beasley

Herald of Health and Naturopath, XXIII (1), 69-72. (1918)

At a Symposium, held on Tuesday evening, November 9, 1917, by the Philadelphia Branch of the American Pharmaceutical Association, at the Temple University School of Pharmacy, 18th and Buttonwood Streets.

As Doctor Wadsworth, in his remarks just finished, characterized the anti-vaccinationists as being *ignorant*, as *using underhanded methods of fighting*, and as *championing the cause of pestilence*, I think that it is only fair that the audience should have a look at an anti-vaccinationist, for inspection purposes, to see whether we have horns or not, and also to hear the arguments that come from such *crazy* people.

Doctor Wadsworth says that there is only one side to the vaccination question. I say in reply to this what John Stuart Mill says: "He who knows only his own side of the case, knows little of that."

The great obstacle that stands in the way of every attempt to secure, by intelligent discussion, a settlement of the vaccination question, is that the vaccinationists do not meet our objections with scientific data. Mere epithets and assumptions prove nothing.

The vaccination question has its historical and political, as well as its scientific, aspects. It is historical, in the sense that it involves consideration of the experience of communities with smallpox epidemics; and it is political, in that an influential element of the medical profession has caused compulsory vaccination to be put into the statute law, which is enacted by the legislative representatives of the people.

The greatest smallpox epidemic in history, both in the number of cases and in the proportion of deaths, occurred, not in pre-vaccination times, but in 1872, after more than half a century of well-nigh universal vaccination. It has been conclusively proved that of the more than 44,000 deaths from smallpox that occurred in England and Wales in 1870-1872, at least 90 percent occurred in vaccinated persons, and the experience of Prussia and other German States, in the same epidemic, was similar. This failure of vaccination to protect the world from the furious smallpox epidemic of 1872 turned the minds of men toward more thorough investigation than has before been undertaken, of the protection that vaccination was alleged to afford to communities against epidemics of smallpox.

Jenner assured the English House of Commons, in his petition for remuneration, presented in 1802, that cowpox "admits of being inoculated on the human frame with the most perfect ease and safety, and is attended with the singularly beneficial effect of rendering through life the

person so inoculated perfectly secure from the infection of the smallpox."
This was soon shown by actual experience to be a false promise.

Cowpox virus contaminated with the virus of smallpox, Jenner
denounced as spurious.

Now, the medical profession has almost entirely discarded the cowpox, and only smallpox is generally used for the propagation of vaccine
virus. In other words, the members of the medical profession have thrown
overboard their vaccination hero, Jenner. They have put Jenner's cowpox
virus into the scrap heap, and have substituted for it the matter of human
smallpox.

Another dead-surely-right cult, arm-to-arm vaccination, which was
upheld by the members of the medical profession for nearly a century, they
finally discovered to be a mistake; and this, also, they have thrown overboard. In fact, they have now thrown overboard nearly everything, nearly
every alleged fact, nearly every argument, upon which, in the beginning,
they induced the governments of the leading civilized nations of the world
to endorse vaccination, and subsequently, to force it upon their people by
the instrumentality of statutory compulsion.

Arm-to-arm vaccination* was found to be a mistake because it was
dangerous to health and life. It was proved that by it many diseases had
been transmitted from one arm to another. It was, therefore, discarded.

Anti-typhoid serum is a sterile substance made of dead typhoid fever
germs; so, also, is diphtheria antitoxin a sterile substance. But vaccine
virus is not sterile. It is decaying living matter derived from suppurating
sores on diseased beasts. The introduction of such diseased matter into
the human circulation is denounced by true biologists, except when vaccination against smallpox is concerned. Why the introduction of diseased
living matter is always dangerous, except when vaccination against smallpox is concerned, is as yet unexplained.

Something has been said of the safety of which the public can rest
assured because of laboratory inspection, not only by the vaccine manufacturer, but also by representative of the United States Public Health and
Marine Hospital Service. When we recall, however, that for five or six
years several vaccine farms in this country propagated vaccine virus contaminated with the foot-and-mouth disease of cattle, and that this contamination escaped discovery during that time, causing hundreds of thousands of diseased vaccine points to be used for the vaccination of children,
we can gather some ideas of what the so-called laboratory inspections
amounts to from the standpoint of public safety.

Tetanus germs exist in soil and in hay, and in the alimentary canal, the

---

*Arm to arm vaccination was the practice of inoculating people using only one needle
for all. —Ed.

hair, and the manure of the calf. We can easily realize, therefore, that the very origin of vaccine virus is in an environment of tetanus. And when we recognized, further, that tetanus in the form of spores is apt to elude discovery, and further, that tetanus spores require for their development only just such a favorable culture medium as the vaccination sore furnishes, we may conclude, by reasoning from analogy, that these facts are in favor of the theory that the germs of tetanus implanted in the vaccination sore are derived from the vaccine matter rather than the theory that they are acquired from extraneous infection.

It has been asserted here to-night that Doctor Anderson's tests have shown that when tetanus germs were mixed with vaccine matter for the purpose of experimentally determining whether such matter could produce tetanus, this matter failed to produce tetanus in guinea pigs inoculated with it. If this is so, why does it happen that these same germs cause tetanus when they are directly introduced into the vaccination wounds, from outside infection, although they do not cause tetanus when they are directly introduced into the vaccination wound in the experimental inoculation of guinea pigs?

The spores of tetanus cannot grow into adult tetanus germs and produce their specific toxin except in the absence of oxygen, and this is aided by the presence, also, of pyogenic organisms. As long as the vaccination sore is open and discharging its pus outwardly, there is little likelihood of the tetanus spores developing, but when, after the scab begins to form, the air is excluded, and the affected tissues are deprived of oxygen, the medium provided by the vaccination sore and produce their appropriate toxin, and the disease tetanus results. These conditions and the time required for the tetanus spores to develop into full-grown tetanus organism account for the prolonged incubation period that usually characterized cases of vaccinal tetanus. Indeed, Dr. Joseph McFarland, in his paper on "Tetanus and Vaccination," read at the Second Annual Meeting of the American Association of Pathologists and Bacteriologists on March 28, 1902, in speaking of severe local lesions following vaccination, says: "Lastly, and I think truly, it may mean that it is only when such local lesions occur that the implanted tetanus bacilli can find conditions suitable for their development." And Doctor McFarland adds, as one of the conclusions that he thinks seems justifiable from the facts stated in his paper: "The tetanus organisms may be present in the virus in small numbers, being derived from the manure and hay."

Dr. Robert N. Willson, of Philadelphia, while making bacteriological examinations of the contents of glycerinated vaccine points, found pus-organisms, the streptococcus, the staphylococcus, and the pneumococcus. Dr. Willson says that glycerine "would tend to accelerate rather than to retard the action of the tetanus process." Doctor Willson inoculated a white mouse with a culture of vaccine virus, with the result that one minute later the mouse died in convulsion. This culture was derived from a glycerinated point purchased in the open market and ready for use.

Thus, it has been shown that vaccine virus itself, and the vaccination sore, furnish the best possible media for the adult germs of tetanus, resulting in the disease itself. And in the fact of these facts, it is idle to declare that it is proved that cases of tetanus following vaccination must necessarily be due to some outside infection. This is especially so as Bolton states, in William's *Manual of Bacteriology*, that "the toxic substance of tetanus appears not to be a ptomaine, as was at first supposed," and that "its exact nature is not determined." As the very nature of the toxic substance of tetanus is unknown, and positive statements, such as have been made here to-night, about the virus used in vaccinating not being the infective agent, are manifestly unwarranted by the facts.

What the anti-vaccinationists want is to receive satisfactory answers to all these questions, such as will clear up all the doubtful points concerning vaccination, and not mere dogmatism and mere assertion. Present experience proves that smallpox can be kept out of a community or kept under control by quarantine and isolation and other sanitary measures, without vaccination. In England and Wales, vaccinations have decreased in number nearly 50 percent in recent years, and smallpox has been kept down to the lowest point it has reached there during the last four hundred years. The medical profession will have to deal more frankly with the public in this matter, if it expects the confidence of the public. Utah has expressly prohibited compulsory vaccination, and various other States of the Union have done away with the general enforcement of vaccination; and Great Britain has [relieved parents by simply requiring them to provide] a written declaration, and the child is left unvaccinated, and no increase of smallpox has followed among its great unvaccinated population.

The vaccine virus now most generally used in humans [is] smallpox matter modified by passage through lower animals and by mixture with glycerine. In the original preparation of seed virus, the most satisfactory material was found to be pulp taken from the vesicles on the corpses of persons that had died of smallpox. This material was inoculated into the monkey, on whose body it makes a sore and sometimes an eruption. After passage through several monkeys, the resulting decayed and diseased matter from the sores of the monkey is in turn inoculated into the calf, when another kind of sore is produced, resulting from the diseased tissues of the monkey; and then the process in completed by the addition of impurities derived from cultivation of this diseased matter in the skin of a series of calves. Such an origin for any substance to be introduced into the human circulation is abhorrent to both reason and science.

Continued inoculation of the seed virus, from calf to calf, in time produced a still further modified virus, which loses the power to make a satisfactory sore. The vaccine manufacturer must then get something to start with again that is sufficiently impure to last for a while. Finding themselves in this predicament some years ago, propagators of vaccine virus sent to Japan and procured some seed vaccine virus from that country. What it was, was unknown. It seemed, however, to be of sufficient impurity and disease-producing character to start a new strain of vaccine virus in the United States. For five or six years, this virus was sent out, and then it was discovered that in spite of the Federal inspection, this seed virus was matter either derived from, or contaminated with, foot-and-mouth disease. Meanwhile, many hundreds of thousands of children had been inoculated with the vile stuff, and what disease is left in its train is not known.

The great obstacle that stands in the way of every attempt to secure, by intelligent discussion, a settlement of the vaccination question, is that the vaccinationists do not meet our objections with scientific data. Mere epithets and assumptions prove nothing.

The greatest smallpox epidemic in history, both in the number of cases and in the proportion of deaths, occurred, not in pre-vaccination times, but in 1872, after more than half a century of well-nigh universal vaccination. It has been conclusively proved that of the more than 44,000 deaths from smallpox that occurred in England and Wales in 1870-1872, at least 90 percent occurred in vaccinated persons, and the experience of Prussia and other German States, in the same epidemic, was similar.

When we recall, however, that for five or six years several vaccine farms in this country propagated vaccine virus contaminated with the foot-and-mouth disease of cattle, and that this contamination escaped discovery during that time, causing hundreds of thousands of diseased vaccine points to be used for the vaccination of children, we can gather some ideas of what the so-called laboratory inspections amounts to from the standpoint of public safety.

The vaccine virus now most generally used in humans, smallpox matter modified by passage through lower animals and by mixture with glycerine.

Editorial, Influenza, Immunization

by William Freeman Havard, N.D.

Herald of Health and Naturopath, XXIII (11), 865-867. (1918)

The most alarming epidemic in years has spread over the country like a prairie fire.* Practically every community will be visited. The present figures show an abnormally high death rate.

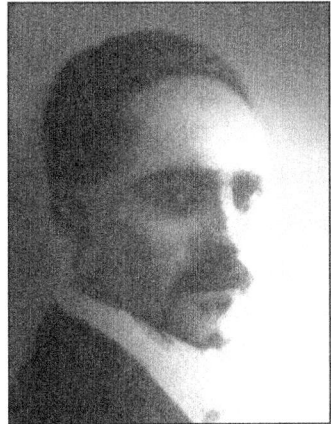

William Freeman Havard, N.D.

It is the same thing as the old grippe with which we have become quite familiar, only in a more violent form. It starts with an inflammation of the nose, throat and lungs. The onset is very sudden with pains over the body and extreme headache. The accompanying prostration is great and out of all proportion to the symptoms pointing to a high degree of toxicity. Deaths occur as a result of the pneumonia which is likely to develop under improper treatment, and failure of the right side of the heart. Of the cases we have so far handled, only one developed into pneumonia, and none have terminated fatally.

We desire to warn against some of the recommendations of our health bureaus in the treatment of influenza. **Abundant food** is one, and Dover's powder, a preparation of ipecac and opium, is another. Both will swell the death rate. Also fight against the use of any serum they may develop. Every doctor and laboratory man is anxious to make a name for himself at a time such as this and there is no doubt many "bug juice" preparations will be tried.

Keep cool; do not be alarmed. There is no cause for fear in those who know how to handle these conditions.

The proper treatment is rest in bed, plenty of fresh air, absolutely no food except fruit juices, cool sponge baths and alternate full sheet packs and trunk packs. At the beginning of treatment the bowels should be emptied, using enemas if necessary. Give light abdominal massages. If the headache is very severe, use cold compresses to the head and apply a throat pack.

Full sheet packs are applied by dipping a sheet in cold water and

---

*The Spanish Flu of 1918 brought WWI to an abrupt end killing an estimated 35 – 50 million people. —Ed.

enveloping the entire body, with the exception of the head. The patient is then wrapped in several layers of blanket and allowed to remain thus until a good reaction is secured. This will reduce the temperature by causing skin action (perspiration) but should not be pushed too far. If the temperature is 103° F/39° C before the pack is applied, remove it when the temperature falls to 101° F/38° C, which may take anywhere from one-half hour to an hour and a half. Sponge the patient, cover him warmly and allow him to rest for a half hour to an hour, and then apply a trunk pack. For this, a piece of linen is dipped into cold water, and applied around the trunk of the body, and a piece of blanket is wrapped securely around it several times. This pack may be left on a longer time than the other. Your temperature is your indicator. If within an hour to two after the body pack is removed the temperature rises again, revert to your full sheet pack. Continue this procedure until all symptoms have abated and the patient begins to convalesce. Do not resort to feeding until the temperature has remained normal for at least a day. Then begin with fruit, milk and gruels.

The condition usually runs a rapid course and terminates in recovery in three or four days.* Some of our cases have completely recovered in forty eight hours.

If pneumonia develops, continue the same treatment with packs and the other measures recommended until all symptoms subside.

Follow these directions and there will be no after effects to deal with.

IMMUNIZATION

Ever since Natural Therapists have realized the true function of so-called acute disease, they have warned against their suppression, pointing out that such a procedure would lead to the establishment of a chronic disease process. We cannot state too often nor too emphatically that *acute diseases* are forms of the reaction which the body makes to poisonous or irritating substances and are in themselves healing efforts of nature.

Encumbrance of the body with foreign matter leads to an interference of physiological function and when this interference becomes too great the resistive forces of the body manifest themselves in reaction increasing circulation and oxidation and resulting in increased elimination.

This encumbrance may be the result of autotoxemia (poisons generated in the body) or of poisons accidentally or willfully introduced into the body. This latter class includes drugs and serums, but whatever the

---

*In 2010, I had been exposed to the H1N1 flu and was bedridden with severe symptoms. I used the wet sheet wraps and recovered within 3 to 4 days while others with this flu suffered for several weeks. —Ed.

character of the poisonous substance the body must make a supreme effort to throw it off.

All acute diseases are for this identical purpose, and will only occur in a body containing foreign substance. To endeavor in any manner to suppress the reaction would be working counter to nature's method of destroying and eliminating the trouble maker, and will either cause death or at the least serious impairment of organic function and lay the foundation for chronic disease.

Any substance eliminated from a body undergoing a reaction is poisonous to any other body into which it may be introduced. If the second body has the power to react, an acute disease will be produced. The degree of toxicity of the substance and the degree of body resistance will determine the degree of reaction.

Serums taken from diseased animals are toxic (poisonous) products, and no amount of treatment in the laboratory has been able to rob them of their poisonous character. To be considered minimizing agents they must be poisonous, otherwise they will not produce a reaction. The theory of immunity from violent acute disease is based on the idea that a person can have such conditions but once, and it is supposed that a body while undergoing a reaction generates a substance which renders the disease toxin neutral. The theory then, of serum immunization is that by giving an individual a mild form of the disease it will prevent a recurrence of that particular disease in his body. If the individual does not contract that particular disease during his life time, it is considered proof that the theory is correct. In other words a specific serum is supposed to raise the resistance of the cells of the body and fortify them against the attacks of a particular disease.

Another theory of immunity through inoculation is that the blood is at once charged with the anti-bodies of the disease poison which has been generated in another body. This might be true [if] the serum consists only of antibodies, but an analysis shows them to contain live and dead germs and their toxins, as well as the antitoxin.

Someday our wise and learned will realize that there is a heap of difference between preventing disease and preventing or suppressing reactions. A body encumbered with morbid matter must either react, thereby relieving itself of its accumulations or rot in its own pollutions.

All acute reactions (we must stop calling them diseases) such as measles, scarlet fever, typhoid fever, pneumonia, etc., are means of relieving the body of poisons. They are self-limiting, run a natural course, and terminate in recovery when the patient is properly cared for. Any doctor who tells you that recovery from one of these conditions was due to a drug or a serum is self-deluded. These conditions are a blessing in disguise, and after such a reaction a person should take a new lease on life.

These acute reactions are contagious, infectious or epidemic because under our present unhygienic methods of living all persons are more or less encumbered with morbid matter. Natural immunity is with the individual who has a pure blood stream and such cannot be maintained or acquired on a diet of animal foods, white bread, devitalized sugar, pastry, coffee, tea, alcohol and tobacco with bad air, overindulgence and lack of exercise as side partners of bad diet.

Immunity from acute reactions cannot be brought nor transported from one body to another by so simple a process as a squirt in the arm. It may prevent an individual from reacting in a certain manner, but if an individual is ripe for a reaction what is to prevent its taking another form?

Since the war we have had a splendid opportunity to study the action of serums for never before have they been administered in so many varieties and such great quantities. Procure this false immunity from one form of reaction and it takes another form. The serums themselves are an added encumbrance.

If only someone in authority would stop long enough to reason, but that in itself would endanger his authority. There is absolutely no hope from that quarter.

But you and I can reason on this subject. There are hundreds of kinds of pathogenic germs, bacilli and bacteria, every variety of which is capable of producing disease in some specific form. Suppose we would grant that serumizing were the only means of procuring immunity and suppose that a specific serum had been developed for every disease, what would it mean to gain perfect immunity? From earliest childhood till your last breath you would be busy immunizing against something. Doctors would then be forced to specify the causes of death as *heart failure*, *lack of breath* or *accidental*.

But how long do you suppose a body could stand such repeated pollution? When do you suppose our health authorities will see this point? When do you suppose they will begin teaching people the way to natural immunity through right living?

The answer is plain—when the people compel obedience to their will and no longer, through ignorance, submit to abuse because they do not understand.

Teach them that they may know the truth.

The proper treatment is rest in bed, plenty of fresh air, absolutely no food except fruit juices, cool sponge baths and alternate full sheet packs and trunk packs.

Ever since Natural Therapists have realized the true function of so-called acute disease they have warned against their suppression, pointing out that such a procedure would lead to the establishment of a chronic disease process. We cannot state too often nor too emphatically that acute diseases *are forms of the reaction which the body makes to poisonous or irritating substances and are in themselves healing efforts of nature.*

To endeavor in any manner to suppress the reaction would be working counter to nature's method of destroying and eliminating the trouble maker, and will either cause death or at the least serious impairment of organic function and lay the foundation for chronic disease.

All acute reactions (we must stop calling them diseases) such as measles, scarlet fever, typhoid fever, pneumonia, etc., are means of relieving the body of poisons. They are self-limiting, run a natural course, and terminate in recovery when the patient is properly cared for.

Someday our wise and learned will realize that there is a heap of difference between preventing disease and preventing or suppressing reactions. A body encumbered with morbid matter must either react, thereby relieving itself of its accumulations or rot in its own pollutions.

Natural immunity is with the individual who has a pure blood stream and such cannot be maintained or acquired on a diet of animal foods, white bread, devitalized sugar, pastry, coffee, tea, alcohol and tobacco with bad air, overindulgence and lack of exercise as side partners of bad diet.

There are hundreds of kinds of pathogenic germs, bacilli and bacteria, every variety of which is capable of producing disease in some specific form. Suppose we would grant that serumizing were the only means of procuring immunity and suppose that a specific serum had been developed for every disease, what would it mean to gain perfect immunity? From earliest childhood till your last breath you would be busy immunizing against something. Doctors would then be forced to specify the causes of death as heart failure, lack of breath or accidental.

1919

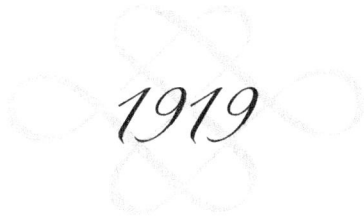

THE DOPING MEDICAL DOCTOR'S SQUIRT-GUN SCIENCE
E. H. JUDKINS, M.D.

The Doping Medical Doctor's Squirt-Gun Science

by E. H. Judkins, M.D.,

Herald of Health and Naturopath, XXIV (4), 200-201. (1919)

The eager college student always starts reading Rollin's *Ancient History*; and the first volume is well worn—often has to be rebound; but rarely does the third show use. Medical Science, so-called, is like this dry history, but in the third volume, Book VI, Chapter 11, we read, "The two armies were a long time coming into action, because the soothsayers and diviners, inspecting the entrails of their victims, foretold both parties equally they should be victorious only upon the defensive! Otherwise defeated if either made the first attack."

The Doctor's Dilemma, the five-act play by George Bernard Shaw, recently on at Copley Theatre, Boston, wherein physicians and surgeons discuss each other's theories, is nothing to the real dilemma of doctors whose expert *entrails diviners* cannot tell them what course to pursue, or even *practice*, in the present medical chaos. Their *scientific* soothsayers, seeing the immunity of savages, with their snake venom inoculations, originated serum treatment; but it was mixed with the use of offal and fecal matter of both human beings and animals during the Middle Ages; and then displaced when blood-letting, mercury and opium became the fads. Protesting with Prof. Waterhouse of Harvard against *learned quackery*, Dr. O.W. Holmes (*Border Lines of Knowledge,* p. 70) says: "The system of self-deception, in obedience to which foul veins have been emptied, entrails of animals taxed for impurities, poison-bags of reptiles drained of their venom, and all these inconceivable abominations thrust down the throats of suffering human beings."

But then doctors say: "You don't have to swallow these things now: a scratch of the knife, a jab of the hypo and a shot of serum, what's that to having the disease?" Let results answer: *Bulletin 12, Hygienic Laboratory*, Washington, "found tetanus spores on dry vaccine points, alive and virulent, after 295 days and in glycerinated (tubes) virus 355 days". Besides, pus cocci and bacteria of skin of cow, calf and horse are more or less mixed with all vaccine; and the cell of these animals grows nine times to one of human; hence, Drs. Snow and Bell show seven-tenths of all cancer and consumption is caused by vaccine serums, 225 percent increase in cancer (New York) causing 80,000 deaths, and 2,500,000 consumptives in this country, 70,000 British soldiers sent back from Gallipoli with tuberculosis after treatment for typhoid immunity. Paratyphoid fever (human hog cholera) was unknown until soldiers in India were inoculated with Wright's anti-typhoid serum, and it occurs only in those inoculated. Thousands of our soldiers suffered from same virus and other sera {serum}.

In one camp, 85 young men were inoculated with a certain virus and 82 fell down on the floor from its effects. One who refused vaccination was sent to Fort Leavenworth Prison, in Kansas, for 15 years. One out of every 20 of these heretofore healthy young men died from "Influenza"; but, if the truth be told, more from virulence of vaccines and the treatment of *regular, dominant, official* medicine. The half cannot be told, even with this paper filled three times over; nor in three times three." Dr. Peebles says: "Medical men have a habit of covering up when the facts look ugly." Professor Wallace gives a list of 785 deaths "directly due to vaccines, yet which were officially returned as deaths from erysipelas". Dr. H. May, health officer, admits: "To reserve vaccination from reproach, I omitted all mention of it from the certificates." (Read the book, *Quacks and Grafters*; also *Debates in Parliament*, and those coming in Congress—unless the Medical Lobby objects—as they did to the last clause of first draft of U.S. Constitution, providing for political, religious and medical freedom.

Recent epidemics of foot and mouth disease started from vaccine virus. (Bureau Animal Industry, 147, *Farmer's Bulletin, No. 666*) Infantile Paralysis followed vaccination; and serums to cure that, as in one city hospital, caused 14 out of 15 deaths! No wonder nearly a million children under ten years annually perish. During the last *plague* of infantile paralysis Johns Hopkins experts and doctors of the Baltimore Health Board found by many autopsies the disease was due neither to adenoids nor tonsils as first *theories* supposed; but in every case the intestines were affected and an effective *entrail* serum was hoped for. They would better use the colon bath! Wide use of diphtheria antitoxin neither lowers the number of cases, nor the deaths. (*Special Report, N. Y. Health Dept.*) Unfavorable to influenza sera, also.

While the present writer was House Surgeon at a Maine Infirmary, Dr. Crothers, of Hartford, Connecticut, stated that 21 percent of physicians suffered from their narcotic drugs and drink. To-day, in this country, there are 1,500,000 drug addict victims. (Revenue report now in hands of Congress.) Chinese have similar records; and for centuries used serum via the septum of the nose. But doctors cannot *ring* the American people that way; at least, *not all the time.*

—*Cosmopath*

But, then, doctors say: "You don't have to swallow these things now: a scratch of the knife, a jab of the hypo and a shot of serum, what's that to having the disease?"

Bulletin 12, Hygienic Laboratory, *Washington*, *"found tetanus spores on dry vaccine points, alive and virulent, after 295 days and in glycerinated (tubes) virus 355 days".*

Dr. H. May, health officer, admits: "To reserve vaccination from reproach, I omitted all mention of it from the certificates."

No wonder nearly a million children under ten years annually perish.

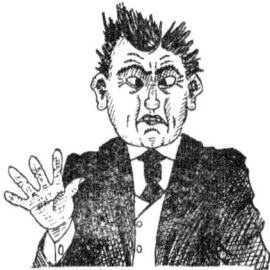

In the following year of the 1918 Spanish Flu, books and products were ready to inform and help alleviate fears of impeding infections and flus.

1920

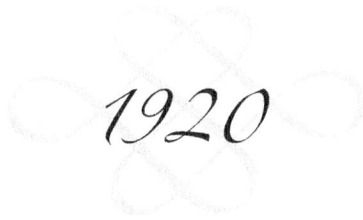

Naturopathy Versus Medicine
Per Nelson, N.D.

Naturopathy Versus Medicine (Continuation)
Per Nelson, N.D.

Get Together Or "Take Your Medicine"
Bernarr Macfadden

An ad appearing in 1921 announcing Benedict Lust's new schools, American School of Naturopathy and America School of Chiropractic located in the elegant neighbourhood of Central Park.

Naturopathy Versus Medicine

by Per Nelson, N.D.

Herald of Health and Naturopath, XXV (2), 78-82. (1920)

One need not use lanterns or field glasses to discover the many defects of the so-called science of medicine, neither does one need to waste any time in constructing arguments against the drug system, for the reason that this system itself furnishes us with the best of arguments; living arguments, if you please.

Look around in any community and what will you find? You will find hundreds, yes, thousands of so-called incurables or chronics—men, women and children. You will meet them on the street, in the trolley cars, churches and everywhere. You will see thousands of crippled and defective people, sounds of nervous wrecks; yes, and their dull eyes, their bent backs, their deformed bodies, their shaky limbs and their pale faces will tell you a story, not only of the inefficiency of the drug treatment, but of malpractice, the thousand time damnable malpractice that is going on.

Visit the hospitals, the insane asylums, the institutions for dope fiends, the colonies for epileptics, the homes for defective children.

Do you wish for any more evidence? Do you want any sharper arguments against the system of medicine? Can you help wondering why we have so many defectives? Haven't you read in the Sunday paper about the advance in medical science? What is the matter with this crazy world, anyway? Why all this suffering?

Haven't we got Health Boards in every city and town? Haven't we a dozen doctors—highly educated, college-bred and dignified men—in every city building? Haven't we a drug store on every street corner, each one with barrels of specific drugs?

Let us calm ourselves. Let us stop asking questions. Let us try to reason out what is wrong with medicine, and also what we can do to alleviate all this suffering. The history of medicine will help in this respect, and we will therefore consult her pages. She tells us, among other things, that there was a time when disease was looked upon as something mysterious or supernatural that no human being could explain; something frightful that had to be fought with all kinds of weapons. Yes, the belief at that time was that evil spirits entered the bodies of persons who were sick, and that these had to be driven out by forcible means. It was, therefore, a common practice, a few hundred years ago, to tie the sick person to a tree, and to torture him or her until the evil spirits had left the body. Others used milder means for driving out evil spirits, such as, for instance, prayer, temple, sleep, etc.

The very same idea, but in somewhat modified form prevails in the science of medicine of our day. The evil spirits of today are the germs, and the whip that is used in driving them out are the drugs and these germs, according to medical science, are lurking around everywhere to find those "whom they may destroy." In other words, medical science attributes the various diseases to the presence of specific disease-producing micro-organisms, some of which have been discovered and classified into *family groups*, others, again, that have escaped the eyes of the bacteriologists, and who, therefore, work on our destruction like thieves at night. These germs, according to medical science, are carried around by flies, mice, mosquitoes, dogs and cats, and also according to the latest fad, by *human germ carriers*.

Germs are supposed to be equally dangerous to each and every one of us, and no matter how strong and healthy we are, if it should happen that they get into our systems, they will at once begin to raise *cane* with us especially so if we haven't had all of the 59 varieties of artificial antitoxins injected into our blood.

With the above conception of disease, we can readily grasp the reason why practically all of the research work conducted in medical circles today is concentrated on the discovery and production of serums or antitoxins that will kill off these germs, and, as shown during the recent influenza epidemic, they have succeeded in this respect so remarkably well, that not only the lives of the germs, but in many instances also the lives of the patients were taken.

In contrast to the medical men, the Naturopaths do not blame disease on external causes, which are not under our control, but claim that disease is merely the result of bad habits or wrong modes of living, which have to be corrected before a cure is possible. We claim that all persons born from healthy parents have a certain amount of vitality. This vitality or force controls and enables all organs and parts of the body to function. If vitality is good, the skin, bowels, kidneys, lungs and every organ in the body will function properly. The food we eat will be transformed into heat, energy and tissues, and the gases that are set loose in this chemical process, as well as the waste materials given off from the cells, will be expelled from the body through the four channels mentioned above (the skin, kidneys, bowels and lungs). But should we abuse ourselves in any manner, so as to lower our vitality, (this can be done in hundreds of ways, such as, for instance, through sexual abuse, over-eating, lack of sleep, overwork, etc., etc.,) the organs of excretion will at once become impaired, and poisonous gases and waste products that under normal conditions would leave the body, will begin to collect. When this has been going on for some time, Nature will be forced to try a house cleaning, and this she performs in the form of acute disease. Thus it will be seen that acute disease is nothing more than an outbreak of morbid matter that has accumulated in the system, hence the bad odor you always find in the sick-room.

Acute disease may be compared with a thunderstorm on a hot summer day. When the air is loaded with foreign substances, the thunderstorm is bound to come and clear the atmosphere. But what would happen if we, through some artificial means, could suppress or hinder the thunderstorm from breaking? Simply this: the air would become so fouled that we could hardly breathe. And this is just what takes place when we suppress the body's thunderstorm, the acute diseases, and here lies the terrible crime that has been, and is being committed daily, and the very cause that has produced our chronics, our invalids and nervous wrecks. Here is the cause that has filled our hospitals, insane asylums and homes for defective children.

The recent influenza epidemic has probably more than anything else proven the Naturopathic conception of disease to be correct. What was the cause of the so-called Spanish influenza? Let us see. We all know that the American nation is a wheat-eating nation. Being wheat-eaters, our systems have been accustomed and are quite able to neutralize and to get rid of the waste products of wheat; but owing to war conditions, the government deemed it necessary to substitute wheat with barley and corn-meal. Now, everybody knows that barley and corn-meal ferments very readily, and as our systems were not used to handling these *sticky* substance, their waste products began to clog our cells and tissue-spaces. Well, everything went fine until the leaves started to fall from the trees and ferment. During that time of the year the air is always full of fermented substances, and as we inhaled these substances, as the air in the sick-room of those who had this disease, the barley and corn-meal products, which loaded our systems, were set into fermentation, and here is the whole *mystery* of the Spanish influenza, which seemed to puzzle especially our medical men so very much.

As a contributing cause, we can mention that early in the fall, we had a short spell of very cold weather, which scared a number of people into heavier underwear. After this short spell of cold weather, we had about two months of very warm weather, but many of those who had put on heavier underwear during the short cold spell, continued to wear it during the two warm months that followed, and in this manner interfered with the skin elimination. Sorrow, caused by loss of relatives and friends in the Great War, also undermined the body vitality, and in this manner made the population more susceptible to disease. Overwork, which was very common during the war, may also be regarded as a contributing cause.

The causes of other acute diseases are identical with influenza, in that they always constitute Nature's efforts to eliminate waste material from the system. An individual description of each and every one of them would be superfluous. We will, therefore, leave the subject of acute diseases in order to describe chronic disease.

What is a chronic disease? A chronic disease is a condition where the body is so loaded with waste material that Nature cannot arouse herself in an active reaction, or produce the *thunderstorm* that would rid the system of poisonous waste material, and this accounts for the heavy dragging feeling always connected with chronic disease. The cause has already been explained; it was simply due to the suppressing of the acute diseases by means of strong drugs, which rendered the poisonous waste material in the body latent, instead of expelling it through the body's natural channels. These waste products, after being sealed up in the body inhibited Nature's functions, and attacked the cells and structures, sometimes only causing function disturbances, but more often causing pathological changes in the tissues themselves.

Insanity and mental diseases are but another form of chronic disease, and very similar to all other chronic ailments. One need not be a philosopher to understand that if a human brain is built up on pure blood alone, and if only pure blood is circulating through its vessels, that no insanity can exist unless caused by external traumatic conditions.

If, on the other hand, the brain is built up on abnormal and poisonous blood, and if only poisonous blood circulating through the vessels, constantly irritating the cells and structures, then, of course, insanity or other mental diseases must necessarily be the logical outcome, and here again the blame is to be played on the suppressive methods used by the medical profession.

When knowing the nature of disease, i. e., that acute diseases are simply Nature's way of expelling poisonous waste matter from the system, and that chronic disease is caused by the sealing up in the body of these same substances, it is easily reasoned out that elimination must necessarily be the keynote to the treatment of all diseases, and here is where the Naturopath comes in with his hydrotherapy and massage, his light treatments and electricity, his chiropractic stimulation and concussion, his diet and mental suggestion, his herb and bio-chemical remedies. In other words, the Naturopath simply assists Nature in her efforts to eliminate waste material through the body's natural channels, by improving and equalizing the body fluids, and by stimulating the lungs, kidneys, bowels and skin to normal activity, and this is the reason why Naturopaths are able to cure diseases after all other systems have failed to do so.

But the Naturopath goes even further than to merely cure disease. Knowing that transgression of Nature's laws lies at the root of all human ills, he also considers it his duty to teach humanity how to follow these laws, thereby making it possible for them to avoid disease. The Naturopath is, therefore, not only a healer who is able to cure disease, but also a reformer and preacher in the true sense of the word, and he believes in his system not only as a science and an art, but as a religion that will, if followed, lead humanity to heaven of health and happiness.

As I have not, in the above description of disease been mentioning the germs at all, someone may ask: What about the germs? Is it not possible that they cause disease, or if they do not, what then is their function, and in what way are they related to disease?

In order to answer these questions, it is necessary to make a comparative study of germs and their functions in all Nature, not only in the bacteriological laboratories, and perhaps if we find out what their function is outside of our bodies then we can probably be in a better position to draw our conclusions as to their function in our interior during acute disease.

As far as we can make out at the present time, and as we will try to prove in the following, the function of germ life in all Nature is to split up complex chemical compounds into simpler ones. Let us begin with a few illustrations from farm life. When the farmer or gardener sows his vegetable seeds in the ground, these seeds are at once attacked by thousands of germs, and their albuminous matter is through this germ action softened and broken up into simpler chemical substances, which the young seedling is able to use for its nourishment.

The same happens when fertilizer is put into the ground. Here again the germs have to split up the complex material of the fertilizer into simpler substances, which can be used as a food for the plants. Indeed, manure which has not been acted upon by bacteria is practically useless. The up-to-date farmer knows this. He therefore always puts the manure in heaps for ripening, as he calls it. During this ripening process, the manure is attacked by billions and billions of germs, and all complex materials are thus converted into simple chemical substances.

Let us take another illustration from germ life, which will perhaps be a little different from the previous two. We all know that when a tree falls in the forest, it does not forever stay on the top of the ground. After a short while we find that its bark loosens from the wood and falls off. A while longer and we find that the whole tree has been reduced to a powdery mass, which is finally absorbed by the soil. What has happened in this case? The same as happened to the vegetable seed and the fertilizer. Here again the germs have been at work and reduced its solid mass into substances which can again be used in Nature's cycle.

Hundreds of illustrations, similar to the ones spoken above, could be given to prove our assertion that the function of germ life in all Nature is to split up complex matter into simpler chemical substances, but they would in the main be the same story repeated, and as my article has already lengthened to a greater dimension than was intended at its start, I shall give just one more example, taken direct from the greatest laboratory in the world—the human body.

We are often told that millions of germs are lodged in our intestines, but we are very seldom told what their function is. Needless, however, to say that their function there is the same as everywhere else in all Nature—to split up complex chemical compounds into simpler ones. Foods that have escaped the digestive fluids are thus acted upon by various kinds of bacteria. Proteins are broken up into peptone amino-acids and ammonia, starches into sugars, fats into valeric and butyric acid, cellulose into carbonic acid and methane, etc., etc.

Now, if we use a little logic and reasoning, what conclusions can we form from the foregoing? Must we not necessarily be led to the belief that if the germ-function everywhere else in Nature is to split up complex compounds into simpler ones, that that most likely also is their function during acute diseases, and when we furthermore know, as stated in the beginning of this article, that acute disease is merely an outbreak of morbid matter, then it seems so much more logical that the germs must be present during an acute attack in order to split up or decompose the complex colloid material which otherwise would remain too complex to be eliminated.

The Naturopath, therefore, holds the view that the germs are the result of the disease, and not its cause, and that germ action during acute disease (the splitting up of complex pathogenic material into substances which the body is able to eliminate) is beneficial, not harmful.

Now, someone may ask: "Is it not possible that there are harmful germs also, as well as useful ones, inasmuch as in animal life we have poisonous snakes and reptiles, and in vegetable life poison ivy, etc., and if that is the case, is it, then, not proper to kill off these dangerous germs with strong drugs?"

To this we answer: Yes; it is quite true that there are a few species of dangerous germs—for instance, the tetanus germ (Bacillus tetani); but these dangerous germs are in a very small minority compared with the thousands of different species of useful germs, and do not affect the body unless there is a medium in which they can live—an accumulation of foreign matter, in other words. But in the treatment, the Naturopath again holds the trump card, as the danger from these germs lies in the fact that they produce poisonous toxins which affect the body structures. It, therefore, stands to reason that elimination, the great principle on which Naturopathy is founded, is again the proper measure to employ—indeed, elimination is the only salvation in these cases, as pathogenic germs show a very high resistance to poisonous drugs. The problem of killing pathogenic germs inside of our bodies with strong drugs is identical to killing ourselves, and has, therefore, no therapeutic foundation whatsoever.

But the world slowly but surely keeps on moving, and old theories everywhere are forced to make room for new and more advanced ones, and this holds true in the science of medicine also, despite all efforts, conscious or unconscious, to hold back the wheels of progress; and as a result of this, we find broadminded men in the medical profession also—men who dare to think for themselves, and who are not afraid to let the world know their thoughts.

When knowing the nature of disease, i. e., that acute diseases are simply Nature's way of expelling poisonous waste matter from the system, and that chronic disease is caused by the sealing up in the body of these same substances, it is easily reasoned out that elimination must necessarily be the keynote to the treatment of all diseases, and here is where the Naturopath comes in with his hydrotherapy and massage, his light treatments and electricity, his chiropractic stimulation and concussion, his diet and mental suggestion, his herb and bio-chemical remedies.

In other words, the Naturopath simply assists Nature in her efforts to eliminate waste material through the body's natural channels, by improving and equalizing the body fluids, and by stimulating the lungs, kidneys, bowels and skin to normal activity, and this is the reason why Naturopaths are able to cure diseases after all other systems have failed to do so.

But the Naturopath goes even further than to merely cure disease. Knowing that transgression of Nature's laws lies at the root of all human ills, he also considers it his duty to teach humanity how to follow these laws, thereby making it possible for them to avoid the disease. The evil spirits of today are the germs, and the whip that is used in driving them out is the drugs and these germs, according to medical science, are lurking around everywhere to find those "whom they may destroy."

We are often told that millions of germs are lodged in our intestines, but we are very seldom told what their function is. Needless, however, to say that their function there is the same as everywhere else in all Nature—to split up complex chemical compounds into simpler ones.

The Naturopath, therefore, holds the view that the germs are the result of the disease, and not its cause, and that germ action during acute disease (the splitting up of complex pathogenic material into substances which the body is able to eliminate) is beneficial, not harmful

Naturopathy Versus Medicine (Continuation)

by Per Nelson, N.D.

Herald of Health and Naturopath, XXV (3), 134-138. (1920)

Such a man is John B. Fraser, a prominent physician from Toronto, Canada. Dr. Fraser has probably done more than anyone else in wrecking the theory of germs as a cause of disease, a work for which we Naturopaths are greatly indebted to him, as it proves our theories to be correct. For several years Dr. Fraser, assisted by a number of Canadians, carried out the most painstaking experiments, which prove, first, that germs are not present at the onset of acute diseases; and second, that germs do not cause disease. To avoid misrepresentation, I shall let Dr. Fraser himself relate his experiments. He wrote about them as follows in the *Truth Teller* of February 1st, 1918:

> (a) A man crossing a river broke through the ice, was rescued, later became ill, and the doctor, fearing pneumonia, tested for pneumococci—there were none present; when the pneumonia developed, they appeared.
>
> (b) After an oyster supper some men had cramps and diarrhea, followed by typhoid fever—no Eberth bacilli were present in the first stools, but were present later.
>
> (c) Hurrying, a girl arrive at her shop sweating; as the shop was cold, she became very chilly; next day complained of a sore throat, but no Klebs-Loffler bacilli were found; later, when a diphtheritic patch appeared, the bacilli were present.
>
> Here in each case the bacilli followed the onset of the disease.
>
> Believing that the above germs were the result and not the cause of the diseases, tests of the germs of diphtheria, typhoid and pneumonia were made.
>
> The first test was whether the Klebs-Loffler bacilli would cause diphtheria, and about 50,000 were swallowed without any result; later 100,000, 500,000, and a million more were swallowed and in no case did they cause any ill-effect.
>
> The second series of tests was to decide whether the Eberth bacillus would cause typhoid, but each test was negative; even when millions were swallowed. The third series of tests, showed that one could swallow a million (and over) pneumococci without causing pneumonia, or any disturbance.
>
> In testing typhoid germs, 45 experiments were made in which water, milk, bread, cheese, meat, fish, potatoes, headcheese, butter, porridge, etc., were infected with millions of fresh, vigorous typhoid germs; this food containing the germs was used in the ordinary way;

and, as the Bio-Chemics expected, there was not a single instance of any sign of typhoid. Here we have 45 facts—not assumptions—to build on.

In this series of 19 experiments, milk, water and food were infected with millions of pneumonia germs, and although no precautions were taken to prevent the disease no sign of the disease developed.

A total of forty experiments were made with germs of diphtheria, in which they were not only taken in water, milk, bread, porridge, potatoes, cheese, butter, etc., but other millions of germs were swabbed in the nose and throat, and every facility given them to develop, but in spite of all efforts they refused to develop, although they would grow rapidly on nutrient agar. These tests were made scientifically and part of the germs were grown from stock tubes furnished by one of the best known laboratories in North America. These are facts, not opinions.

In this series of tests, 19 experiments were made; special attention was paid to thoroughly infect milk, water, bread, meat, potatoes, etc., with millions of germs, fresh and vigorous, but in spite of every effort to get them to develop, they were positively inert. The germs used were human (not bovine) tubercule bacilli germs.

As these are the dreaded germs supposed by some to cause infantile paralysis, and believed to germinate in the nasal mucous membrane, especial pains were taken to infect nostrils and throat with fresh colonies of germs; they were swept over the turbinated bones, pushed into sinuses, swabbed over the floor of the nostrils, rubbed on the tonsils, placed beneath the tongue, taken in milk, water and food; but in spite of coaxing, coddling and urging, they refused to produce a solitary sign of meningitis in the eleven tests made.

Ten experiments were made with germs, viz.: Typhoid and pneumonia, typhoid and tuberculosis, diphtheria and meningitis, typhoid and meningitis, diphtheria and pneumonia, etc., but all failed to produce any effect.

For the benefit of bacteriologists we enumerate the germs used in the tests mentioned: Eberth bacilli, Klebs-Loffler bacilli, tubercle bacilli (human), diplococcus pneumoniae, and diplococcus intracellularis meningitidis—all well known to bacteriologists.

It is, however, not only from the other side of the Canadian border that we find broadminded medical men.

Our own United States have several of them, among whom we can mention R. L. Alsaker, M.D., of New York City, as one. Dr. Alsaker has for years, in common with the Naturopaths, advocated the theory that germs are the result of the disease, not its cause. We quoted the following from an article by his pen, which appeared in the *Physical Culture Magazine,* a short while ago.

Germs are present in disease, but they do not cause disease. If germs really produced disease there would not be a warm-blooded being alive on earth. For germs are everywhere. They are in food and water; they are in the air; they are in the ground. Every place fit for human habitation is populated by germs—germs by the million and germs by the billion.

You and I have the pneumococcus with us at various times —sometimes for weeks. All of us carry around some thousand pneumonia germs—so-called—at times. Why don't we get pneumonia? Because the pneumococcus is not the cause of pneumonia. The pneumonia comes first, and then the conditions in the lungs are just right for the multiplication of germs. Ask those who examine the sputum in pneumonia if the pneumococcus is the only germ found. They will tell you that numerous strains of germ life are present. The congestion of the lungs and the presence of excessive waste is a condition upon which numerous germs thrive. The pneumonia comes first, and then there is a great multiplication of germs. In other words, the germs are an effect, not a cause, of the disease.

Then there is tuberculosis. No civilized human being can possibly live to maturity without eating or drinking or breathing tubercular germs. About one-seventh of the human race dies of tuberculosis, but if the tubercular germs could produce consumption, not one of us could live to be thirty-five years old. The bugs would get us long before that time. Tuberculosis is almost entirely a disease based on bad blood, and the bad blood is based on poor air, food and drink principally. When the body has time to degenerate, some kind of disease must take place, and then the individual gets tuberculosis or some other ill. Surely, there are lots of tubercular germs in these cases, as well as an excess of other germs. But again the germs are not the cause of the disease; they are the effect of a degenerated body, or in other words, they are the effect of the disease.

I have been right in the midst of typhoid epidemics and have drunk the water from the same faucets that was said to cause the typhoid fever. Why did not those who drank this water escape the fever? Because the typhoid germs do not cause typhoid fever, and are absolutely harmless to those who keep their bodies in good condition. To get typhoid fever, it is necessary to allow the body to deteriorate (get into a run-down condition) and then one can get typhoid fever or any other disease.

Germs are scavengers. Their duty is to break down substances in the body that need to be removed. So long as we live according to the laws of nature, no germ will or can injure us. If we live so as to cause deterioration of the structures of the body, allowing them to fill with waste, the germs come upon the scene as scavengers. They try to break down the parts that are already diseased, so that they can be carried out of the body.

A boil is a simple illustration. The average doctor says that germs cause the boil. This is putting the automobile before the engine. For the boil causes the multiplication of the germs. How does the boil happen? Some part of the body is weakened through abuse or bruising or other injury. The circulation is disarranged and stagnation takes place; deprived of pure blood, a small part of tissue dies, and the germs which thrive on unhealthy tissue come, multiply and break down the dead tissue, so that it can be thrown out of the body.

When an animal dies in the open, buzzards gather about. Did the presence of the buzzards cause the death of the animal? Quite the reverse. The dead animal caused the gathering of the buzzards, and they gather to dispose of the carrion—they don't cause the carrion.

Those of us who live according to the laws of nature are not sick—never! Yet we breathe germs, and drink germs and eat germs every day. This is proof in itself that germs are not the real cause of disease.

Learn how to live according to the laws of nature, and you will have absolutely nothing to fear from germs.

Not even the Allopathic journals have of late been absolutely *immune* from the belief that germs do not cause acute diseases. During the recent influenza epidemic a series of experiments were carried on among naval men. In Boston, Massachusetts, no less than 68 volunteers were subjected to an attempt to transmit influenza to them, after being informed of the *risk* incurred. All these experiments, however, proved negative, as not a single case of influenza appeared among all these men. Similar experiments were made in San Francisco by Drs. McCoy and Richey, and with similar results.

The *Journal of the Florida Medical Association* in its issue of July, 1919, wrote as follows about the methods of inoculation, used in the above mentioned experiments:

A freshly isolated culture of B. influenzae was instilled in the noses of three non-immunes, and in three controls who had had influenza in the recent epidemic. No cases developed. Later, ten non-immunes were inoculated with negative results.

Thirty men were subjected to inoculation by means of spray, swab, or both, of the nose and throat, with secretions both filtered and unfiltered from the upper respiratory tract of typical cases of active influenza, but the results were negative. Ten volunteers who had been subjected to inoculation with secretions were allowed to come in contact with fresh influenza patients, who were made to cough in their faces, but no cases developed. In ten cases secretions of influenza cases were injected by needle into the volunteers, but no cases developed.

Even the *Journal of the American Medical Association* acted *surprised* about the outcome of these experiments, as the following clipping taken from its issue of Jan. 25th, 1919, will prove. This journal wrote as follows:

Two extensive attempts have been made under the auspices of the United States Public Health Service and the United States Navy—one at Boston and one at San Francisco—to transmit influenza experimentally. Sixty-eight men from the naval detention camp at Deer Island volunteered for the experiment at Boston. These volunteers had been exposed in some degree to influenza, but most of them gave no history of any illness suggestive of an attack of influenza. Inoculations were made of pure cultures of the influenza bacillus, of secretions from the upper air passages of persons in the early state of influenza, and of blood from typical cases of influenza. Suspensions of freshly isolated bacilli were introduced into the nose. Both filtered and unfiltered secretions from the air passages of typical cases of influenza in the active stages of the disease were inoculated by means of spraying and swabbing of the nose and throat. Volunteers were placed in very close association for a few minutes with each of ten selected influenza patients, who were instructed to cough directly into their faces. Filtered secretions and the blood from influenza patients were injected subcutaneously into a group of volunteers. In San Francisco the volunteers had not been exposed to influenza at all in the present epidemic, but they had been vaccinated with large doses of a mixed vaccine of influenza bacilli, pneumococci and hemolytic streptococci. In view of the negative results, however, of such vaccinations in controlled experiments it is believed that this vaccine may be regarded as having no influence. Here also suspensions of influenza bacilli were introduced into the nose. In one group the suspension was first filtered through a Berkefeld candle. Filtered, as well as unfiltered, emulsions of respiratory secretions from active cases of influenza were introduced into the nose. Filtered emulsion was dropped into the eye and injected subcutaneously. Blood taken during the active stages of influenza was injected subcutaneously.

Not one of the many volunteers developed influenza. Three volunteers who received the filtered secretion developed acute tonsillitis, and in two, cultures gave almost pure growths of hemolytic strep-tococci. That so many attempts to transmit influenza should fail is a great surprise and disappointment in view of the positive results reported by Nicolle and Le Bailly.

The results of these experiments may naturally be the subject of much speculation. However, it is certain that the cause of influenza remains a mystery to be solved only by continued experiment. In the meantime, we must not relax our effort to control the disease and its complications according to the principle that both are droplet injec-tions, with special attention to the probabilities that uncomplicated influenza is infectious in the earliest stages of the attack.

It is, however, not only the medical journals that begin to show symp-toms of distrust in the germ theory, but also the lay press. The following clipping is taken from the *St. Louis Times*, where it appeared at the time of the "Waite murder case," which I believe is still fresh in the memory of readers of this magazine.

Waite, the New York murderer, fed his father-in-law, the late Mr. Peck, quantities of germs of deadly disease. He placed in the alimen-tary canal of the late Peck large colonies of bacilli of diphtheria. He fed his wife's father a swarm of tuberculosis germs. He gave the old gentleman a dose of tetanus, otherwise lockjaw.

He passed the dessert in the way of smallpox, with an interven-ing entree of leprosy, and for a side dish a garnish of bubonic plague. Other dainties in the way of hook worm, sleeping sickness, meningitis and scarlet fever were administered with a lavish hand. And still the old man continued to be well and hearty.

He fattened on the plague and grew gray on diphtheria. Indeed, the only effect of the combined disorders seemed to be a new lease of life and a sort of Ponce de Leon recuperation. When all of these germs failed to do their work, chloroform and a pillow, after the Des-demonean manner, brought the desired quietus.

What, then, is science to say of the germs? What if, after all, the germ 'isolations' have been mere scientific myths? The world has accepted the statement that this or that germ would do this or that thing, and that cultures injected into the veins of guinea pigs and white rabbits proved it.

What if, after all, the guinea pigs merely died following the injec-tion of foreign matter into their circulatory system? What, indeed, are we to say to a lot of what science has taught us, if a pint of germs had no effect whatever when swallowed by old man Peck? Of course, we look for a scientific and highly acceptable explanation, but mean-while. . . .

Hundreds of clippings from medical journals as well as from newspapers could be given to prove my assertion that the people in general—the medial men included—begin to doubt the theory that germs cause disease, but I consider the ones given above to be sufficient.

I have intentionally dealt with the germ theory at considerable length, as that is the very foundation of medical science, and if this theory is done away with, then the science of medicine has hardly a leg to stand on.

Naturopathy, on the other hand, has come to stay, and we predict that the time is not far distant when the people will realize that natural living and healing are the only solution of the world's health problems. The barbarous system of poisonous medication will then be a thing of the past, and as a result we will have a happier and healthier race. Friends of Naturopathy, have you in the past and will you in the future put your shoulder to the wheel, and help us to speed that day—the day when tears and suffering are banished from this world, and the paradise on earth is regained?

For several years Dr. Fraser, assisted by a number of Canadians, carried out the most painstaking experiments, which prove, first, that germs are not present at the onset of acute diseases; and second, that germs do not cause disease.

Germs are present in disease, but they do not cause disease. If germs really produced disease there would not be a warm-blooded being alive on earth. For germs are everywhere. They are in food and water; they are in the air; they are in the ground.

Germs are scavengers. Their duty is to break down substances in the body that need to be removed. So long as we live according to the laws of nature, no germ will or can injure us.

I have intentionally dealt with the germ theory at considerable length, as that is the very foundation of medical science, and if this theory is done away with, then the science of medicine has hardly a leg to stand on.

GET TOGETHR OR "TAKE YOUR MEDICINE"

by Bernarr Macfadden, Editor, *Physical Culture*
Herald of Health and Naturopath, XXV (8), 405. (1920)

The American Medical Association (monopoly) has determined to abolish all medicine (health building) measures not fathered by their professional members.

Forty million people of this land of the free and the brave opposed to allopathic principles are about to be deprived of their physical liberties, and are to have the privilege of being taxed forty million dollars to help pay for this enslavement.

The officials of this powerful medical organization seem to think that they have reached the peak of all knowledge appertaining to the healing art—that there is nothing more to learn outside of that which can be garnered by the members of their own profession.

All other practitioners are mere pretenders—the worst of ignoramuses.

And with the above aim in view they (the A. M. A.) have introduced into the House of Representatives and the Senate at Washington seven separate bills. These bills propose to establish a Federal Department of Health. They have not mentioned therein that the special object is to protect the financial interests of the graduates of their school of medicine.

And if these bills pass, may God help the citizen who refuses to have his children vaccinated, or allows himself to have any conscientious scruples as to the treatment of himself or family when attention of this sort is needed.

Notwithstanding the fact that many of the greatest discoveries of medical science have been made by laymen, the A. M. A. believes that the *health* opinions of those outside of their ranks is not worth considering.

And all doctors not in the A. M. A. have received specially significant attention in these bills!

Many of these pioneer martyrs think they have gone through *some* persecution, but when the bills referred to begin to *work*, if they ever do, our practitioner friends of progressive healing will consider their former experience heavenly in nature when compared to the *hades* of torment that has been prepared for them in these aforementioned bills.

If the doctors who have been brave enough to follow the bent of their conscience and intelligence do not become *feverishly* active and do something BIG to defeat these enslaving bills they will go on to a richly deserved fate.

And the same can be said of the forty million Americans whom this bill will force to accept conservative medical treatment whenever they or the members of their families are ill.

Therefore, GET TOGETHER, or be prepared to *take your medicine* literally and figuratively as prescribed by the allopathic doctors.

If we do not defeat these bills we will deserve to die in the festering pus of the vaccination and serum poisons which these monopolistic doctors maintain is the accredited method of treating all disease.

The progressive doctors, non-drug and otherwise, have been *making good*. Conventional medicine is fighting for its life, and with its gasps for breath it is making this attempt to fetter intelligence; to enslave the bodies of American citizens from the cradle to the grave.

Will they do it? Let time decide.

As a means of cementing the forces arrayed against the compulsory medication referred to above, a number of believers in medical freedom made a covenant between themselves, and it appears herewith.

Sign it and get the signatures of your friends.

Mail to us and ask for more copies, that you may help in the fight against medical imposition. We want a million names.

Donations for distributing this literature acceptable.

OUR COVENANT

We, and each of us undersigned, agree and stipulate that we will not by ourselves, or by our representatives, be a party to securing the passage of any legislation, State or National, that may in any manner affect any doctor in the practice of his profession, or any citizen in his choice of a practitioner, and we hereby bind ourselves at all times to use every legitimate and legal means within our power, and within the power of each of us, to secure the amendment and repeal of any laws, State or National, now in force that in any way prohibits or abridges the rights or privileges of any doctors or physicians in the practice of their several professions, or any citizen in his choice of a practitioner, and we further agree, in so far as we justly and legally may, to assist in preventing undue prosecutions of respectable non-drug and liberal doctors or laymen under existing state laws.

Dated and signed in the United States of America, this ....
day of..........nineteen hundred and twenty. ....
....

1921

THE "UNVACCINATED" DEATH RATE
ALFRED RUSSEL WALLACE

THE "UNVACCINATED" DEATH RATE

by Alfred R. Wallace

Herald of Health and Naturopath, XXVI (3), 134-138. (1921)

> *"Here in the natural smallpox but one in 49 died; and I can assure the reader than upon a strict review of thirty years' business and more, not one in forty of smallpox patients of the younger life died, that is above five and under 18."*
>
> —Isaac Massey, 1727
> Writing of pupils of Christ's Hospital, London.

If I were an aviator or a pigwidgin and laid claim to having made in private trial certain flights of a very astonishing character, but upon saying such flights in the full glare of pre-arranged publicity, lamentably failed to equal even the mediocre achievements of some of my aerial compeers, what in all probability would be the verdict?

If an enterprising laboratory chemist in realms of the organic should get up a serum for typhoid fever, and announce a reduction in the death-rate per million, as evidenced in the statistics promulgated by some experimental sanitorium of from 175 to 25, how should we regard him, if, upon the general introduction of his specific throughout large populations, the death-rate, instead of decreasing were found to remain perversely stationary?

Or take cerebral-spinal meningitis. Some Flexnerian savant skilled in evoking whimsical signs and wonders from the animal economy distills a remedial injection. He volubly protests that in some spatially and temporally circumscribed hospital practice of his the deaths have been reduced from ninety out of every hundred attacked to a paltry twenty or thirty, with the vanishing point almost in sight down the resplendent vistas of the coming years. But unfortunately, when his concoction has attained an orthodox mode over wide areas, the mortality, as revealed by official governmental returns, is shown to have fallen off by not so much as a degenerate iota. In what light, then, as a simple matter of unadorned fact, is mankind to view the validity of the new medical largess?

Coming down to the plain logic of things as regards these last two supposititious cases, we surely know that in some way or other a grave and grievous mistake must have managed to creep into the statistical functioning's of our serumists. One supposes that perchance the prismatic "will-to-believe" or the obfuscating goggles of expectant attention have induced a seriously errant excursion from the realm of prosaic factual verities, and that the trip has ended in cloudlands of the subjective vision. Something has been overlooked, something added, something minimized, something magnified, something invented, something shuffled out of sight, something guessed at, something seized upon and bent and shaped to suit the ideas of a pre-conceptual and substantially farcical investigation.

With this investigation, let us to the main matter, and inquire how things lie in the rather threadbare, and to a certain extent, analogous question of vaccination and smallpox. Time after time without number and decade after decade stretching back into dead centuries, we have regaled with classical recitals to the effect whereas the unvaccinated customarily insist on dying at the discreditable rate of thirty, forty, fifty and sixty in every hundred, the vaccinated are held by the supreme potency of their prophylactic sheet-anchor to the very gratifying and suggestive rates of five, ten and fifteen per hundred. We are invited to scrutinize the frightful, indeed quite impassable, gulf between these two camps. It is borne in upon us by triumphant grimaces that there is no case against vaccination—none at all.

Pro–vaccinal Humpty–Dumptyism, slightly regal in its poses, says with comfortable finality that the fanatical "Anti" is out of court with men that know; that it is "all over but the shouting"—which, by the way, to those who pass at all near the beshingled offices of scratching and scraping, appears rarely or never to subside.

And yet, all the while, one simple fact, historical and contemporary in its facets, and granolithically authenticated, is sufficient to overthrow the whole romancing fabric thus reared with such grandiose certitude. That fact is that the total death-rate from smallpox of all classes lumped together, vaccinated and unvaccinated, now approximates almost identically the figure clearly established by the returns of the prevaccinal eighteenth century—that is to say, about 15 or 20 percent.

The trained statistician must of course throw out of account unverified ancient tourist tales and old wives' fables from Kamschatka, Madagascar, the Arctic Circle, the Aborigines and the Antipodes, and confine himself to some comparatively stable section of the earth's civilized surface where mortuary figures have been conscientiously kept for a number of centuries. One or two continental countries are fairly good in this respect; and to the Continent and England we will go for the great body of evidence.

Comparing these authoritative summaries with those of modern times, we immediately find that, once persons contract the disease of smallpox, no difference in aggregate fatality-rate worth the snap of the fingers can be discerned between the eighteenth, nineteenth and twentieth centuries.

Year	Place or Authority	Cases	Deaths	Rate
1696	Martin Lister, *Tractaties of Varioles*			2.50
1721	Boston, North America Review, 1821	5,889	844	14.30
1723	Dr. Jurin, Quoted by Dr. Duvillard	18,066	2,986	16.53
1746-63	London Smallpox Hospital	6,456	1,634	25.30
1752	Boston	5,400	539	10.00
1763	Lambert, quoted by Duvillard	72	15	20.00
1763	Tissot, the eminent French Inoculationist			14.20
1773	Tissot			15.30
	A. De Haen, an opponent of Inoculation *Refutation of Inoculation*			14.20-20.00

Year	Place or Authority	Cases	Vaccinated	Deaths	Rate
1836-51	Marson's Hospital Report	5,652	3,094	1,125	19.72
1870-72	Metropolitan Hospitals	14,808	11,174	2,764	18.66
1876	Metropolitan Hospitals	1,470		338	23.00
1871-77	Homerton Hospital (Gayton)	5,479	4,236	1,065	19.43
1876-80	Dublin Hospital (Grimshaw)	2,404	1,956	523	21.70
1876-80	Metropolitan Hospital (Jebb)	15,171	11,412	2,677	17.60
1908	German Empire	434		65	14.90

Singular Death Rate Among the Modern Unvaccinated	
Marson's	35.00
Metropolitan Asylums Board Hospitals, 1870-1872	40.84
Hampstead, 1876-1878	46.60
Homerton, 1871-1877	53.00
Fulham, 1878	46.20
Fulham, 1880	40.32
Fulham, 1881	44.28
Deptford, 1878-1879	47.20
Stockwell, 1879	38.70
Homerton, 1880	32.00
Deptford, 1881	47.40
Sheffield, 1884	28.47
Western, 1885	61.00
Board's Hospitals, 1888	33.33
Rochdale, 1881-1882, Home	51.00
Rochdale, 1881-1882, Hospital	68.00

In the light of these illuminating comparisons the observer must be exceedingly mystified at the pleasant simplicity of doctors who in the year A. D. 1913 blithely ask us to think that the unvaccinated have turned over a new and terrible leaf, and are now habitually dying under the hands of up-to-date practitioners at the portentous and unaccountable rate of 50 per cent; while, as is indisputable, even in the unsanitated noxiousness and immature therapeutic socialism of two hundred years ago the unvaccinated ensemble—for all were unvaccinated in ante-Jennerian then—passed away at a rate of only 15 to 20 percent in 1800; 50 percent now.

What is the crux of this amazing embarrassment? Where lurks the irisated fallacy? For the very simpleton-in-reasoning cannot fail to understand, however feebly, that somewhere and in some manner an unpropitious Pandora's Box—or at any rate a paralogism—must have entered.

This is the crux and this is the fallacy. In the eighteenth century the unvaccinated included all, without a solitary exception—not alone, as now, the impecunious, quickly succumbing strata of populations, but the rich, and the great vigorous millions making up the ever more dominant middle classes. It included the most vital along with the least vital. To-day, from obvious reasons, it is principally the least vital of the least vital who remain in unvaccinated aloofness wherever vaccination laws are in force. Today, when in company with numerous other medical conventionalisms of the moment, vaccination is embraced without much question by virtually all those superior tiers of society formerly one and all numbered among the comparatively healthy unvaccinated, it is among the poor and outcast and low-living and untutored proletarians possessing a sadly depleted, patriomonially transmitted vital resistance that the unvaccinated ranks are almost exclusively drawn. The filthy 50 percent people—who, from causes easily recognizable, chance in our day to be unvaccinated, as they also chance not to have their hair combed—may die at that startling rate, it is true. No less true is it that two hundred years ago the very same class, if socially demarcated in the statistics as at present, would have been found to be dying at exactly this same frightful rate of 50 percent. And write it in eternal fire across the escutcheon of time: This class died at that rate, and to-day die at that rate, and two hundred or two thousand years in the future will be found, in the absence of improved environing fundamental conditions of life and light, to be dying at that same old historically declared rate, whether vaccinated or unvaccinated, inoculated or uninoculated, Theist or Atheist, bond or free. Not failure to be pussed, not failure to be poxed, but failure to be decent and failure to live right—that is what sends men to the grave at 50 percent, in this age and in every age, now and forever. To die at 5 percent have a good grandfather. Be a pariah, and you die at 50.

The medical necromantist, then, has simply been juggling confusedly with social strata in the body politic. Lately he has been blunderingly segregating into layers, remarkably convenient for his purpose, a humanity that in the mass always has died of smallpox at the rate of 15 to 20 percent. Foolishly he flounders about, infallible, impeccant. He has succeeded in setting in statistical opposition through the adventitious touchstone of a medical conformity (whether the conformity be that upper-class conformity known as Vaccination or that upper-class conformity known as footing the bills necessary to being examined by a physician two or four times a year makes no earthly difference) wholly distinct types of citizenry—distinct to a certain extent in age, distinct in occupation, distinct in habitat, distinct in social level, distinct in condition of general health, distinct in sanitation, distinct in all the wide-swinging influences of heredity and environment.

And his name is Ichabod. His myopic conclusions are hopelessly and everlastingly vitiated at the ultimate bar of prevailing reason.

The English city of Leicester, in which nowadays nearly all escape the vaccinating rite, has proved to be a veritable clamp of remorseless steel around the coffin of Vaccination; for in this unvariolous and unbovinated city where of necessity the unvaccinated comprise rich as well as poor and bourgeois as well as pauper, the unvaccinated, mulishly oblivious to the demands of our doctoral vaccinating science, emphatically refuse to pass away at the hackneyed rate of 50 percent—or at 40 percent, or at 30 percent, or 20 percent. They cross the Styx at a rate less even than that of the vaccinated as found to prevail elsewhere throughout the kingdom. The *Majority Report of the British Royal Commission on Vaccination* had to present in one of its tables a statistic showing that out of 107 unvaccinated subjects attacked by smallpox during a certain epidemic at Leicester, only 15 (or 14 percent) perished. More than this, the same is lately becoming true of other unbogied English municipalities, which, emancipated from the pall of medieval medical cant, have followed in the pioneer wake of Leicester. Nelson and Northampton in 1903, Loughborough in 1904, Kneighley in 1903 and 1905, and Oldham in 1906—all anti-vaccinationist centres—returned 645 cases of smallpox without a death.

Nobody under the stars of heaven ever did or ever can present so much as a single numeral to show that class for class, primary conditions of life being similar, lack of Vaccination has operated to reduce by one scintilla the chance of recovery of any human being, living or dead.

Let us repeat. The utterly destitute of the Whitechapel's, those in reduced circumstances and of irregular wage, the teeming millions hovering insecurely on the lower fringes of economic existence, from whose wretched ranks, constituting as they do an indelible stain on a supposedly civilized age, are recruited the preponderant mass of the coroner's "unvaccinated," are doomed with the calamitous and mighty diathesis of fatality, not only as to smallpox, but as concerns everything else that menaces the life of the human race on this planet. From malaise, to pneumococci and from pole to pole, the inexorable "survival-of-the-fittest" does not grant favors to poverty and filth—no, not one. Take the very identical ill-fated beings, man for man, woman for woman, child for child and babe for babe, who have gone under from the black curse of smallpox, since time began at 50 percent; collect them, to the chant of the Miserere, in one pitiful Grand Army of the Oligarchy of sodden sin and uttermost grovelling want from the four quarters of the globe; and give them not smallpox, but any or every other disease known to the pharmaceutical complexes of to-day,—and those who died at 50 percent from smallpox would nevertheless be seen to pass down and out into the great unknown at equally disproportionate and exaggerated rates, as compared with Dives, whether vaccinated or unvaccinated, saint or sinner, bronze, yellow, white or black.

The casualty, the fortuity, of Vaccination has no more to do curatively with the recovery of any patient at any time from any disease than the superstitious terpsichorean antics of Tottipottymoy Patagonians with the terrific rush of our solar system toward the constellation of Orion, far, far away in the blue distance.

Not a particle.

In the hospital statistics of today you generally find that the unvaccinated people die at the rate of from 30 to 60 and even 80 percent, or higher; and yet when we come to look at the fatality of the last century amid the horrible condition of things which I have mentioned to you, we find that the fatality was only 18 percent. If therefore, the fatality of the unvaccinated people last century was only 18 percent, and the average fatality of the present day amongst the unvaccinated runs from 30 to 80 percent, I want to know, like Trelawney's Cornishman, 'the reason why'. I do not believe the doctors of the present day are less competent than those of a hundred years ago; and therefore why double and treble the number of unvaccinated patients who are slipping through their fingers as compared with a century before?

> —W. R. Hadwen, M.D., L.R.C.P., M.R.C.S., L.S.A.,
> Speech at Gloucester, Jan. 25, 1896.

In spite of fatal cases, an advantage was claimed for inoculation, in that it had been calculated, that of all those affected with smallpox in the ordinary way, about one in six died, whereas the deaths from inoculation contended for by the anti-inoculators amounted to not more than one in fifty.

> —Edgar M. Crookshank, M.B.,
> *History and Pathology of Vaccination*, p. 42.

Epidemics of smallpox, slight and severe, give mortality of about 13 percent, or one death out of eight attacked.

> —Tissot, the famous Swiss physician (1728-1797).

The total death-rate from smallpox in modern times is almost the same as it was in the 18th century.

> —Charles Creighton, *Encyclopedia Britannica*,
> article on Vaccination.

Dr. Jurin, writing early in the last century, laid it down as the result of his investigation that of persons of all ages taken ill of natural smallpox, there will die of that distemper one in five or six.

> —Dr. Seaton, *Handbook of Vaccination*, 1868, p. 191.

When we consider all the sources of error to which we have alluded we are led to conclude that the difference in fatality between the vaccinated and unvaccinated smallpox patients is not as great as is sometimes contended, and that so far as it exists it cannot be merely to the effect of vaccination, while the fact that the fatality of all cases lumped together is practically the same now as it was in the unvaccinated of last century, when large numbers are taken for comparison, strongly suggests that of the inclusion of a large contingent of vaccinated persons has not exerted a mitigating effect on the average fatality of the whole.

—*Minority Report of the British Royal Commission on Vaccination*, paragraph 110.

Tous les ouvrages a qui le zele de l'inoculation a donne l'etre, fourmillent de temoinages qu'on dit etre les plus exacts et les plus propres a demontrer, que de cinq a six personnes, ou de sept, tout au plus et par grace, qui ont la petite verolle naturelle, il en meurte une." (i. e. an eighteenth century rate of 14.2 percent)

—A. de Haen,
Professor of Medicine, the University of Vienna, 1759.

Now an immense body of statistics of the last century compiled by disinterested persons who had no interest to serve by making the severity of smallpox large or small, gives an average of from 14 to 18 percent as the proportion of smallpox deaths to cases; and we naturally ask, how is it that, with so much better sanitary conditions and greatly improved treatment, nearly half the unvaccinated patients die, while in the last century less than one-fifth died? It is, however, a most suggestive fact that, considering smallpox mortality **per se**, without reference to vaccination—the records of which are, as have been shown, utterly untrustworthy, we find the case-mortality to agree closely with that of the last century. Thus, the figures given in the *Reports of the Hampstead*, Homerton, and Deptford smallpox hospitals at periods between 1876 and 1879, were 19.0, 18.8 and 17.0 percent respectively (*3rd Report*, p. 205). If we admit that only the worst cases went to the hospitals, but also allow something for better treatment now, the result is quite explicable; whereas the other result, of a greatly **increased** fatality in the unvaccinated so exactly balanced by an alleged greatly **diminished** fatality in the vaccinated is not explicable, especially when we remember that this diminished fatality applies to all ages, and it is now almost universally admitted that the alleged protective influence of vaccination dies out in ten or twelve years."

—Alfred R. Wallace, *The Wonderful Century*, pp. 240-241.

Comparing these authoritative summaries with those of modern times, we immediately find that, once persons contract the disease of smallpox, no difference in aggregate fatality-rate worth the snap of the fingers can be discerned between the eighteenth, nineteenth and twentieth centuries.

In the light of these illuminating comparisons the observer must be exceedingly mystified at the pleasant simplicity of doctors who in the year A. D. 1913 blithely ask us to think that the unvaccinated have turned over a new and terrible leaf, and are now habitually dying under the hands of up-to-date practitioners at the portentous and unaccountable rate of 50 per cent; while, as is indisputable, even in the unsanitated noxiousness and immature therapeutic socialism of two hundred years ago the unvaccinated ensemble—for all were unvaccinated in ante-Jennerian then—passed away at a rate of only 15 to 20 percent in 1800; 50 percent now.

Nobody under the stars of heaven ever did or ever can present so much as a single numeral to show that class for class, primary conditions of life being similar, lack of Vaccination has operated to reduce by one scintilla the chance of recovery of any human being, living or dead.

"When we consider all the sources of error to which we have alluded we are led to conclude that the difference in fatality between the vaccinated and unvaccinated smallpox patients is not as great as is sometimes contended, and that so far as it exists it cannot be merely to the effect of vaccination, while the fact that the fatality of all cases lumped together is practically the same now as it was in the unvaccinated of last century, when large numbers are taken for comparison, strongly suggests that of the inclusion of a large contingent of vaccinated persons has not exerted a mitigating effect on the average fatality of the whole."

1922

DR. KATZOFF ON VACCINATION
BENEDICT LUST, N.D.

This announcement was made in May, 1921.

Dr. Katzoff On Vaccination

by Benedict Lust, N.D.

The Naturopath and Herald of Health, V (5), 230-231. (1922)

"Vaccination never did prevent smallpox." Thus declares Louis Simon Katzoff, M.D. in the *Bridgeport Sunday Post* for January 15, 1922. Dr. Katzoff, who is president of the Bridgeport Philosophical Society, in response to the Post's invitation to give its readers his views on the subject of compulsory vaccination wrote:

> I shall present at this time a few points of importance based upon an impartial study of the subject for the past fifteen years.

> After having believed in vaccination as a preventive for smallpox, after having vaccinated many children and after having studied the subject from both standpoints, I finally learned to realize that vaccination was useless as a preventive of smallpox. Upon observation and reflection I soon realized that smallpox is an illness which has its origin in filth, that it follows closely upon flagrant violations of the laws of hygiene and sanitation. Clean water, unadulterated food, sanitary and modern lavatories, good plumbing and good sewage are the greatest enemies to smallpox and all filth diseases.

In speaking of epidemics Dr. Katzoff stated: "The occurrences of *epidemics* or *scares* have coincided with periods of sanitary neglect accompanied by fatigue, anxiety and fear." The recent Flu pandemic was due to the enervated condition of the whole world, from fear, worry, anxiety, etc., connected with the war. Flu we have with us every year but seldom does it assume epidemic proportions. In the recent pandemic, however, the people were in a condition to come down under the epidemic influence, which was probably atmospheric, in large numbers: the fear that the disease and doctors created probably added many more victims than would otherwise have been.

In the days prior to vaccination, smallpox devastated whole cities; today smallpox is comparatively rare. The pro-vaccinationist credits vaccination with having given smallpox the knockout blow. But we think we can account for it in another way.

In those days the towns and cities were devoid of any sanitary or sewage systems and were surrounded by high walls and a moat of stagnant water. The streets were narrow, and served as dumping grounds for the kitchen wastes, dead animals, garbage and refuse of all kinds. The small one and two room houses were equipped with dirt floors covered with straw and boughs, a hole in the roof to permit the smoke to escape, and one small window. Piles of straw served for beds. Bones and scraps of food fell from the table into the straw on the floor and there it lay until picked up by the cat or dog. The people lived in constant fear of marauding knights that roamed the country. Bath-tubs were unknown.

Under such unhygienic and unsanitary conditions plagues of many kinds swept over the country and killed thousands.

About the time vaccination was introduced into practice, gun powder came along and battered down the city walls and dried up the moats of stagnant water. Bathing began to be popular, sewage systems and sanitary systems came into use. People began to build better houses and the standard of living was raised. The plagues passed away—all but smallpox—and these all went without the aid of any vaccines.

Smallpox, too, would have gone with the other plagues had it not been that vaccination kept it alive. Dr. Katzoff says: "The truth is that we have epidemics of vaccination and not of smallpox. Very few, comparatively, die of smallpox, but many die, or remain diseased and weakened from this pus-compound called *vaccine*."

Another interesting feature about the history of vaccination to which Dr. Katzoff called special attention is the way in which the period of immunity afforded by vaccination became progressively shorter. "Once," he writes "the pro-vaccinationists claimed that vaccination gave immunity or prevention for the life time. Later when they saw the many who were vaccinated got smallpox they began to claim that it is good only for 21 years. When the 21 year theory failed they began to claim that it was *good* for only 14 years. After they find that many get smallpox within the 14 year limit they claim it is *good* for only 7 years. Their very latest *style* about immunity period now is that it is good for 4 years. Some who notice poor results during this period are beginning to advocate the vaccination every year; that the vaccine will protect only one year." The doctor might have mentioned that many provaccinationists now claim that vaccination does not prevent smallpox at all but only makes it less severe—the vaccinated get varioloid rather than variola. At least the term has been modified.

"Compulsory vaccination" he says, "ranks with human slavery and religious persecution and is one of the most flagrant violations of the rights of the human race. If people are forced to submit to compulsory vaccination for smallpox, why not be inoculated for typhoid fever, diphtheria, tuberculosis, pneumonia, measles, hay fever, cancer and the like—and by force?"

"Thomas Jefferson well expressed it: "Compulsory vaccination is an outrage and a gross interference with the personal liberty of the people in a land of freedom." It is unnecessary to actually set up one disease in a healthy organism (as vaccination does) with an idea in view of avoiding another. Such a procedure is an appalling violation of the basic principles of hygiene and sanitation.

The doctor calls attention to the fact that the medical professions themselves are divided on the subject, that many of our most eminent scientists, physicians, teachers, educators and thinkers in general throughout the world are opposed to vaccination. He claims, also, that many physicians who vaccinate the children of others never vaccinate their own. He points to the record of death from vaccination, of smallpox after vaccination, of the disease, like measles, diphtheria, enlarged tonsils, pneumonia, weak hearts, and mental derangements that often follow in the wake of *cowpox* infection. We use the term infection advisedly for the smallpox vaccine is pus of a septic nature; it represents animal matter undergoing retrograde metamorphosis—and is either septic or inert when it reaches the victim. It is, indeed, a crime to force such stuff into the bodies of our children. It is a violation of the cardinal principles of health and hygiene which demand purity of blood and lymph. It is a slap in the face of asepsis which demands that poisons etc., be taken from or withheld from the body and not introduced into it—forcibly or otherwise.

Dr. Katzoff gives us his views on ways to prevent smallpox in these words: "The only immunity—the only way to prevent developing smallpox—is to be healthy. And the only way to be healthy with good vitality and clean blood is to have plenty of fresh air, sunshine, good food, and interest in one's work. These are Nature's remedies and cannot be improved by arrogant conceited man, no matter how he may vainly try."

Any finally he says, in speaking of further proofs that can be offered that vaccination is both useless and harmful; "I would also refer to the lists of deaths from this superstitious rite, which will be relegated to the dusty attic of oblivion when we mortals become truly civilized and live according to Nature's laws instead of living the abnormal life of haste, hate, ignorance, and fear, including the fear of two or three individuals who bring into existence, the iron heel, the last of the Siberian Cossacks, and the spirit of the Spanish Inquisition—for it robs the people of their fundamental liberties as guaranteed by our federal and state constitutions."

"The only immunity—the only way to prevent developing smallpox—is to be healthy. And the only way to be healthy with good vitality and clean blood is to have plenty of fresh air, sunshine, good food, and interest in one's work. These are Nature's remedies and cannot be improved by arrogant conceited man, no matter how he may vainly try."
—Dr. L. S. Katzoff, M.D.

The truth is that we have epidemics of vaccination and not of smallpox. Very few, comparatively, die of smallpox, but many die, or remain diseased and weakened from this pus-compound called vaccine.

It is unnecessary to actually set up one disease in a healthy organism (as vaccination does) with an idea in view of avoiding another. Such a procedure is an appalling violation of the basic principles of hygiene and sanitation.

1923

The Schick Test For Diphtheria
London And Provincial Anti-Vivisection Society

Fallacy Of Drugs
Benedict Lust, N.D.

Not to take a back seat on the issue of compulsory vaccination, in 1927 Benedict Lust published a monograph, *The Crime of Vaccination*.

The "Schick Test" For Diphtheria

by London and Provincial Anti-Vivisection Society

Naturopath, XXVIII (3), 124. (1923)

What It Is And What It Is Not?

The Test

This consists of the injection of a solution of diphtheria toxin (poison) into the skin of the forearm. If certain signs of irritation appear around the point of injection it is claimed—not, be it noted, that the individual has contracted diphtheria—but *is liable to do so.*

The Next Step

That involves further inoculations—this time with toxin, antitoxin—by which it is claimed that the individual treated is rendered immune, i.e., is no longer liable to contract diphtheria.

THE FACTS OF THE CASE are that perfectly healthy persons are thereby subjected to the dangers of successive involutions for a disease which they may never contract. In many cases, e.g., in Poor Law Schools, etc., *this is done at the expense of the taxpayer.*

THE MINISTRY OF HEALTH in its official pamphlet advocating the *Schick Test* admits that the results are not always satisfactory, and that the resulting *re-action* may be *decidedly severe.*

SEVERAL CHILDREN DIED in Texas, U.S.A., directly as a result of this treatment. (Attention has called to this fact in the House of Commons during the early part of this year.) Legal proceedings were instituted against the company who manufactured the toxin, antitoxin and heavy damages were awarded to the parents of the children. It was claimed in extenuation that the preparation supplied must have been faulty in these particular cases, but—and here is the important point—*these supplies had all been submitted to the necessary Government tests and had been passed for use.*

THIS IS ONLY ONE INSTANCE of the dangers of these so-called preventive treatments by ANTITOXINS, SERUMS, VACCINES, ETC., whose only certain value is that they are *money-getters* for their producers.

London and Provincial Anti-vivisection Society,
22a Regent Street, London, S. W. 1.

Fallacy Of Drugs

by Benedict Lust, N.D.

Naturopath, XXVIII (10), 579-580. (1923)

> *"Drugs are poisons that shorten life."*
> *"Almost every virulent poison known to man is found in allo-pathic prescriptions."*
>
>   —Dr. Henry Lindlahr

> *"The man who pretends to heal by means of drugs or surgery does not possess even rudimentary knowledge of the nature and cure of disease."*
>
>   —Dr. Reinhold

In the United States alone, more than five hundred million dollars are spent each year for drugs. A million and a half a year are spent for one particular laxative. Drugs and drug signs meet us on every hand. Everywhere we go, we find such ads as "Mr. E. Z. Mark, of Ohio, owes his wonderful health to shumac. Over ten million bottles sold already."

Due to this active propaganda by patent medicine fakers, the craze for drugs is increasing at an alarming rate, and drug manufacturers and drug-shops are doing their utmost to keep the supply equal to the

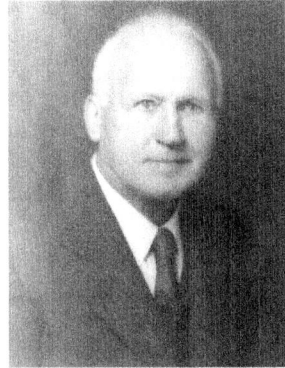

Benedict Lust, N.D..

demand. This makes it all the more interesting to observe what some of our leading medical authorities say as to the value of drugs in the treatment of disease. Dr. J. F. Baldwin, President of the Ohio State Medical Association, in June, 1920, said:

> The ordinary physician who successfully treats pneumonia or typhoid fever, or any other self-limited disease, to say nothing of the host of functional diseases, is very apt to assume that the treatment which he has been given has been instrumental in effecting the recovery of the patient. He may even get a little chesty over the results, as he calls them. He ignores the fact that all these diseases tend to get well, and that, as a matter of fact, none of these diseases are in the slightest degree affected beneficially by any drug treatment.

Could the public become fully aware of that which all intelligent physicians are familiar, namely, that the fact that a patient recovers is no evidence whatever of the value of the medication, and that he might have recovered quicker, indeed, if he had had no medication, then the evidence afforded by quacks and patent medicine fakers will be recognized as entirely valueless.

As to the value and need of drugs, Dr. O. W. Holmes, a prominent member of the Medical Faculty of Harvard University, once said before his medical class: "The disgrace of medicine is that colossal system of self-deception, in obedience to which mines have been emptied of their cankering minerals, the vegetable kingdom robbed of its growth, the entrails of animals taxed for their impurities, the poison bags of reptiles drained of their venom, and all the conceivable abominations thus obtained thrust down the throats of individuals suffering from some fault of nourishment or of vital stimulation."

The famous Dr. Wm. Osler, considered as the world's greatest authority on drugs, in an article entitled "Modern Medicine," in the *Encyclopedia Americana*, says:

> The new school does not feel under obligation to give any medicine whatever, while a generation ago not only could few physicians have held their practice unless they did, but few would have thought it safe or scientific. Of course, there are still many cases where the patient or the patient's friends must be humored by administering medicine, or alleged medicine, where it is not really needed, except where the buoyancy of mind, the real curative agent, can be created only by making the patient wait hopefully for the expected action of the medicine; and some physicians still cannot unlearn their old training. But the change is great. The modern treatment of disease relies very greatly on the old so-called 'natural' methods, diet and exercise, bathing and massage—in other words, giving the natural forces the fullest scope by easy and thorough nutrition, increased flow of blood, and the removal of obstruction to the excretory systems, or the circulation in the tissues.

So at last Medical Science has openly but reluctantly confessed that there is no healing power in drugs. This is a constrained confession, forced by the remarkable records being made by Naturopathic Physicians, who are employing "the old so-called *natural* methods," as mentioned by Dr. Osler, and curing patients given up by Medical Science as hopeless and incurable.

But the astute Medical Profession does not propose to relinquish so readily its grip on the public purse. When one theory has been in practice so long that the people learn it is only an empty sound, some new discovery is duly made. Medical Science has passed through the stages of incantation, blistering, and bleeding. Then came vaccines, serums, and antitoxins. Now that people are waking up to the fact that these last methods are not only worthless, but the most dangerous of all to health and life, we are furnished with a new discovery, that is being praised to the skies as the long sought for panacea for all ills. We refer to the transplantation from monkeys or goats of living sex glands into the bodies of human beings. As to this fad one enthusiastic Allopath says: "So far, it is certain that no practical or lasting results have been achieved; but," he hastens to add, "nevertheless, the secret of longevity and the perpetuation of our powers may eventually be found in that direction."

In view of what our foremost medical authorities say as to the worthlessness of drugs in the treatment of disease, how strange it is that any number of people will continue to believe that they can abuse their organs until they cease to function normally, and then when they are worn out make them over with drugs or have new ones to replace them. But this is the whole scheme of Medical Science. People look to it, because they think that they can neglect and violate all the rules of hygiene, and then, when their bodies break down from abuse, have them repaired with a bottle of medicine or a gland operation. When will we learn that we may be able to fool ourselves, but that we cannot hoodwink Nature?

"God never made His work for man to mend."

Therefore, to believe that one had only to find the right drug poison to put into his body and so banish his ills is a fallacy so foolish as to be perfectly ridiculous, and could have had its origin only in some diseased mind. Yet this stupid belief has been instilled into the mind of medical science so long that to the Disciples of Drugs and Dogmatism, and all their adherents, it is a positive reality. Should this seem strange? No. If we are thoroughly taught a theory, it becomes our fixed belief, no matter how false or farcical it may actually be.

Health is the most precious heritage of man. It can be had by strict observance of and obedience to the law of his being, and in no other way. The body of man is governed by Natural Law, which is just as positive in its operation and requirement as the man-made law governing the mechanism of a watch.

No man can violate this unfailing and unalterable law of Nature, which is older than the race itself, and expect to escape suffering the penalty by simply swallowing some poison drug. If we could do that, then the law of God would be completely subservient to the caprice of the will of man, and the price of drugs would soar so high that only the rich could afford to buy them.

"The man who pretends to heal by means of drugs or surgery does not possess even rudimentary knowledge of the nature and cure of disease." —Dr. Reinhold

Due to this active propaganda by patent medicine fakers, the craze for drugs is increasing at an alarming rate, and drug manufacturers and drug-shops are doing their utmost to keep the supply equal to the demand.

Medical Science has passed through the stages of incantation, blistering, and bleeding. Then came vaccines, serums, and antitoxins. Now that people are waking up to the fact that these last methods are not only worthless, but the most dangerous of all to health and life, we are furnished with a new discovery, that is being praised to the skies as the long sought for panacea for all ills.

In view of what our foremost medical authorities say as to the worthlessness of drugs in the treatment of disease, how strange it is that any number of people will continue to believe that they can abuse their organs until they cease to function normally, and then when they are worn out make them over with drugs or have new ones to replace them.

The body of man is governed by Natural Law, which is just as positive in its operation and requirement as the man-made law governing the mechanism of a watch. No man can violate this unfailing and unalterable law of Nature, which is older than the race itself, and expect to escape suffering the penalty by simply swallowing some poison drug.

EPILOGUE
by Jared L. Zeff, ND

This book on the early naturopathic view of immunization begins with a series of quotations from the writing contained in the subsequent chapters. I want to begin with a reflection upon one of these statements:

> Vaccination represents an honest effort on the part of the medical profession to find a preventive for a simple, yet loathsome disease. This effort, however, like many others of its kind, has not only failed to meet the expectation of its discoverer, but has left in its wake, a blighting curse which it will require many generations to remove. Were it not for the fact that vaccination has been enforced by legislation, we would not now be discussing it except as an antiquated medical experiment akin to leeches and blood-letting.
>
> —Charles W. Littlefield, 1912, 12

One of the oldest precepts in medicine is *to do no harm*. In naturopathic medicine this is a guiding principle, and the Naturopath takes special care in this regard. It is with this precept firmly in mind that I, as a naturopathic physician, consider the risks and benefits of immunization. I believe that physicians who choose to immunize do so assuming that vaccines are harmless and effective, or they do not really think about this question. But I believe that this question demands examination.

The day before I was invited to write this, a mother brought her young son into my office. She told me that he had been perfectly normal in all respects, but within 24 hours of receiving an immunization from his pediatrician he began to lose the ability to speak. She took him back to the pediatrician, who told her that this was not uncommon, she had seen this reaction to immunization before, and that he would probably recover over time. Rather than reassured, the mother was astonished at this revelation. He recovered the ability to speak over the next several months; however, his personality changed. Eventually he was diagnosed as OCD, ODD, and ADD: "obsessive-compulsive disorder", "oppositional-defiance disorder", and "attention deficit disorder". It was for these problems that she brought him to my office. This case was not reported to the VAERS: Vaccine Adverse Event Reporting System.

Last year a 53 year old man came into my office. He worked in the hospital system as an accountant. During a routine medical examination, his doctor said that she wanted to give him a TDaP immunization (tetanus, diphtheria, and acellular Pertussis), because, "you haven't had one in a while". Five days later he noticed bruising all over his body. He went back to his doctor, who eventually diagnosed ITP, "Immune Thrombocy-topenia", a failure of the body to produce thrombocytes, or blood clot-ting cells, following an immune hyper-stimulation. He asked his doctor whether the TDaP caused this. She said that it could not have, because only MMR (measles-mumps-rubella) vaccine can cause this. A simple search of the medical literature demonstrated that TDaP has been known to cause ITP, though MMR is a more common cause.[1] She began treating him for this life-threatening problem, first with a massive dose of steroids. He had a bad reaction to the steroids, which brought him into my office. I have been treating him for the past year for the ITP. This case was also not reported to the VAERS, because the doctor who administered the vac-cine would not attribute the vaccine as the cause. Basing my treatment in part on the use of a homeopathic preparation of the DTaP, to counter its effects, the platelets have attained a normal range, at least for now.

I am not opposed to immunization. When two of my children, in their early twenties, undertook emergency medical technician training, they were required to get Hepatitis B immunizations. I did not object. Their work as EMTs would bring them into contact with blood under dif-ficult circumstances, and this was a reasonable precaution to take to pre-vent a difficult disease they were likely to encounter. Thirty-five years ago, shortly after I had begun my practice and fresh out of medical school, an old friend called me and asked whether he should have his young children vaccinated. I saw no reason why not. We had studied the mechanism of immunization in school, but discussions of harm had not been a part of my education. Since he had asked me, however, I began to ponder the question.

Later that year a woman brought me her baby. He had received a set of vaccinations a few months prior. In those days there were only seven vaccines administered to children: DPT, MMR, and Polio. Two weeks later she noticed that he was losing skills: the ability to walk and to talk, eye contact was changing, and he was becoming less responsive. She took him back to the pediatrician, wondering whether the immunization had caused this, and asking what could be done about it. He told her that it was not the immunization because she noticed it more than a week after the immunization and therefore it was not considered related to the immunization and thus he would not report it. But she told him that nothing else had occurred. He told her that this was just a coincidence. This incident, nevertheless, brought back to mind my friend's inquiry con-cerning the safety of vaccination. I had presumed them to be safe because they were recommended by the CDC, the federal government's Center of Disease Control, an agency charged with the highest level of monitoring and controlling disease in the United States.

I tended to believe the MD, but I wondered. Then I had a similar case brought to me some months later. And then another. And then another.

None of these cases was reported to the VAERS because in each case the mothers were told by an MD that this was just a coincidence. A pattern was emerging for me and motivated my looking more closely. I found very little research on the subject. There were almost no safety studies on the vaccines, and those that were available were cursory. There was an assumption that vaccines were safe and effective, but little corroborated "evidence" supported this assumption. I could not find what I thought would have been the most obvious studies, having presumed that such studies existed. One could simply inject one hundred baby monkeys with the vaccines, and compare their development to one hundred unvaccinated monkey babies over several years. One could compare a population of vaccinated children with a similar cohort of unvaccinated children and see what differences existed over time, if any. Not finding references to such simple studies, I began to wonder why not.

Several years ago I bought a puppy. When he was six weeks old I took him to the vet for immunizations. I presumed he needed a rabies shot, etc. The vet lectured me, informing me that the puppy was too young to immunize; and that this could damage him neurologically. They did not vaccinate puppies until they were six months old and their neurological systems were more mature. I was stunned. Who would consider a puppy's brain is more sensitive than that of a human infant? What do veterinarians know that pediatricians do not? Since that time I have learned that a puppy's first vaccines are recommended at between 12 and 16 weeks, but human infants are vaccinated at the time of their birth. This makes no sense.

A perusal of international statistics shows that there is not one other nation that immunizes as frequently or with as many vaccines as the US. Similar research reveals a high statistically significant correlation between increasing number of vaccine doses and increasing infant mortality rates.[1] Although such correlation is not proof of a causative relationship, it should at least cause substantial research to occur, and it has not.

The rumor that vaccination was causing the autism epidemic became increasingly common. Prior to 1980 the incidence of autism was about 1:10,000 in the US population. Last year it was 1:68, and 1:42 among boys. And this number is increasing. One in six children in the US is now diagnosed with some form of neurological disturbance.[2] It used to be fewer than 1:1,000. What is causing these disturbances in the brains of our children?

In 1999 there was a secret meeting of a committee of the CDC and vaccine manufacturers, known as the "Simpsonwood Conference". During this conference, Dr. Thomas Verstrataen, a CDC researcher, presented research data demonstrating a very strong causative relationship between vaccination, especially the MMR, and the growing incidence of autism. He came to the inescapable conclusion that vaccination was causing autism and other neurological disturbances, and it appeared that the Thimerosal component of the vaccines was the likely cause. Thimerosal is a mercury-based preservative, and mercury is a known neuro-toxin. Although the vaccine manufacturers offered to remove Thimerosal from all childhood vaccines, the CDC declined this offer, and continued to recommend Thimerosal containing vaccines for another 7 years, despite their own research.[3] Thimerosal is still contained in the "flu" vaccine, which is recommended for pregnant women, and for children to receive annually. Knowing of the link between immunization and autism, why has the CDC failed to protect children?

We are told that "the science is settled", that vaccines are safe and effective. Of the 350,000,000 doses of the various vaccines administered annually, an average of only 600 claims are considered by the vaccine court each year, and only 150 are approved for compensation. That suggests that only one person in 2,000,000 is damaged annually, a pretty good safety statistic. But is this a valid assessment of vaccine harm? Not one of the many cases of damage I would attribute to vaccination and that I have witnessed over my professional career has been reported to the VAERS.

Based upon my own experience, I must presume that the vast majority of vaccine injury is not reported as such. If the one-in-six figure for neurological damage and disturbance is due in some measure due to immunization, this question must be more deeply examined. We currently (2015) immunize children in the US with 69 doses of vaccine administered in 50 injections over the course of 12 years. In 1983, the CDC vaccine schedule included 24 vaccine doses administered in 7 injections through childhood. Are all of these 69 doses necessary? Vaccines are currently administered for Chickenpox, Diphtheria, Haemophilus influenza, Hepatitis A, Hepatitis B, Influenza, Measles, Mumps, Pertussis, Polio, Pneumococcal pneumonia, Rotavirus, Rubella, Tetanus, and Human Papilloma virus. When I was a child, we were immunized against Small Pox, Diphtheria, Pertussis, and Tetanus. Polio was added in the early 1950's.

From my clinical experience of 36 years, I have become convinced, both through research into the question and from my clinical observations, that vaccinations harm some children. In considering the logic of immunization I have to ask if the risks outweigh the benefit. In the case of my adult children, I believed that the risk of Hepatitis B for an EMT outweighed the risk of a single immunization against Hep B for an adult with a developed nervous system. But I cannot rationalize the need for so many vaccines in young children and infants against benign illnesses, such as measles, mumps and chickenpox, particularly since measles immunization is implicated more than most in neurological disturbance in children.

A stated goal of the World Health Organization is to immunize more people against more diseases.[4] It is the general belief of the public health community that immunization is a safe and effective means of reducing mortality and morbidity. The effectiveness of the international smallpox vaccination program is the model. By 1980, the entire world had been vaccinated against smallpox, and since that time no case of wild small pox has occurred. An international victory was declared, and was attributed to universal vaccination against smallpox. Smallpox had a high rate of mortality at a time when sanitation, and hygiene were non-existent and poverty rampant. It no longer plagues the human community.

This victory has become a model for the international public health community, to eliminate as many diseases as possible through mass immunization, a worthy goal, and one so worthy that the public health community overlooks the harm of immunization toward the accomplishment of this goal. The victims of this vaccination program were ignored to accomplish this goal, and have been forgotten. The Raggedy Ann doll was a testament to one of the victims of that vaccination program. Marcella Gruelle's death was attributed to the smallpox vaccination by her parents. The doll was created by her father, Johnny Gruelle.[5]

There is a problem with this approach. Not all diseases have demonstrated this kind of susceptibility to immunization. For example, measles outbreaks occur among the immunized.[6] In considering measles, however, there are other considerations that must be made. The recent outbreak of measles in Disneyland infected 113 children. All recovered with no significant sequelae. Some of these children had been immunized. It is a curious paradox that as measles immunization rates rise to high levels in a population, measles becomes a disease of immunized persons.[7] The same thing is true of pertussis.

In the past, measles was common, being the most contagious of human diseases. When I was a child, all children in my community got measles (as well as mumps and chicken pox). It was extremely rare that anyone was harmed, and life-long immunity was created, and reinforced as these diseases ran through the community every few years, re-stimulating our immunity. Before the introduction of the measles vaccine, and even into the 1980's measles was considered to have, "...a low mortality rate and is usually benign...".[8] With the reduction in wild measles outbreaks this natural immune stimulation no longer occurs. The current public health approach to massive immunization against what were considered "benign diseases of childhood" is therefore changing the "immune-biome" in the population, increasing susceptibility to disease, making the community increasingly dependent upon vaccination to maintain immunity, and shifting these diseases from children to adults, in whom they are generally more dangerous.

If vaccination were totally benign, this would be less of a consideration. But let us consider the ingredients of vaccines. Of especial interest is peanut oil and its link to the peanut allergy epidemic that has required the removal of peanuts from classrooms and airplanes.[9]

A review of vaccine ingredients can be obtained on the internet.[10] The list includes aluminum, antibiotics, egg protein, formaldehyde, monosodium glutamate, thimerosal, and many other substances, designed to enhance the immune reaction to the main ingredient, the virus or bacterial remnant, to preserve the active component, or for some other reasons.[11] Several of these ingredients, such as polysorbate-80, reduce the blood-brain barrier, which is the presumed cause of the neuro-degenerative response apparently seen in some children.[12, 13] The problem of vaccine ingredients is compounded by the large and increasing number of vaccines administered to infants and young children, with actively developing brains. This is postulated to be a significant link in the neurological insult that vaccines are apparently capable of. The more vaccines that are administered, the more these toxins accumulate in these developing nervous systems.

Other ingredients mentioned are common allergens in the population. And others, historically, have introduced unexpected viruses into children. An Independent researcher learned of the presence of a monkey virus, SV40, in some of the polio vaccines, that was suspected of causing cancer in humans. She informed the CDC. They decided to be quiet about it and did not recall the vaccines contaminated with it, to prevent public concern about the vaccination. As a result, two million more people were injected with the carcinogenic virus. The researcher that originally discovered and reported this viral contamination lost her job.[14]

A similar thing happened to Andrew Wakefield, MD, a world-renowned gastrointestinal surgeon and researcher who has been accused of fraud and fabricating studies that showed a link between the MMR vaccine, bowel disease, and autism. Dr. Wakefield was a well-published and well-respected researcher, not opposed to immunization. Rather, he was a doctor interested in vaccine safety. His studies and those of other researchers led him to believe that there were problems with the MMR vaccine. He did not advise his patients to stop vaccinating. He advised separating the vaccines for these three diseases, based upon his research. His published research was considered to suggest that there might be a relationship between the MMR vaccine and autism. He was forced out of the British Medical Association, and unfairly denigrated for simply reporting these findings. The journal, Lancet, was forced to retract his article, and he was unfairly charged with fraud in his research. Since that time, at least six other researchers have validated his findings, but he has never been publically exonerated.[15]

The question of whether vaccines cause damage in some persons is clear. A simple examination of the package insert in any vaccine will reveal the answer. For one of the chicken pox vaccines: "Anaphylaxis (including anaphylactic shock) and related phenomena such as angioneurotic edema, facial edema, and peripheral edema, eye disorders, necrotizing retinitis (in immunocompromised individuals), hemic and lymphatic system aplastic anemia, thrombocytopenia (including idiopathic thrombocytopenic purpura (ITP)), infections and infestations, varicella (vaccine strain), nervous/psychiatric encephalitis, cerebrovascular accident, transverse myelitis, Guillain-Barré syndrome, Bell's palsy, ataxia, non-febrile seizures, aseptic meningitis, dizziness, paresthesia, pharyngitis, pneumonia/pneumonitis, Stevens-Johnson syndrome, erythema multiforme, Henoch-Schönlein purpura, secondary bacterial infections of skin and soft tissue, including impetigo and cellulitis, herpes zoster."[16]

For MMR, the list is significantly longer: panniculitis, atypical measles, fever, syncope, headache, dizziness, malaise, irritability, vasculitis, pancreatitis, diarrhea, vomiting, parotitis, nausea, diabetes mellitus, thrombocytopenia purpura, regional lymphadenopathy, leukocytosis, anaphylaxis and anaphylactoid, angioneurotic edema, bronchial spasm, arthritis, arthralgia, myalgia, arthralgia and/or arthritis, polyneuritis, myalgia and paresthesia, encephalitis; encephalopathy, measles inclusion body encephalitis (MIB; subacute sclerosing panencephalitis (SSPE), Guillain-Barré Syndrome (GBS), pneumonia; pneumonitis, Stevens-Johnson syndrome, erythema multiforme, urticarial, rash, measles-like rash, pruritis, deafness, otitis media, retinitis, optic neuritis, papillitis, retrobulbar neuritis, conjunctivitis, epididymitis, orchitis, death".[17]

The public health community and the vaccine manufacturers are apparently severely averse to any findings that may suggest that vaccines are anything but harmless and effective. But, clearly, the risk of harm is real, if low, and is listed on the package inserts. Research is growing, and this is an area of growing controversy.

In the naturopathic profession this is perhaps the most significant controversy at this time. There are Naturopaths who are fully supportive of the CDC schedule of immunization, and see this as a fulfillment of the dictum to prevent disease, one of the philosophical tenants of naturopathic medicine. They believe that vaccines are harmless and effective. But the majority of naturopathic physicians disagree. Some prefer an extended vaccine schedule starting later with fewer vaccines. Some doctors prefer to administer only those vaccines that seem appropriate for a given child's risk, and assess whether a particular child is likely to be damaged by a vaccine. They prepare the child to reduce the potential damage from the vaccine before administration. Some oppose vaccination altogether and promote other means of disease prevention, including greater attention to hygienic measures, the use of homeopathic or other means to stimulate or promote immunity, or even to focus on promoting health and using some of the means discussed in this book to treat these diseases should they occur.

But some of our colleagues believe that it is only through fully embracing the CDC approach to immunization that we can make political progress as a profession. I would argue that the past 30 years demonstrates that we can make great political progress while taking the position that we will support the informed choices of our patients, which may include any of the above approaches to vaccination.

Do vaccines cause autism? Do vaccines cause other neurological damage, or damage to the immune system? The answer to these questions appears to be increasingly "yes", based upon an examination of the literature, briefly discussed above, though certainly not in a majority of children. If so, does the benefit outweigh the damage? I guess this answer depends upon whether it is your child that has been injured. For myself, I choose to err on the side of caution. Most of the diseases that are vaccinated against are benign, or are easily prevented or treated given a healthy milieu of clean water, good food, and appropriate naturopathic health care. Measles vaccination may save lives when administered in refugee camps to children under great emotional and physical stress, though there are other measures that would provide protection. But it makes little sense to me, a physician treating children in an affluent country with clean water and plenty of food for all, to administer potentially damaging substances to children with developing nervous systems and immature immune systems when there are good alternatives that carry no risk.

The question of vaccine safety was raised soon after Jenner began experimenting with vaccination for smallpox over two hundred years ago. His own son apparently died at a young age, mentally and physically damaged by repeated vaccination. The conventional medical profession has consistently downplayed the risks of vaccines and denied what has been obvious to the mothers of the children damaged by them, that sometimes vaccination harms children. The fact that this seems to be a rare occurrence does not justify ignoring or denying it, downplaying it, or denigrating those who are concerned about this fact. We have apparently seen perfidy at the hands of those agencies charged with the safety of medical practice, which have chosen to sacrifice the health of some children for the goals of their vaccination programs.

Accommodation must be made for those who choose not to vaccinate, for whatever reason. The exploration of safer alternatives should be welcomed rather than scorned. And the practitioners of these alternatives should be accorded respect for their conscientious efforts, rather than marginalized. In the same regard, the use of potentially harmful vaccines for relatively benign illnesses, such as measles or chickenpox, should be seriously questioned, not only for their potentially harmful impact on some children, but also for the impact these immunizations are having on the historical adaptation that has evolved in the human community to these illnesses. For all of these reasons, I value the writings that have preceded this "epilogue" as not only historically valuable, but as guides that we can turn to even today for information and inspiration in the quest to improve and preserve the health of our children and our communities.

References:

1. http://www.ncbi.nlm.nih.gov/pmc/articles/PMC3170075/

2. http://www.cdc.gov/ncbddd/autism/data.html

3. Transcript, Scientific Review of Vaccine Safety Datalink Information, June 7-8, 2000, Simpsonwood Retreat Center, Norcross, Georgia., Thomas Verstraeten speaking, page 40, 41.

4. http://www.who.int/immunization/givs/en/

5. https://www.facebook.com/national.vaccine.information.center/photos/a.151705002930.117058.143745137930/10152772910722931/?type=1&theater

6. http://www.ncbi.nlm.nih.gov/pubmed/8053748

7. http://www.ncbi.nlm.nih.gov/pubmed/8053748

8. The Merck Manual, 15th Ed, 1987, pg. 2023

9. http://vactruth.com/2010/07/15/non-disclosed-hyper-allergenic-vaccine-adjuvant/

10. http://www.cdc.gov/vaccines/vac-gen/additives.htm.

11. http://www.cdc.gov/vaccines/pubs/pinkbook/downloads/appendices/B/ excipient-table-2.pdf

12. http://www.ncbi.nlm.nih.gov/pubmed/9098875

13. http://vaccinechoicecanada.com/vaccine-ingredients/when-vaccine-ingredients-cross-the-blood-brain-barrier-a-formula-for-disaster/

14. http://www.theatlantic.com/magazine/archive/2000/02/the-virus-and-the-vaccine/377999/

15. http://www.ncbi.nlm.nih.gov/pubmed?term=%22The+American+journal+of+gastroenterology%22%5BJour%5D+AND+598%5Bpage

%5D+AND+2004%5Bpdat%5D&cmd=detailssearch)(Yazbak   FE. "Measles, mumps, and rubella (MMR) vaccine and autism. MMR cannot be exonerated without explaining increased incidence of autism." BMJ. 2001;323(7305):163-4.

16. http://www.merck.com/product/usa/pi_circulars/v/varivax/varivax_pi.pdf

17. http://www.merck.com/product/usa/pi_circulars/m/mmr_ii/mmr_ii_pi.pdf

AFTERWORD

by Alex Vasquez, DC, ND, DO, FACN

Director International College of Human Nutrition and Functional Medicine
and author of *Antiviral Strategies and Immune Nutrition.*

We receive Dr Czeranko's book, *Vaccination and Naturopathic Medicine*, with urgent necessity as we witness vaccine hysteria rage uncontrolled across the United States and spread by political extension to other countries. Reasoned debate, intellectual discourse, scientific inquiry, and consideration of reasonable and perhaps even synergistic options have all been slashed and burned by politicians, so-called "scientists", and medical organizations, most of whom are paid directly by the drug companies that make the vaccines that are later forced into the bodies and brains of non-consenting children and adults. Without any question, vaccines are the most overused and least studied medical intervention ever devised; the multicomponent vaccine schedule currently enforced on American children has never once undergone a controlled study, and even if it had, the combination vaccine schedule would still have to be tested against alternatives such as combination supplementation with vitamin D, vitamin A, selenium, and N-acetylcysteine before being designated as reasonable, let alone superior (in cost-effectiveness, safety, collateral benefits, etc.). All of these considerations would have to be established and broadly accepted before vaccines could be reasonably mandated.

As patients and physicians alike, we have been sold the idea that vaccination produces immunization and that immunization provides protection against disease; the distinctions among these differing concepts and realities have not been widely discussed, let alone appreciated. Our perception of reality has been obscured; we've been taught and forced to accept that these different things are identical. Vaccination is not immunization, and immunization does not ensure disease prevention. And even if proven, patients and physicians alike still maintain their personal autonomy. As I discussed in my book, *Antiviral Strategies and Immune Nutrition*, we as medical physicians have never been trained to treat and prevent viral infections in a structured manner; our confusion makes us more dependent on vaccines and antiviral drugs, thereby making us endorse and enforce those same treatments. The naturopathic profession is the only healthcare profession that has a structured model of health and disease which allows for a logical approach to the prevention and treatment of viral infections. The chiropractic, osteopathic and allopathic medical professions do not have structured approaches to the prevention of infectious diseases; what they have are loose assemblages of various treatments, thrown together and then thrown at patients. Vaccine regimens and regimes were amassed long before we knew about molecular cross relativity, chemical immuno-toxicity, and glial inflammation that result in neurodegeneration. Looking back, we see that a cautionary resistance against the overuse of vaccines was wholly reasonable, and we also see that the historic precedent to today's current vaccine resistance was established well over 100 years ago.

America's corporate controlled media consistently attempt to paint the picture that vaccine resistance is a fad, sparked recently by isolated individuals, when in fact this movement and its logical basis have permeated American society and medical science, respectively, for generations. We need rational discussion and default use of the precautionary principle for all treatments, especially considering the forced injection of what vaccines truly are: combinations of microbial antigens, microbial contaminants, and inflammatory and allergenic antigens, heavy metals, antibiotics, preservatives and adjuvants. Only with an accurate and contextualized perception can we make the decisions that support the actions that lead us to healthier societies. Sussanna's book is an archive of social context and historical conversations, both of which are of the highest value if we are to avoid the intellectual errors and medical mistakes that currently beset us in the promotion of mandatory vaccination.

References

Anti-Vaccination League of America. (1910). Constitution. *The Naturopath and Herald of Health*, XV (9), 549-550.

Anti-Vaccination League of America. (1912). How vaccine virus is made. *The Naturopath and Herald of Health*, XVII (10), 614.

Antonius F. (1911). Anti-vaccination victory in California. *The Naturopath and Herald of Health*, XVI (7), 429-430.

Beasley, C. O. (1918). Vaccination. *Herald of Health and Naturopath*, XXIII (1), 69-72.

Blue, F. D. (1901). Vaccination. *The Kneipp Water Cure Monthly*, II (4), 116.

Bourden, T. (1911). An open letter. *The Naturopath and Herald of Health*, XVI (5), 303-305.

Bowman, G. (1917). Vaccination and serum treatment. *Herald of Health and Naturopath*, XXII (6), 372-377.

Bradshaw, W. R. (1917). Lecture by Professor William R. Bradshaw at the 21st annual convention of the American Naturopathic Association. *Herald of Health and Naturopath*, XXII (6), 327-329.

Carr, C. S. (1907). Vaccination wholly empirical. *The Naturopath and Herald of Health*, VIII (7), 220-222.

Carrington, H. (1909). The plague. *The Naturopath and Herald of Health*, XIV (6), 353-357.

Clausen J. A. (1901). Address to the people of St. Paul, Minneapolis, on vaccination. *The Kneipp Water Cure Monthly*, II (6), 158-160.

Elfrink W. E. (1908). Anti-compulsory vaccination. *The Naturopath and Herald of Health*, XI (3), 95.

Erz, A. A. (1913). Medical laws vs rights and constitution (excerpt). *The Naturopath and Herald of Health*, XVIII (12), 834-836.

Gentry, W. D. (1909). Brief, regarding vaccination. *The Naturopath and Herald of Health*, XIV (10), 633-635.

Goodell Smith, E. (1906). Vegetarians safe. Are they? *The Naturopath and Herald of Health*, VII (4), 159-160.

Gray, H. S. (1912). Smallpox, the mumbo jumbo of the medical profession. *The Naturopath and Herald of Health*, XVII (6), 381-383.

Havard, W. F. (1918). Editorial, influenza, immunization. *Herald of Health and Naturopath*, XXIII (11), 865-867.

Hodge, J. W. (1910). Tuberculosis and vaccination. *The Naturopath and Herald of Health*, XV (2), 75-77.

Hodge, J. W. (1910). Vaccination villainous, it's compulsion a crime. *The Naturopath and Herald of Health*, XV (8), 465-467.

Hodge, J. W. (1911). How smallpox was banished from Leicester. *The Naturopath and Herald of Health*, XVI (1), 26-33.

Hodge, J. W. (1912). Anent the microbe mania. *The Naturopath and Herald of Health*, XVII (3), 173-174.

Hodge, J. W. (1912). A physician's reasons for having renounced vaccination. *The Naturopath and Herald of Health*, XVII (4), 223-226.

Judkins, E. H. (1919). The doping medical doctor's squirt-gun science. *Herald of Health and Naturopath*, XXIV (4), 200-201.

Katz, (1915). Dangers of contagion. *The Naturopath and Herald of Health*, XX (7), 427-428.

Kneipp, S. (1903). Children's diseases. *The Naturopath and Herald of Health*, IV (8), 237.

Leverson, M. R. (1906). Vaccination: should it be enforced by law? *The Naturopath and Herald of Health*, VII (7), 260-261.

Lindlahr, H. (1910). The anti-vaccination crusade. *The Naturopath and Herald of Health*, XV (3), 129-132.

Lindlahr, H. (1910). The anti-vaccination crusade, II. *The Naturopath and Herald of Health*, XV (5), 257-259.

Lindlahr, H. (1910). The anti-vaccination crusade, III. *The Naturopath and Herald of Health*, XV (7), 385-388.

Lindlahr, H. (1910). The anti-vaccination crusade, IV. *The Naturopath and Herald of Health*, XV (8), 489-492.

Littlefield, C. W. (1912). Does vaccination prevent smallpox? *The Naturopath and Herald of Health*, XVII (1), 12-17.

London and Provincial Anti-Vivisection Society. (1923). The Schick Test for diphtheria. *Naturopath*, XXVIII (3), 124.

Lust, B. (1900). For the little children. *The Kneipp Water Cure Monthly*, I (2), 28.

Lust, B. (1903). Compulsory vaccination. *The Naturopath and Herald of Health*, IV (5), 127.

Lust, B. (1905). Diphtheria. *The Naturopath and Herald of Health*, VI (1), 12-15.

Lust, B. (1907. The whooping cough. *The Naturopath and Herald of Health*, VIII (12), 355-356.

Lust, B. (1910). Public health tracts. *The Naturopath and Herald of Health*, XV (11), 661-662.

Lust, B. (1911). An innocent victim of that medical superstition, vaccination. *The Naturopath and Herald of Health*, XVI (5), 312.

Lust, B. (1922). Dr. Katzoff on vaccination. *Herald of Health and Naturopath*, XXVII (5), 230-231.

Lust, B. (1923). Fallacy of drugs. *Naturopath*, XXVIII (10), 579-580.

Macfadden, B. (1920). Get together or take your medicine. *Herald of Health and Naturopath*, XXV (8), 405.

Miller, C. W. What is their real purpose? *The Naturopath and Herald of Health*, XVII (2), 84-86.

Nelson, P. (1920). Naturopathy versus medicine. *Herald of Health and Naturopath*, XXV (2), 78-82.

Nelson, P. (1920). Naturopathy versus medicine, [continuation], *Herald of Health and Naturopath*, XXV (3), 134-138.

Padelford, F. M. (1910). Vaccination and cancer. *The Naturopath and Herald of Health*, XV (11), 659-660.

Rinn, J. P. (1911). Does vaccination grant immunity from or lessen the severity of smallpox? *The Naturopath and Herald of Health*, XVI (4), 205-211.

Robinson, J. T. (1909). A system of autocracies. *The Naturopath and Herald of Health*, XIV (2), 116-120.

Saloman, S. (1911). Vaccination, a dangerous operation. *The Naturopath and Herald of Health*, XVI (3), 170-173.

Schulze. (1905). Diphtheria and antitoxine. *The Naturopath and Herald of Health*, VI (1), 16-18.

Strueh, C. (1904). On the mechanism of protection in our body. *The Naturopath and Herald of Health*, V (4), 81-83.

Titus, E. D. (1917). The crime of the century. *Herald of Health and Naturopath*, XXII (3), 129-133.

Unknown author. (1911). A doctor's reasons for opposing vaccination. *The Naturopath and Herald of Health*, XVI (7), 449-450.

Wagner, O. (1900). Cure of infantile cholera, in its last stage. *The Kneipp Water Monthly*, I (3), 45-46.

Wallace, A. R. (1912). Alfred Russel Wallace and the vaccination question. *The Naturopath and Herald of Health*, XVII (1), 41-42.

Wallace, A. R. (1921). The unvaccinated death rate. *Herald of Health and Naturopath*, XXVI (3), 134-138.

Weinberger, H. (1914). Vaccination and the law. *The Naturopath and Herald of Health*, XIX (6), 393-395.

Wood A. L. (1902). Influence of water on health and longevity. *The Naturopath and Herald of Health*, III (3), 127-132.

Zurmuhlen, C. (1916). The passing of the serum craze. *Herald of Health and Naturopath*, XXI (8), 537-541.

Name Index

About the Editor, NCNM, NCNM Press

Sussanna Czeranko, ND, BBE, is a 1994 graduate of CCNM (Toronto). She is a licensed ND in Oregon. In the last twenty-two years, she has developed an extensive armamentarium of nature-cure tools and techniques for her patients. Especially interested in balneotherapy, botanical medicine, breathing and nutrition, she is a frequent international presenter and workshop leader. She is a monthly Contributing Editor (Nature Cure —Past Pearls) for NDNR and a Contributing Writer for the Foundations of Naturopathic Medicine Project. Dr. Czeranko founded The Breathing Academy, a training institute for naturopaths to incorporate the scientific model of Butyeko breathing therapy into their practice. Her next large project is to complete the development of her new medical spa in Manitou Beach, Saskatchewan, on the shores of a pristine medical waters lake.

⚭

NCNM (National College of Natural Medicine, Portland, Oregon) was founded in 1956. It is the longest serving, accredited naturopathic college in North America and home to one of the two U.S. accredited graduate research programs in Integrative Medicine. NCNM is also home to one of North America's most unique classical Chinese medicine programs, embracing lineage and a powerful mentoring model for future practitioners.

⚭

NCNM Press publishes distinctive titles that enrich the history, clinical practice, and contemporary significance of natural medicine traditions. The rare book collection on natural medicine at NCNM is the largest and most complete of its kind in North America and is the primary source for this landmark series—*In Their Own Words*—which brings to life and timely relevance the very best of early naturopathic literature.

The Hevert Collection: *In Their Own Words*

A Twelve-book Series

Origins of Naturopathic Medicine

Philosophy of Naturopathic Medicine

Dietetics of Naturopathic Medicine

Principles of Naturopathic Medicine

Practice of Naturopathic Medicine

Vaccination and Naturopathic Medicine

Physical Culture in Naturopathic Medicine

Herbs in Naturopathic Medicine

Water Cure in Naturopathic Medicine

Mental Culture in Naturopathic Medicine

Clinical Pearls of Naturopathic Medicine, Vol. I

Clinical Pearls of Naturopathic Medicine, Vol. II

From the NCNM Rare Book Collection On Natural Medicine.
Published By NCNM Press, Portland, Oregon.

CPSIA information can be obtained at www.ICGtesting.com
Printed in the USA
BVOW08s0111060516

446725BV00002B/99/P

9 780996 986304